What Emergency Physicians are saying about *Bouncebacks! Medical and Legal*

"Bouncebacks is a medical-legal thrill ride! The authors have created a tremendously educational integration of medical facts and legal orientation intertwined with medical expert and deposition testimony, including viewpoints of the actual plaintiff and defense attorneys involved in the litigation. This is a fast, educational and enjoyable read."

Dan Sullivan, MD, JD
Associate Professor of Emergency Medicine, Rush Medical College
Past President, Illinois Chapter of the American College of Emergency Physicians (ACEP)
Editor, ACEP's Emergency Medicine Risk Management, 2nd edition
Founder, The Sullivan Group

Bouncebacks! Medical and Legal is even better than its prior-published companion, *Bouncebacks! Emergency Department Cases*. The cases are engaging, true to life and applicable to emergency medicine physicians everywhere. As a recent graduate experiencing the "real world" for the first time, it is reassuring to know that even the best physicians at times make mistakes, and more importantly, that we are all able to learn from them. This book has made me think differently about the way I practice, the way I document and how I treat patients and their families in the emergency department. Thank you for providing such a dynamic read—you definitely know your audience.

Veronica Vasquez, MD
Assistant Professor of Emergency Medicine
Director, Quality Assurance
Department of Emergency Medicine
LAC+USC Medical Center

"The cases of *Bouncebacks! Medical and Legal* are frightening and feel awfully close. Because each feels like it could be mine tomorrow, the book does much more than entertain. The book is real, it is emotional, it is technical, and it is educational—it should be mandatory reading for every practicing emergency physician. I still feel bad for the patients as well as the doctors in the situations, but hearing their tales made me better. There are lessons that I am taking away.

This is an advanced course, written for skilled doctors who need to identify the unusual cases, recognize the rare events, and make great diagnoses based on subtle symptoms. It is a harsh reminder about how tough and uncertain the malpractice system is, but we do not need a reminder of that—fear is a powerful motivator. Congratulations to the authors for an important book. It is still resonating with me."

James G. Adams, MD
Professor and Chair, Department of Emergency Medicine Feinberg School of Medicine
Northwestern University, Northwestern Memorial Hospital

"'Riveting' is not a term I would typically use in describing a medical text, much less a medical-legal text. However, Weinstock and Klauer have indeed created a book that is not just educational, but also an enjoyable read. The authors do a literal postmortem exam on ten malpractice cases, focusing on medical records, trial transcripts, recollections of patients, family members and physicians, as well as commentaries by involved attorneys and expert witnesses from both sides. In addition, medical and legal experts not involved in the cases provide guest commentary. Although written with emergency physicians in mind, physicians from all specialties would benefit from these in-depth analyses of selected medical malpractice cases."

Richard Nelson, MD, FACEP
Professor Emergency Medicine and Vice Chair, Clinical Affairs
The Ohio State University College of Medicine

"*Bouncebacks! Medical and Legal* is the second offering of lessons in the practice of emergency care. The authors extract the knowledge of a superstar panel of experts to provide insight into bad outcomes on the medical and legal aspects of a variety of malpractice cases. They offer great insight into the anatomy, physiology, and toxicology of emergency medical care. With each case, there is acknowledgment of the breadth and depth of the specialty, the temporal demands of care, and the necessity of an organized approach.

The authors offer fabulous insight into why "bouncebacks" are the friend of emergency care; because the challenges of diagnosis are so profound, the second visit offers an opportunity for the patient to clarify the symptoms and signs, and allow the emergency physician to more precisely determine a safe and effective disposition.

In the world of firefighting, the incident commander is required to take a look beyond the 360 degree approach, and consider the 6 sides of an emergency situation (what is going into the air and what is going into the ground). *Bouncebacks! Medical and Legal* offers the reasons why emergency physicians need to be able to take an equally expansive look into the medical and legal aspects of patient care. This book is a must read for emergency physicians and those who aspire to be emergency physicians."

James J. Augustine, MD
Director of Clinical Operations, EMP Ltd., Canton, Ohio
Assistant Clinical Professor
Wright State University, Department of Emergency Medicine
Executive Editor, *ED Management*
Former Medical Director and Assistant Fire Chief, Atlanta Fire Rescue Department and the
    District of Columbia Fire and EMS Department

"*Bouncebacks! Medical and Legal* offers a novel and compelling method of teaching emergency physicians to identify, prioritize and avoid 'missing' high risk presentations. There are already many highly regarded texts and other curricula focused on the clinical diagnosis and treatment of ambiguous, but potentially lethal, cases, but few deal directly with the psychological environment faced by the emergency physician and staff. These professionals encounter multiple competing agendas for their attention. What can they do proactively to avoid stimulus fatigue and other human heuristic responses that may mask a high risk process?

Weinstock and Klauer address this conundrum with an effective instructional approach—the use of salient, real case studies from the emergency environment. They then extract from these cases a set of prospective actions, thought questions and behaviors to reduce latent diagnostic errors. Their focus is on one major subset of risky presentations—the bounceback, that is, the patient returning to the emergency department after prior discharge. The authors raise the bar by asking the reader to be concerned not just with avoiding litigation, but on becoming a better physician as well. As they remind us, 'just because you didn't get sued, doesn't mean you did the right thing by the patient.'

Any physician desirous of improving patient outcomes while reducing risk will find *Bouncebacks! Medical and Legal* a useful practical acquisition to their training library."

Robert E. "Bob" Sweeney, DA, MS
CEO, Challenger Corporation

"*Bouncebacks! Medical and Legal* is a masterful blend of everyday cases, actual court transcripts, educational pearls and of course, Greg Henry's notorious wit. This is a must read for those of us in the pit. I simply could not put the book down and am already looking forward to the next edition!"

Ghazala Sharieff, MD, FACEP, FAAEM
Director of Pediatric Emergency Medicine
Palomar-Pomerado Health System/California Emergency Physicians
Clinical Professor, University of California, San Diego

"*Bouncebacks! Medical and Legal*, if read periodically throughout one's EM practice career, has the potential to save lives and prevent countless hours of physician angst. As medical record digitalization alters ED team workflow, it also reminds us of the pitfalls of miscommunication and/or obscured communication between the members of the ED team."

Ronald Hellstern, MD, FACEP
Principal & President of Medical Practice Productivity Consultants
  Dallas, Texas

"This is a very readable set of cases that combine real clinical cases with their medical and legal outcomes. The style combines wisdom with medical issues in a format that keeps the reader's attention. These cases nicely combine the inputs into a medical-legal case from the medical, expert review, jury and attorney perspective—a great combination."

Neal Little, MD
Clinical Instructor, University of Michigan Medical School
Co-author, *Neurologic Emergencies: A Symptom-Oriented Approach*, 2nd Ed.
Co-presenter, *Medical Practice Risk Assessment: Continuing Medical Education for Emergency Physicians*

"*Bouncebacks! Medical and Legal* is a fascinating and somewhat terrifying read. This phenomenal work allows you to vicariously experience and learn from some truly sad cases. Will this book help you to keep your butt out of court? Absolutely! But of far more importance, it will help you avoid errors and better protect your patients."

Scott Weingart, MD of the EMCrit Podcast
Associate Professor and the Director of ED Critical Care at the Mount Sinai School of Medicine

"*Bouncebacks! Medical and Legal* is one of the most unique and illuminating books I have read on the subject. The evaluation of both the medical and legal aspects of representative cases will have great value for patients, physicians and lawyers. Science and art may have truth at their base; law is more interpretive and subject to opinion. By combining the two, Drs. Klauer and Weinstock will help reduce malpractice claims while improving medical care and saving lives."

Bruce Hensel, MD, FACEP
Chief Medical Editor NBC 4 LA
Clinical Professor of Medicine at UCLA
Boarded in Internal Medicine and Emergency Medicine

"I loved **Bouncebacks! Medical and Legal**. Not only do the authors provide an education on malpractice law and risk management, but they do it in the way doctors learn best—through the eyes of their colleagues and patients. Each case is a study in humanity, walking in the shoes of both the provider and patient from the first symptom to trial. The commentary by the authors and other noted experts is in the voice of a learned colleague mentoring another. Cases read like a Sherlock Holmes story, and for good reason. Sherlock Holmes was a fictional character invented by a physician who wrote stories to raise money while starting his practice. How the famed detective thinks is how physicians think—sorting through a stream of clues to find which ones are incidental and which ones are critical. Don't forget Sherlock's famous line that when you have eliminated the impossible, whatever remains, however improbable, must be the truth. These cases reinforce that sage wisdom. In the end, we live to do what is best for our patients; knowing how to spot key clues to their illness makes us better physicians."

Ricardo Martinez, MD, FACEP
Associate Professor of the Division of Emergency Medicine, Department of Surgery
Emory University School of Medicine
Former Administrator of the National Highway Traffic Safety Administration (NHTSA)
Past Chairman of the Trauma Care and Injury Control Committee (ACEP)

What Urgent Care Physicians are saying about **Bouncebacks! Medical and Legal**

"Compelling, enjoyable and easy to read. I found myself trying to guess the outcomes as the cases were presented. The teaching points are memorable. This is an indispensable book for any clinician who is responsible for taking care of walk-in patients. Congrats!"

Jill Miller, MD
Board Certified Internal Medicine and Pediatrics
Senior Clinical Instructor Case Western Reserve University
Staff Attending, Chagrin Highlands Urgent Care, University Hospitals of Cleveland

"**Bouncebacks! Medical and Legal** is an absolutely innovative and provocative take on the traditional *morbidity and mortality* conference. The legal analysis is both dramatic and realistic, expertly woven into the clinical discussion. The format demystifies medical liability and highlights the difference between the legal 'standard of care' and a 'guarantee against harm.' Perhaps most important, each case illustrates the perils of judgments and assumptions and their ability to cloud medical decision-making. Just the right amount of humor keeps it accessible and enjoyable to read. Ideal for all urgent care, emergency medicine and primary care providers. Should be required reading for *all* physicians-in-training. Even better than the first **Bouncebacks!** book."

Lee A. Resnick, MD
Editor-In-Chief, *The Journal of Urgent Care Medicine* (JUCM)
National Program Director, Fellowship in Urgent Care Medicine (UCAOA)
Assistant Clinical Professor, Department of Family Medicine
Immediate Past President, Urgent Care Association of America (UCAOA)
University Hospitals Case Medical Center, Cleveland, OH

Enjoy Philip !
Michael

Bouncebacks!
Medical and Legal

Michael B. Weinstock, MD

Kevin M. Klauer, DO, EJD

Case by Case Commentary by:

Gregory L. Henry, MD

Foreword by: Mel Herbert, MD

Illustrations by:

Hudson Meredith & Alyssa Klauer

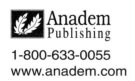 Anadem
Publishing

1-800-633-0055
www.anadem.com

3620 North High Street
Columbus, OH   43214
Tel: 1 (800) 633-0055
www.anadem.com

Bouncebacks! Medical & Legal

Michael B. Weinstock
Kevin M. Klauer
Commentary by Gregory L. Henry

Illustrations by Hudson Meredith & Alyssa Klauer

Bouncebacks! is based upon information from sources believed to be reliable. In developing this book the publisher, authors, contributors, reviewers, and editors have made substantial efforts to make sure that the regimens, drugs, and treatments are correct and are in accordance with currently accepted standards. Readers are cautioned to use their own judgment in making clinical decisions and, when appropriate, consult and compare information from other resources since ongoing research and clinical experience yield new information and since there is the possibility of human error in developing such a comprehensive resource as this. Attention should be paid to checking the product information supplied by drug manufacturers when prescribing or administering drugs, particularly if the prescriber is not familiar with the drug or does not regularly use it.

Readers should be aware that there are legitimate differences of opinion among physicians on both clinical and ethical/moral issues in treating patients. With this in mind, readers are urged to use individual judgment in making treatment decisions, recognizing the best interests of the patient and his/her own knowledge and understanding of these issues. The material in Bouncebacks! is not intended to substitute for the advice of a qualified attorney or other professional. You should consult a qualified professional for advice about your specific situation. Readers are cautioned to use their own judgment in making decisions on the issues covered in this book because there are on-going changes in these matters. The publisher, authors, reviewers, contributors, and editors disclaim any liability, loss or damage as a result, directly or indirectly, from using or applying any of the contents of Bouncebacks!

PRINTED IN THE UNITED STATES OF AMERICA

ISBN 978-1-890018-74-0

PREFACE

The format of *Bouncebacks: Medical and Legal* is modeled on the TV show *Law and Order*; each case starts with a patient's story, then progresses to the attorney's desk. This book is not bathroom reading; ten cases formatted to suck you into the personal experience of both the patient and doctor. As a lengthy medical and litigation process is compressed into a single chapter, we want you to feel empathetic, indignant, scared and humbled.

All of these stories are true; from the 15 year-old girl who presented with a headache hours after the World Trade Centers were hit on September 11, 2001, to the 42 year-old fireman whose symptoms began after walking out of an estate-planning meeting, to the playwright who collapsed on opening night. These cases not only touched the patients and their families, but also their physicians and attorneys; many were a defining time in the provider's and counselor's career. Even years later, my call prompted memories of the most-minute details. One attorney told me he thinks about his experience "at least once a week," and one physician thinks about his patient daily.

How did we get these cases? Well, that's a long and painful story. I spent the first six months in a futile search—it seems no one knows for sure where patient confidentiality ends and medical education begins. I begged insurance companies ("You are doing a good thing, but we don't want to be a HIPPA test case") and searched the net. Finally, I was handed a few appeals decisions by the lead guitar player in my blues band. Oh, he is also an attorney.

Reading through the decisions, it became obvious these were not only amazing medical cases, they were amazing *stories*. Unfortunately, it turns out that complete records are not available on the web; without the actual ED chart and trial testimony, there is no teaching value … another seeming dead end. I eventually realized that I was focusing on the wrong section of the appeals summary, not noticing the answer was right in front of me; the decision began with a listing of the attorneys who had tried the case. On a whim, I cold-called one of the plaintiff's attorneys, Dwight Brannon, and had the strangest experience. He was enthusiastic about the project and told me he was happy to help. A few weeks later, he drove to Columbus and filled my Prius with boxes of hospital records, depositions, 4 × 6 foot posters, and 5,000 pages of trial testimony. Finally, some success … but could it be duplicated?

I called more attorneys, some had heard of *Bouncebacks!* and many had heard of Greg Henry. Most said they were happy to help. Responses ranged from unreturned calls to bits and pieces from different attorneys. For one case I received the emergency department chart from one, the depositions from another and the trial testimony from a third. Dwight even flew to San Francisco to re-try his case in front of hundreds of doctors and a true "jury of our peers" at Mel Herbert's *Essentials of Emergency Medicine* conference this past November.

Compiling each case took about a month, depending on the complexity of the legal process. I read thousands of pages of depositions and trial testimony, sorted through hundreds of folders filled with income estimation, witness statements and sadly, family photos. Some cases required releases from a hospital, others from patients, and some from the State.

We include cases in which the patient was initially seen by a mid-level provider (MLP), a resident in an academic center, or a community emergency physician—all deceived by well-appearing patients who were, in fact, mortally ill. Each chapter has discussion of the presenting medical complaint and final diagnosis by nationally recognized experts in emergency medicine, as well as a legal review by plaintiff and defense attorneys, some who were actually involved in trying the case. Most names have been altered, some abbreviations have been expanded, and lengthy testimony has been compressed.

A final note regarding the legal analysis by Greg Henry: there are several cases where he knew the outcome from prior discussion and one in which I was surprised to discover that he was an expert for the defense (I won't say which side won). On all others, he is blinded to the case outcome, whether settled or jury trial. Calling upon wisdom gleaned from involvement in over 2,000 medical malpractice cases, he opines on the medical management, plaintiff and defense strategy, advisability of settlement and prediction of jury outcome, all in his well-known colorful and animated fashion.

I will close with a quote from Greg's foreword to the first *Bouncebacks!* book:

The smart doctor is not the one who learns from his own mistakes ... it's the one who learns from the mistakes of others. Here's hoping that this book is read by a lot of smart doctors.

Michael Weinstock
Kevin Klauer
September 25, 2011

We must not say every mistake is a foolish one.
Cicero 106-43 BC

"Remember that patient you saw yesterday?" Rarely is this question followed by "Good job! They did great!" Is there any other statement in the practice of Emergency Medicine that creates such a swirling pit of angst? You are left to wonder how bad the return visit was, did the patient live or die, and whether or not you are going to be sued. *Bouncebacks* confronts these dark encounters and drags them into the light.

It was Greg Henry that first taught me, "nothing focuses the mind like someone else's screw-up!" This is the essence of *Bouncebacks*. It is hard to believe that it's been five years since the first book in this series was published. Not only one of the most innovative and successful textbooks in Emergency Medicine of the last decade, *Bouncebacks* has also become a "radio show" and a live event at some of Emergency Medicine's most prestigious CME meetings.

Using real cases and expert commentary by some of the most well-known and influential educators in the field, Drs. Weinstock, Klauer, and Henry have spared no effort in creating a unique and exceptionally educational textbook. The cases are compelling, common and "real world." The reader has that sinking feeling in the stomach; "Hell! I would have sent that patient home too!"

Bouncebacks should be required reading for all residents, mid-levels and attending physicians. Anyone can look after the "clearly sick" patient, but more importantly, it is the clinician's approach to the "not obviously sick" that sorts the wheat from the chaff. Learn from others' "mistakes" and absorb the educational pearls from the expert faculty. Immerse yourself in other peoples' "bouncebacks," and spare yourself the same fate. This book is a treasure—read it!

Mel Herbert, MD

ABOUT THE AUTHORS

Michael B. Weinstock, MD

Michael and Beth Weinstock and their four children, Olivia (12), Eli (10), Theo (7), and Annie (4) live in Columbus, Ohio. Michael is a Clinical Associate Professor in the Department of Emergency Medicine at The Ohio State University College of Medicine, Attending and the Director of Medical Education with Immediate Health Associates (IHA) in the Emergency Department at Mt. Carmel St. Ann's, and Medical Director of the Ohio Dominican University Physician Assistant Studies Program. He is risk management section editor for the CME program Emergency Medicine Review and Perspectives (EM RAP), as well as the author of *Bouncebacks!* and *The Resident's Guide to Ambulatory Care*, currently in its 6th edition. Interests include international medicine, having practiced in Papua New Guinea, Nepal, and the West Indies, as well as being an avid traveler, skier, and blues guitar and harmonica player, currently the leader of a foot-stompin', harmonica playing group, The Big Rockin' Blues Band.

Kevin M. Klauer, DO, EJD, FACEP

Kevin Klauer is an Assistant Clinical Professor of Emergency Medicine at Michigan State University College of Osteopathic Medicine; Chief Medical Officer for Emergency Medicine Physicians in Canton, Ohio; Board member for Physicians' Specialty Limited Risk Retention Group; Board member for Emergency Medicine Physicians, Ltd.; Editor in Chief, Emergency Physicians Monthly; and Director, High Risk EM course. Dr. Klauer is an attending at Summa Health System, working at Barberton Citizen's Hospital and Wadsworth Rittman Hospital. In 2011, he completed his Executive JD degree with honors.

Gregory L. Henry, MD

Gregory L. Henry is a Clinical Professor in the Department of Emergency Medicine at University of Michigan Medical Center. He was the President of the American College of Emergency Physicians (ACEP) from 1995–1996 and is currently the President and CEO of Medical Practice Risk Assessment, Inc. and President of Savannah Assurance Limited, LTD. He is on the editorial boards of *Emergency Medicine Practice, Emergency Department Management, Foresight* and recently of the *Emergency Department Legal Letter*. He is the recipient of numerous awards including the "Over the Top" lecturer award and the "Outstanding Speaker of the Year" award from ACEP. He is the author of *Neurologic Emergencies: A Symptom-Oriented Approach, 2nd ed.* Greg is a jazz musician, columnist for Emergency Physician's Monthly (EPM), raconteur, bon vivant, and all around good guy.

To my lovely wife Beth, my amazing kids Olivia, Eli, Theo, and Annie, and parents Frank and Saragale, who have inspired me and instilled the creativity and drive to complete this project. May the good times continue to roll …

Michael

To my beautiful wife Tamara. Thank you for your understanding and patience. To my children, Alyssa (the creative one), Ross (the determined one) and Sam (the pinball wizard), you are a constant source of inspiration for me. To my Father who taught me perseverance and my Mother who taught me to always pursue my dreams. I love you all.

Kevin

To my grandchildren Elle and Cole. This is what the Doc does when he is not busy hugging you guys. If I'm lucky some other children will be better off because a young doctor read this book. En vino, en oculi et enfants veritas est.

Greg

We would like to also thank the many people who contributed, reviewed, encouraged and inspired us for the last two years: Elliot Nipomnick, for obtaining data for several of the cases; Jerry Hoffman, for structural suggestions (which he gave in the most untimely manner as the first book was going to the printer); Rob Crane, for the original idea of calling the book *Bouncebacks!*; and editors Beth Weinstock (the best medical editor in the world), David Sharkis, Carrie Schedler and Alison Barrington. Thanks to Mel Hebert, for a companion Bouncebacks! and providing the opportunity to present many of these cases on EM RAP, and to the many attorneys who took time to provide depositions, trial testimony, and commentary on their cases. A debt of gratitude to Hudson Meredith and Alyssa Klauer, who brilliantly captured the essence of these encounters with their illustrations. Thanks to David Schumick for the cover design (…*love* the bouncing "B"). To Helen, Mike, Will and Clay from Anadem Publishing for the editing, layout and the patience to accept all of our last minute changes. And a huge shout-out to Scott Weingart (of the EMCrit podcast), who helped set up our website/blog so that readers can contribute to an ongoing discussion—visit us at: embouncebacks.com

Michael, Kevin and Greg

TABLE OF CONTENTS

Preface iii

Foreword by Mel Herbert v

About the Authors vi

Dedication, Thanks, Acknowledgements vii

How to Spot the Well-Appearing Patient Who Will Soon Be Dead 1

Michael B. Weinstock, MD
Clinical Associate Professor, Division of Emergency Medicine
The Ohio State University, College of Medicine, Columbus, Ohio
Attending ED physician, Director of Medical Education
Mt. Carmel St. Ann's Emergency Department, Columbus, Ohio

Case 1: A 39 Year-Old Woman with Multiple Complaints: Coughing
during Cold and Flu Season 13

- **Medical**

Amal Mattu, MD, FAAEM, FACEP
Professor and Residency Director
Department of Emergency Medicine
University of Maryland School of Medicine

Emilie Cobert, MD, MPH
Department of Emergency Medicine
University of Maryland Medical Center

- **Legal**

Mark Jones, JD
Roetzel and Andress, LPA, Cleveland Ohio
(Actual defense attorney for this case)

Case 2: A 42 Year-Old Fireman with Shoulder Pain: When a Lifeline
Becomes a Noose 37

- **Medical**

David Andrew Talan, MD, FACEP, FIDSA
Professor of Medicine, UCLA School of Medicine
Chair, Department of Emergency Medicine and Faculty, Division of Infectious
Diseases, Olive View-UCLA Medical Center

Editorial boards: Annals of Emergency Medicine, Emergency Medicine News, and Pediatric Emergency Care
Reviewer: Clinical Infectious Diseases, JAMA, and The Medical Letter
(Actual expert witness for this case)

- **Legal**

Jennifer L'Hommedieu Stankus, MD, JD
Former medical malpractice defense attorney and military magistrate
ACEP Medical-Legal Committee and Ethics Committee
Contributing writer for ACEP News

Case 3: A 15 Year-Old Girl with Headache: A Grandmother's 9/11 Story . 71

- **Medical**

Jonathan Edlow, MD, FACEP
Associate Professor of Medicine, Department of Emergency Medicine, Harvard Medical School
Chair, American College of Emergency Physicians (ACEP) Headache Clinical Policy Task Force

- **Legal**

William Bonezzi, JD (Actual defense attorney for this case)
Bonezzi, Switzer, Murphy & Polito, Cleveland, Ohio

Case 4: A 36 Year-Old Man With Chest Pain: The Double Bounceback 95

- **Medical**

David Sklar, MD, FACEP
Professor of Emergency Medicine University, New Mexico School of Medicine
Associate Dean & Designated Institutional Officer Graduate Medical Education
Author, *Unanticipated Death After Discharge Home From the Emergency*
Department, Annals of Emergency Medicine, June 2007

Rob Rogers, MD, FACEP, FAAEM, FACP
Associate Professor of Emergency Medicine, Department of Emergency Medicine, The University of Maryland School of Medicine
Director of Undergraduate Medical Education

- **Legal**

Diane Sixsmith, MD, MPH, FACEP
(Actual NY State Medical Board reviewer for this case)
Chairman, Dept. Emergency Medicine, New York Hospital Queens
Asst. Professor of Emergency Medicine,
Weill Medical College of Cornell University

Greg Rankin, JD
Managing partner at Lane, Alton, & Horst, Columbus, Ohio
The Best Lawyers in America, Medical malpractice, 2009

Case 5: A 38 Year-Old Woman with Abdominal Pain: CT out of Proportion to Examination 121

- Medical

    Peter Rosen, MD, FACEP
    Senior Lecturer, Emergency Medicine, Harvard University School of Medicine
    Attending, Emergency Medicine Beth Israel/Deaconess Medical Center
    Founding editor, Rosen's Emergency Medicine: Concepts and Clinical Practice

    Gillian Schmitz, MD
    Emergency Medicine Faculty, Georgetown University/Washington University
    2010 AWAEM Early Career Faculty Award from the Academy for Women in
        Academic Emergency Medicine
    (physician who actually cared for this patient)

- Legal

    Karl Schedler, JD
    Principal Attorney, Office of the Attorney General of Ohio
    Court of Claims Defense Section, The Ohio State University

Case 6: A 32 Year-Old Woman with Headache: We *Own* this Diagnosis. 141

- Medical

    Jonathan Edlow, MD, FACEP
    Associate Professor of Medicine, Department of Emergency Medicine,
        Harvard Medical School
    Chair, ACEP Headache Clinical Policy Task Force

- Legal

    Robert Bitterman, MD, JD, FACEP
    President, Bitterman Health Law Consulting Group, Inc.
    Chairman, ACEP Medical Legal Committee
    Contributing Editor, Emergency Department Legal Letter

Case 7: A 52 Year-Old with a Cold: Why Vitals Signs Are Vital 173

- Medical

    David Andrew Talan, MD, FACEP, FIDSA
    Professor of Medicine, UCLA School of Medicine
    Chair, Department of Emergency Medicine and Faculty, Division of Infectious
    Diseases, Olive View-UCLA Medical Center
    Editorial boards: Annals of Emergency Medicine, Emergency Medicine News,
        and Pediatric Emergency Care
    Reviewer: Clinical Infectious Diseases, JAMA, and The Medical Letter

- **Legal**

> **Daniel Malkoff, JD**
> Senior Assistant General Counsel, Attorney General of Ohio
> Ohio State University Medical Center

Case 8: A 15 Year-Old Girl with RLQ Abdominal Pain: It *Is an* Appy ... *Right?*. 191

- **Medical**

> **Ryan Longstreth, MD, FACEP**
> Attending ED physician, Immediate Health Associates, Columbus, Ohio
> Co-author, Bouncebacks!

> **David Andrew Talan, MD, FACEP, FIDSA**
> Professor of Medicine, UCLA School of Medicine
> Chair, Department of Emergency Medicine and Faculty, Division of Infectious
>   Diseases, Olive View-UCLA Medical Center
> Editorial boards: Annals of Emergency Medicine, Emergency Medicine
>   News, and Pediatric Emergency Care
> Reviewer Clinical Infectious Diseases, JAMA, and The Medical Letter

- **Legal**

> **Karen Clouse, JD**
> (Actual defense attorney for this case)
> Partner with Arnold, Todaro & Welch, Columbus, Ohio

Case 9: A 46 Year-Old Male with Neck Pain: Pounding a Square Peg into a Round Hole 223

- **Medical**

> **Stephen Colucciello, MD, FACEP**
> Clinical Professor, Emergency Medicine, University of North Carolina Medical
>   School, Chapel Hill, North Carolina
> Assistant Chair, Director of Clinical Services, and Trauma Coordinator
> Dept. of Emergency Medicine, Carolinas Medical Center
> ACEP's National Speaker of the Year, 1992

- **Legal**

> **Jennifer L'Hommedieu Stankus, MD, JD**
> Former medical malpractice defense attorney and military magistrate
> ACEP Medical-Legal Committee and Ethics Committee
> Contributing writer for ACEP News

Case 10: A 26 Year-Old Woman with Weakness and Falls: A Rough Life, a Tough Prognosis 241

- Medical

    Michael Redd, MD, FACEP (name changed)
    Emergency Physician
    (Actual plaintiff's expert witness in this case)

    Jerome Hoffman, MA, MD, FACEP
    Professor of Medicine and Emergency Medicine, UCLA School of Medicine
    Associate editor, Emergency Medical Abstracts

    Michael Weintraub, MD, FACP, FAAN, FAHA
    Clinical Professor of Neurology, Clinical Professor Internal Medicine
    New York Medical College, Valhalla, NY

- Legal

    Rich Milligan, JD
    Medical malpractice defense attorney
    Buckingham, Doolittle & Burroughs, LLP, Canton, Ohio

    Mark Kitrick, JD
    Medical Malpractice plaintiff's attorney
    President of Kitrick, Lewis & Harris Co., LPA, Columbus, Ohio
    Past President, Ohio Association of Trial Lawyers

Epilogue 281

Legal Considerations: Help! I Am Being Sued 283

Kevin M. Klauer, DO, EJD, FACEP
Chief Medical Officer, Emergency Medicine Physicans, Ltd.
Director, Center for Emergency Medical Education
Board member, Physicians' Specialty Limited Risk Retention Group
Board member, Emergency Medicine Physicians, Ltd.
Editor in Chief, Emergency Physicians Monthly
Director, High Risk EM course

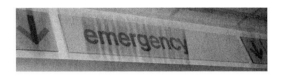

HOW TO SPOT THE WELL-APPEARING PATIENT WHO WILL SOON BE DEAD

Michael Weinstock, MD

I. Deceptively Well Patients 3

II. Bounceback Literature Review 4

III. Law and Order 5

IV. Is There a Way to "Game the System" to Improve Patient Safety and
    Decrease Legal Risk? 6

V. The Rule of Two's: An Approach to Recognizing Subtle Patterrns of
    Severe Ilness in Well-Appearing Patients 7

VI. A Two Minute Legal Primer 8

    A. Burden of Proof... 8

    B. Standard of Care 9

    C. Proximate Cause 9

VII. Approach to the Bounceback Patient 9

VIII. Conclusion 10

INTRODUCTION

HOW TO SPOT THE WELL-APPEARING PATIENT WHO WILL SOON BE DEAD

I. Deceptively Well Patients

Who is the scariest patient? It's not the 80 year-old with an acute MI, the septic dialysis patient or the even full cardiac arrest—in these patients the diagnosis is clear. Contrary to what I feared as a medical student, the sick, well-appearing patient is the most frightening: the 22 year-old woman with a cough and blood tinged sputum in the middle of cold and flu season, the 38 year-old with recurrent headaches and pressure from the staff to "treat and street," the multiple-complaint patient with fibromyalgia who says "everything hurts … and my pain doctor is in prison!"

We can simplify and assign three categories of ED patients:

1. **The straightforward patient:** Our easiest and least-satisfying encounter— an easy diagnosis in a healthy patient (ankle strains and corneal abrasions). It is unlikely we will miss serious illness, but this is not why we chose emergency medicine.
2. **The sick patient:** Our *raison d'être*, the critically-ill patient who can actually be helped. We act quickly, perform procedures and affect lives in a positive manner; it is the patient with a ruptured AAA that makes it to the ED alive, the crashing MVA victim with a tension pneumothorax, the hypotensive STEMI patient.
3. **The patient with diagnostic uncertainty:** The most difficult, frustrating and riskiest; a cadre of unclear diagnoses in patients with poor access to the medical system. The worried-well who tell you the diagnosis, as well as the therapy. The "frequent flier" who wrote a complaint at the last visit. These dispositions can be influenced by bias, "He's back *again?*"

Clearly, this last patient will be our focus. While dissecting each of the following ten cases, we concentrate on two of the most risk-fraught areas of emergency medicine: diagnosis and documentation. Both are important for our patients, while the latter is the cornerstone of our defense when something goes wrong.

Ours is a strange profession, where physician error rate is several numerals to the right of the decimal point, but we are subject to litigation when an adverse outcome occurs. With a sick ED population, often underserved, and previously unknown to us, it's surprising that things don't go wrong more often. During residency, I cared for a 16 year-old pregnant patient with no prenatal care who presented crowning and screaming her head off. The OBs were freaking out: "we don't know her rubella titer, has she been taking Folate?" This is our quintessential ED patient and where our expertise shines. We are experts in making diagnoses and stabilizing sick, undifferentiated patients.

As human beings, we are comfortable recognizing patterns. As ED physicians, the ability to rapidly categorize *life-threatening* patterns, such as respiratory distress or toxidromes, enables us to provide emergent life-saving interventions. However, these very skills, which normally serve us well, can also fool us easily in healthy-appearing patients with serious illness. We find ourselves swimming in a sea of the worried-well, which paradoxically causes us to worry *less*.

Is there a way to create a recognition pattern for this "time bomb" subset? Examination of the bounceback data and ED litigation analysis provides some clues.

II. Bounceback Literature Review

A. **What is the incidence of ED bouncebacks?**
   - Using the commonly-accepted time frame of an ED return within 72 hours, the incidence is about 3%[1-3]
   - For an average provider, this is approximately one patient per shift
   - Significance: Out of 115 million ED visits in 2005, there were 3.4 million bouncebacks

B. **What is the incidence of patients who bounceback and are admitted?**
   - Answer: About 0.6%[4,5]
   - High-risk features for readmission include: age over 65, mental disorders, alcohol-related complaints and abdominal and chest pain
   - Significance: Out of 115 million ED visits in 2005, over 650,000 patients were sent home, returned to the ED within 72 hours and were admitted

C. **What is the incidence of bouncebacks due to medical errors?**
   - Answer: 18–30% (over 30,000 patients studied)[6]
   - Significance: Out of 115 million ED visits in 2005, there were between 600,000 and 1,000,000 patients who returned to the ED due to a medical error

D. **What percentage of patients die with one week of ED discharge?**
   - Kefer found an incidence of 9/100,000 visits[7] and Sklar found 30/100,000 visits,[8] both using a time frame of death within seven days of initial ED visit.
   - Sklar's study is likely more accurate due to examination of almost 400,000 ED visits to the University of New Mexico Health Sciences Center over a 10 year time span, providing a unique geographic analysis as the only level I trauma center for the state and the only public hospital in two counties, likely best able to capture almost all return visits
   - Possible error cases comprised about 30% of the total deaths (for Sklar's patients, this is nine possible error deaths per 100,000 visits)

E. **Sklar found four main themes in the possible error cases:**[8]
   1. Atypical presentation of an unusual problem
   2. Chronic disease with decompensation (e.g., CHF)

3. Mental disability, psychiatric problem or substance abuse (making the history and ability to follow-up less reliable)
4. Abnormal vital signs
   - 71% had tachycardia on ED discharge
   - 83% had abnormal vital signs on ED discharge
   (See Case 4 for a discussion by Dr. Sklar of his study and how it specifically relates to the patient presented)

F. **Bringing it home (to *your* home)**
   - If you see just over three patients per hour and practice 30 hours per week for 30–35 years, you will see over 150,000 patients in your career
   - *During this time, you will send home 17 patients who will die an avoidable death within seven days of ED discharge*

III. Law and Order

A. There are several important points to be made up front regarding the legal aspect of work in the ED:
   - Just because you didn't get sued, doesn't mean you didn't screw up. Of the 35 "possible error" cases in Sklar's study, none resulted in a lawsuit—despite the fact that all the patients died.[11]
   - Our goal is not to merely avoid being sued, but to make patients safer—can awareness of potential litigation improve patient care?

B. Consider these numbers gleaned from the recently published study by Brown, et al., *An Epidemiologic Study of Closed Emergency Department Malpractice Claims in a National Database of Physician Malpractice Insurers*.[9] The authors analyzed data from the Physician Insurers Association of America (PIAA) databank, a trade association whose participating malpractice carriers insure over 60% of physicians in the U.S. They reviewed 11,529 claims originating from the ED from 1985–2007. ED physicians were the principal defendants in about 2,000 of the total.
   - The number one source of suit was error in diagnosis (failure to diagnose and/or incorrect diagnosis), representing 37% of the cases.
   - The three most common conditions misdiagnosed were fracture, including vertebral/cervical fractures (6%), acute MI (5%) and appendicitis (2%). Others included symptoms involving the abdomen and pelvis, injury to multiple body parts, aortic aneurysm and pulmonary embolism.
   - Acute MI (AMI) was associated with the highest ratio of payments (42%) and the highest average indemnity ($317,000), with the majority being error in diagnosis. AMI was the most common claim involving a patient who died.
   - 80% of the total indemnity was associated with severe injury, including loss of sight, amputation, quadriplegia, brain damage, and death.
   - Of the total number of claims:
     o 70% closed without payment to the claimant
     o Only 7% went to jury verdict—of these 85% found for the defendant ED physician

C. Kachalia, et al., examined the causes of missed and delayed diagnosis and found multiple breakdowns in the system including failure to order an appropriate diagnostic test (58% of errors), failure to perform an adequate H&P (42%), incorrect interpretation of a diagnostic test (37%) and failure to order an appropriate consultation (33%).[10]

IV. Is There a Way to "Game the System" to Improve Patient Safety and Decrease Legal Risk?

If you are sued, one approach is just to *stick it out*; if you can make it to a jury verdict, you have an 85% chance of winning. However, we do not recommend this approach; as Greg Henry has often said, "In a lawsuit there are two losers: one loser, and a bigger loser."

Short of investing four to five years of your life to await the "probable" jury verdict, not getting sued in the first place is our recommended policy. If you want to put the book down and stop reading now, here is a little secret: the easiest way to do avoid a lawsuit is to just "be a nice guy." Seriously. Screw up all you want—just don't be a jerk! There are a lot of mistakes we have all made, surely too many to fill the pages of thousands of these books, and we all have stories of an avoidable error we have committed: "Remember that patient you saw last night? Well, he bounced back this morning … horizontal." Most "malpractice" does not result in a legal action.

For those who already are kind, compassionate doctors and still want to avoid misdiagnosis … *is there a way to use the results of bounceback studies and malpractice numbers to improve patient safety?* Are we able to recognize the well-appearing patient who will soon be dead?

- Martin-Gill (bounceback admissions study above) wrote, "by identifying high risk patients prospectively, physicians will be better able to make informed decisions when considering the depth of evaluation, timing of discharge decisions, and extent of follow up care."[5]
- Sklar (bounceback death study above) wrote, "Recognition of the presence of abnormal vital signs and a cautious assessment of these patients offer an opportunity to prevent bad outcomes."[8]

At an M&M conference, where 50 people are focused on diagnosing one patient they know had a bad outcome, it does seem primary. But during a busy shift, where you are being assaulted by 15–17 patients at a time and reinforcements are not arriving for three hours, a father of the three year-old with otitis media is standing at the door tapping on his watch while the squad-bay doors open with paramedics bagging a trach patient, the subtleties of these deceptive patients can easily slip through your fingers.

V. The Rule of Two's: An approach to recognizing subtle patterns of severe illness in well-appearing patients

    A. There are two rules and each has two parts:

        1. Rule #1: Recognition: Recognize patients at high risk for bouncing back with a poor outcome

            a. The patient is tachycardic

            b. *You* are tachycardic (or should be)

        2. Rule #2: Re-evaluation: Re-visit the evaluation before the patient leaves the ED

            a. Review the documentation and re-evaluate the patient at the bedside

            b. Record a progress note

    B. It does seem cursory—don't we do this with each patient? Let's look at the technique in more depth.

        1. Rule #1: Recognition: Recognize patients at high risk for bouncing back with a poor outcome

            a. The patient is tachycardic (or has unstable or worsening vital signs)

                • Tachycardia

                • Hypotension

                • Repeated vital signs which are not improving

            b. *You* are tachycardic (or should be)

                • Diagnostic uncertainty with high-risk complaints (e.g., chest pain, shortness of breath, abdominal pain, headache and fever)

                • Difficulty in obtaining an adequate history or multiple-complaint patients

                • Elderly patients

                • Patients with chronic medical problems with high likelihood of deterioration

                • Discrepancy between the physician and nurse notes

Rule #1 can be shortened to *any patient* you would worry about on the drive home. We estimate this would account for 3–5 patients per shift. When these patients are identified, what should be done?

        2. Rule #2: Re-evaluation: Re-visit the evaluation before the patient leaves the ED

            a. Review the documentation and re-evaluate the patient at the bedside

               i. Documentation:

                • Ensure that you have addressed all documented complaints (by all providers)

                • H&P reflects consideration of life-threatening processes (think worst first)

               ii. Re-evaluation at bedside

                • Confirm that the history is accurate and complete

                • Focused re-examination of presenting complaint (repeat the abdominal exam, reassess the mental status, watch the patient walk, etc.)

Summary: Perform an "eyes-on" evaluation of the patient just before discharge, "as if" you could foretell a bounce back visit

b. Document a progress note
- Record a brief progress note focusing on why the most serious diagnoses are *not* occurring
- An additional "not so obvious" advantage of writing a progress note is that it forces you to review your own documentation and record an explanation of your thought process. If you can't even convince *yourself* that the medical decision-making is appropriate, it is unlikely that you will be able to convince a jury

Consider this: Would you be comfortable defending your documentation and evaluation at your department's M&M conference or from the witness stand?

As you proceed through the following ten cases, consider if the evaluation would have changed by using these two simple rules. Then, as you report for your next shift, consider whether your thought process can be extrapolated from your documentation and if patients with concerning stories or vitals have been evaluated for the worst-case scenario. Our patients give us a lot of slack; most elderly with back pain do *not* have a ruptured AAA, most headache patients with fever do *not* have meningitis. But just because the patient didn't die, doesn't mean you did a great job ...

VI. A Two Minute Legal Primer

We all fear malpractice litigation, and emergency medicine is one of the highest litigation specialties. What a bizarre field we inhabit, where a seemingly routine evaluation today can morph into a four-year legal ordeal regarding a patient we don't even remember! Can you imagine a schoolteacher enduring a multi-year lawsuit because a student did not graduate or get a good job? How about a dog trainer who goes through years of interrogatories, depositions and court proceedings because his "pupil" bit the mailman years after graduation?

Can you the threat of a lawsuit make patients safer? This seems counterintuitive, but the threat of legal action often results in a more cautious clinician, sometimes over testing, but also with better documentation and a more thorough evaluation. The trick is to walk the tightrope between fear and concern while maintaining a balance between speed and vigilance. *Don't practice defensive medicine, but evaluate patients and document in a way which is defensible.*

May we all be blessed with grateful patients who present with textbook symptoms. For all the rest, the following legal terms are defined when bedside care progresses to the courtroom.

Burden of proof: The plaintiff must prove by the greater weight of the evidence that the defendant was negligent, that the defendant's negligence was a direct and proximate cause of the plaintiff's injuries and that the plaintiff was damaged by the defendant's negligence.

Standard of care: The standard of care is to do those things which a reasonably careful physician would do and to refrain from doing those things which a reasonably careful physician would not do.

Proximate cause: To prevail, the plaintiff must not only prove that the physician fell below the standard of care and was therefore negligent, but that the negligence was a direct and proximate cause of injury to the plaintiff. This includes failure to provide therapy (or provide it in a timely manner) which may have proximately improved the patient's symptoms.

As the ten cases in this book unfold, it will become apparent there is a highly subjective interpretation of the above terms. For example, the First Amendment to the Constitution of the United States is only two sentences long, but the Supreme Court often splits 5–4 in its application. So it is not surprising that standard of care and proximate cause can mean different things to different people, especially if they don't have prior medical training … or couldn't get out of jury duty.

VII. Approach to the Bounceback Patient

Are bounceback patients annoying or are they giving us a second chance? Is there a way to approach these high-risk patients which improves patient safety?

Top ten list for handling bounceback patients:

1. Thank the patient for returning
2. *Sit down* when taking history
3. Specifically ask the *main reason* for the return visit
4. After history is taken, verbally repeat it back to the patient
5. Ensure all documented complaints are evaluated (including nurse/triage notes)
6. Review the documentation from the *previous visit*, looking for:
   a. Symptoms that were not evaluated
   b. Abnormal findings or abnormal vital signs not addressed
   c. Accuracy of initial diagnosis
   d. Appropriateness of treatment
   e. Life-threatening conditions which were not considered
7. Document a progress note explaining the medical decision-making process
8. Address concerns with family members
9. Inform patients of diagnostic uncertainty and ensure the patient understands he or she is welcome to return if the symptoms progress or do not resolve
10. Provide action- and time-specific aftercare instructions
    a. Call the primary care provider (PCP)
    b. Give the patient focused instructions, including specific reasons to return

Summary: Perform a fresh evaluation with each visit—do not be misled by *diagnosis momentum*.

VIII. Conclusion

As we proceed through our careers, sometimes tired, sometimes cynical, our challenge is to maintain a high vigilance for the patients who appear well but are soon to decompensate. Like an airport screener, we can become inoculated by the "narcotizing effect of obvious,"[12] but approaching each presentation with a thorough evaluation and defensible documentation will not only be legally protective, but also medically protective, due to improved patient safety.

The following cases are all real. They reflect the pulse of life-in-the-ER. We have included the actual documentation of the provider, deposition testimony from families and physicians, attorney opening and closing statements, direct and cross-examination of expert witnesses, physician testimony, the judge's instructions to the jury and, at the end of each section, the verdict.

One final question before embarking on this journey; what's the best way to learn from case studies? It's easy to look back at a case that has gone bad and to find areas to criticize and to imagine that we would have done things differently. But this strategy may be backward.

Wears and Nemeth suggest the opposite approach: "Questions such as 'How could they not have noticed?' and 'How could they not have known?' often arise in retrospective examinations of adverse events. These questions arise not because people were behaving bizarrely but rather because we (the reviewers) have chosen the wrong frame of reference to understand their behavior. We do not learn much by asking why the way a practitioner framed a problem turned out to be wrong. We do learn when we discover why that framing seemed so reasonable at the time."[13]

Enough said! It's time to report for your next shift, put on your white coat, hang a stethoscope over your shoulders, walk through those double doors, turn the page and get ready to see ten well-appearing patients.

References

1. Wilkins PS, Beckett MW. Audit of unexpected return visits to an accident and emergency department. Arch Emerg Med 1992; 9:352-6.
2. O'Dwyer F, Bodiwala GG. Unscheduled return visits by patients to the accident and emergency department. Arch Emerg Med 1991; 8:196-200.
3. Pierce JM, Kellermann AL, Oster C. "Bounces": an analysis of short-term return visits to a public hospital emergency department. Ann Emerg Med 1990; 19:752-7. (over 30,000 patients studied)
4. Gordon JA, An LC, Hayward RA, et al. Initial emergency department diagnosis and return visits: risk versus perception. Ann Emerg Med 1998; 32:569-73.
5. Martin-Gill C, Reiser RC. Risk factors for 72-hour admission to the ED. Am J Emerg Med 2004; 22(6):448-53. (almost 200,000 patients studies)

6. Nunez S, Hexdall A, Aguirre-Jaime A. Unscheduled returns to the emergency department: an outcome of medical errors? Qual Saf Health Care 2006; 15(2): 102-8. (over 30,000 patients)

7. Kefer MP, Hargarten SW, Jentzen J. Death after discharge from the emergency department. Ann Emerg Med 1994; 24:1102-7.

8. Sklar DP, Crandall CS, Loeliger E, et al. Unanticipated death after discharge home from the emergency department. Annals of Emergency Medicine 2007; 49(6):735-45.

9. Brown TW, McCarthy ML, Kelen GD, Levy F. An epidemiologic study of closed emergency department malpractice claims in a national database of physician malpractice insurers. Acad Emerg Med 2010; 17(5):553-60.

10. Kachalia A, Gandhi TK, Puopolo AL, et al. Missed and delayed diagnoses in the emergency department: a study of closed malpractice claims from 4 liability insurers. Ann Emerg Med 2007; 49(2):196-205.

11. Personal communication, David Sklar, 2010.

12. Ronald Hellstern, Bouncebacks testimonial, 2006.

13. Wears RL, Nemeth CP. Replacing hindsight with insight: toward better understanding of diagnostic failures. Ann Emerg Med 2007; 49:206-9.

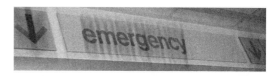

CASE1

A 39 YEAR OLD-WOMAN WITH MULTIPLE COMPLAINTS: COUGHING DURING COLD & FLU SEASON

Primary case author Michael Weinstock

PART 1—MEDICAL

    I. The Patient's Story 15

    II. The Doctor's Version (the ED Chart) 16

    III. The Errors—Risk Management/Patient Safety Issues 17

    IV. The Bounceback 19

PART 2—LEGAL

    I. The Accusation/Cause of Action 21

    II. What Would Greg Do (WWGD)? 21

    III. Deposition/Trial Testimony 22

    IV. The Verdict 29

    V. The Appeal 30

    VI. The Twist 31

    VII. Legal Analysis—Mark Jones, JD (Interview) 31

    VIII. Medical Discussion—Emilie Cobert, MD and Amal Mattu, MD 32

    IX. Authors' Summary 35

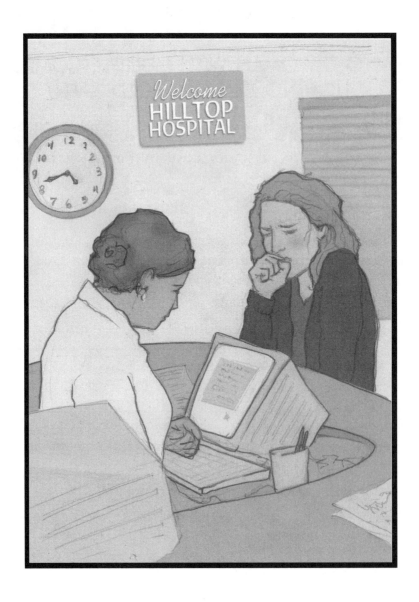

A 39 YEAR-OLD WOMAN WITH MULTIPLE COMPLAINTS: COUGHING DURING COLD & FLU SEASON

Why do so many bounceback patients with poor outcomes have an initial diagnosis of gastroenteritis or receive a prescription for a Z-pack? It *is* a coincidence ... right?

Deep thoughts:

1. *How do we streamline our evaluation to keep patients safe without over-testing?*
2. *How should we approach the "positive review of systems" patient?*
3. *Does our "index of suspicion" decrease in the early morning hours of a night shift?*
4. *Who wins when the nurse and doctor disagree on the chief complaint?*

PART 1—MEDICAL

I. The Patient's Story

In 1979, at the age of 16, Anna marries her high school sweetheart, Mike. Through the years, they raise three boys, always making time for baseball games, despite each working full-time.

As a family, they do not have much. Mike works on an hourly basis for Nebraska Milling, and Anna works at "Barb's Burgers and Such," a low priced restaurant off the highway. For her, it is not just another job; she has established a first-name relationship with her customers, working as waitress and cashier. She is a warm and inviting person. Neither have health insurance.

For the last 10 years Mike has been the little league coach. The year 2002 marked a special occasion for the Kamianka family; after years of watching their kids play baseball, Coach Mike takes the little leaguers to play a tournament game at Jacobs field. Anna has never been to a professional baseball stadium, she has never seen the Cleveland Indians play. She poses for a picture in the dugout with a player on each side.

Anna is generally healthy, but moderately overweight. She is a smoker who has unsuccessfully struggled to quit on several occasions. On September 5, 2002, she is at work and doesn't feel well. She calls her primary care physician, Dr. Brian Rembrandt, for a "sick visit" appointment and is told that if she can make a payment on the balance of her bills, she will be seen. The bill is paid and she arrives at 3:00 in the afternoon. The exam is routine, a CXR is normal, she is diagnosed with bronchitis and she is prescribed antibiotics. A later review of the records shows that this is not a unique occurrence; she has been treated each of the last six years for upper respiratory infections.

Anna is not the type to complain. Despite feeling bad, she does not miss a day of work. After taking her medication, her symptoms are improved, and she is well until the morning of November 6, when she is awakened by a pain between her shoulder blades. The pain is so bad, she throws up. She takes two ibuprofen, without improvement. Mike wakes up to see his wife up and putting her coat on.

She says, "I'm going to the hospital."

"Do you want me to take you?"

"No, you stay here and get the kids to school."

"All right, but I'm going to wait for you; I won't go to work until you get home."

At 4:42 AM, Anna Kamianka walks into the emergency department at Hilltop Hospital.

II. The Doctor's Version (the following is the actual documentation of the provider)

Chief complaint per RN (05:05): "Back pain, chest pain, vomit, arm pain"

Date: November 6, 2002

```
VITAL SIGNS
Time    Temp(F)   Pulse   Resp   Syst   Diast   Pain Scale
05:07    97.4      72      18     138     93       8/10
```

TRIAGE (05:05):

> Woke up from sound sleep c̄ above sx. Took TT Motr Ø relief. Most pain between shoulder blades radi— down Ⓡ arm. ⊖ numbness/tingling chest midsternal pressure. ⊖SOB ⊖ n ⊕ v x1

Chief complaint (physician): Chest pain, coughing, and vomiting

HISTORY OF PRESENT ILLNESS: The patient is a 39-year-old female who approximately one month ago started developing a cough and congestion. She was seen [by her PCP] and started on an antibiotic. She started improving, but after going off the antibiotics, the cough came back and she has been coughing up yellowish sputum. She had post-tussive vomiting today. She indicates that when she coughs, she gets very sharp pain both in the front of the chest and the back. Those are the symptoms that she has been having. She denies any fever or SOB.

PAST MEDICAL HISTORY:
  Allergies: NKDA
  Meds: Birth control pills
  PMH/PSH: Negative
  SH: Smoker 1½ PPD. Drinks 6 pack daily

EXAM:
   CONSTITUTIONAL: She is alert. She does not appear to be in any distress at this point
   HEENT: Mouth and pharynx are clear
   NECK: Supple; no adenopathy of JVD
   LUNGS: Some wheezing in both bases but otherwise clear
   CHEST: She is tender over the anterior chest wall
   CARD: Regular rate and rhythm, nl. S1 S2
   BACK: Non-tender
   EXT: No cyanosis, edema, swelling

ED COURSE:
   05:20 – Pt. ambulatory to XR. **CXR results:** Interpreted by myself is normal without infiltrate or edema. Heart size is normal. [The reading is later confirmed by radiology over-read.]
   05:45 – Pt. medicated with acetaminophen 975mg PO. Albuterol aerosol
   06:15 – Pt. reports pain decreased to 5/10

PROGRESS NOTE: The patient felt much better after the aerosol. Her lungs are completely clear

DIAGNOSIS: Acute bronchitis

DISPOSITION (06:35): Azithromycin for 10 days. Hycodan. Follow up with Dr. Rembrandt in 5-7 days.

Timothy Madison, MD

III. The Errors—Risk Management/Patient Safety Issues

➤**Authors' note:** What could possibly be wrong? Our patient gets bronchitis every fall, and this year is no exception. After two months of being asymptomatic, was this a new infection, an incompletely treated infection, or perhaps something else?

Risk management/patient safety issue #1:

Error: Inadequate history of chest pain.

Discussion: Here is the history recorded for chest pain: "She indicates that when she coughs, she gets very sharp pain both in the front of the chest and the back." No one is recommending a cardiac cath with this presentation, but how about asking some basic questions such as:

- Is it worse with exertion?
- Is there radiation?
- Is this the first time you had it or has this been ongoing?
- Do you have *any* chest pain when you are not coughing?
- Is there associated diaphoresis?

✔ **Teaching point:** All evaluations begin with a good history.

Risk management/patient safety issue #2:

Error: Poor correlation between doctor and nurse notes.

Discussion: Buckle up for the ride; this is the first play-through of a soon-to-be broken record. It is well-known to medical students that attendings will often get a different story; is this because they are better historians, because patients change their tune or because medical students are slackers? In all fairness to the patients, many feel that once their story has been told (to the nurse, registration person… the guy sitting next to you in the lobby…) it is recorded in the chart, and the doctor is able to see it. This is why it is so frustrating to be walking out of the room after explaining the diagnosis only to hear, "but doctor, what about my chest pain … headache … fever …?"

✔ **Teaching point:** Though time-consuming, all complaints documented need to be addressed.

Risk management/patient safety issue #3:

Error: Poor explanation for back pain.

Discussion: Why did she have back pain? Was it because of a muscular strain from the coughing and vomiting, was it worse with movement? There was no back pain to touch. However, her chest did hurt with palpation. Did the chest pain radiate to the back? If her chest was strained from the vomiting, maybe she strained her back also; but it didn't hurt with palpation? Could this be a PE? How about Boerhaave's syndrome? Could a patient living in Cleveland have an aortic dissection and concomitant URI?

✔ **Teaching point:** When multiple complaints are present, a viable explanation for each should be present.

Risk management/patient safety issue #4:

Error: Not exploring cardiac risk factors.

Discussion: I have mixed feelings about this one. When a 17 year-old presents with a sudden onset of reproducible chest pain after lifting a refrigerator, I don't *want* to know that his grandmother had an MI at the age of 25. However, how firm is the diagnosis in *our* patient? The doctor's chart as a "stand-alone" seems quite convincing; a productive cough with sharp chest pain when coughing sounds like bronchitis. But read the nurse's notes and a different story emerges; chest pressure with radiation down the right arm with associated vomiting severe enough to wake her from sleep and prompt a 5 AM visit to the ED. Risk factors? If Anna would have been asked about her family history, she would have relayed that her brother died at the age of 32 from a MI. Coupled with smoking, use of oral contraceptives and moderate obesity, this *could* paint the picture of heart disease or PE.

✔ **Teaching point:** Sometimes, risk factors matter …

Risk management/patient safety issue #5:

Error: Not getting an ECG.

Discussion: Though the nursing protocol at Hilltop Hospital required an ECG be performed on all chest pain patients (this was brought out during the legal proceedings), I do have an issue with this. The true cost of the test to society is really only the electricity used and the ink and paper it is printed on. But is there a greater cost? If she would have had flipped "T-waves" in II, III and aVF, she would have been admitted, contracted a hospital-acquired infection and died. OK. Probably not. But, there is certainly a cost to a false positive result in an uninsured patient struggling to buy her kids Christmas presents, especially when you won't believe the results … or would you?

Teaching point: An ECG is a simple, inexpensive test, which can be helpful when excluding heart disease.

Risk management/patient safety issue #6:

Error: What's the deal with Zithromax?

Discussion: This patient didn't just get one Z-pack; the doctor "doubled-down" and gave her two! This reminds me of the Monty Python skit where the King built his castle on a swamp. It sank, but he would not be deterred and built another and another. Though the Z-pack is a great virus-killer, thrombolytic and aortic sleeve, it still was not indicated for this patient.

✔ **Teaching point:** Zithromax is a great drug, but it does nothing for viral bronchitis.

IV. The Bounceback

Anna arrives home between 7:00 and 7:30 and tells her husband, "Mike, I've got bronchitis. I'm going to lie down." Mike is relieved his wife is OK; he leaves for work and Anna spends most of the day laying around. When he arrives home at 4PM he asks his wife how she is doing. "So-so. I still feel rotten like I did in the morning. The medicine hasn't helped."

One hour later, the boys have eaten, and Anna has fixed dinner for her husband. After they eat, she picks up a glass of water and walks into the kitchen, but Mike is startled to hear her fall to the ground, water glass crashing to the floor. He and his sons rush in to find her unresponsive on the floor. One son calls 911, and Mike does what he can to revive her.

Per Cleveland EMS:
   17:17 – 911 call is received; nature of call from dispatch: "choking"
   17:21 – EMS arrive on the scene to find pt. "lying supine on the floor, unresponsive." They record: "Husband states she choked on food."
   17:23 – Asystole. CPR is initiated. Pt. is intubated
   17:38 – Pulse -0-, resp -0-, BP -0-
   17:40 – Monitor confirms coarse v-fib → shock 200-300-360 without improvement
   18:01 – Arrival at Hilltop Hospital: (documentation per physician)
      • Chief complaint: Full arrest
      • HPI: 39 year-old female intubated with CPR in progress. [EMS] have given several rounds of epinephrine and electrically cardioverted for a run of ventricular fibrillation. I talked

with the husband and he states she had been seen this morning around 5 AM. She had a cough and in general, complained of not feeling well. She had gotten a piece of cube chicken and was eating that when they heard her hit the floor.

- ED course: ET tube is pulled back slightly to account for right main stem intubation and now there are bilaterally equal breath sounds.

18:09 – Code called. The patient is pronounced at 1809 hours. The case is discussed with her husband in the presence of Father Patrick. A call will be placed to the PCP, Dr. Rembrandt and to the coroner.

ED DIAGNOSIS: Cardiopulmonary arrest, questionable etiology

➢**Authors' note:** What *was* the etiology of the arrest? The husband thinks she choked on chicken, but just because she was eating it when she collapsed does not prove cause and effect. Similarly, just because she had a cough earlier in the day does not mean her two previous diagnoses were necessarily from an URI. Is there a way to know if she really had an URI on September 5th? Enter the coroner…

AUTOPSY DIAGNOSIS:

The coronary arteries are patent except for a focal area of the LAD which shows 99% luminal narrowing by gray-tan material. There is focal grey scar tissue in the interventricular septum. Aorta shows mild atheromatous streaks and plaques.

Coronary atherosclerotic heart disease
- Acute thrombosis in left anterior descending coronary artery
- Intramyocardial arteriosclerosis
- Remote, organizing and acute myocardial infarcts

FINAL DIAGNOSIS: Acute myocardial infarction

➢**Authors' note:** So now the diagnosis is clear. No PE. No aspiration. No pneumonia. No dissection. The patient had a small septal MI in September. She didn't improve *because* of antibiotics, but improved *coincidental* with the prescription of antibiotics. She then awoke around 4 AM with symptoms of her acute MI (AMI), including chest and back pain from an acute thrombus in the LAD, the "widow maker." At her first ED visit, an ECG would likely have shown STEMI and there was plenty of time for revascularization or thrombolysis.

This was not an easy diagnosis. She did have symptoms typically seen with bronchitis and associated chest-wall strain reproducible with palpation. But some aspects of the evaluation did not make sense for URI. A previously well person who had never missed a day of work woke up on a cold November morning at 4AM, left her husband and children at home and drove herself to the ED for chest pain, back pain, vomiting, arm pain and cough. That must have been *some* URI … Would you have done an ECG? Should the nurse have automatically done an ECG per the hospital protocol? Does a complaint of chest pain require at least a few questions as to exacerbation (exertion) or associated symptoms (diaphoresis)?

The doctor was aware of the chest pain and did mention that in the HPI, but his impression was certainly different than the nurse's. His documentation suggested a musculoskeletal etiology. This was a *tough* diagnosis. Did the lawyers agree? What did *they* think of the doctor's evaluation?

PART 2—LEGAL

I. The Accusation/Cause of Action

The accusation here is pretty clear: failure to diagnose. For a legal action to be successful, the plaintiff must also prove "causation;" in other words, that the alleged negligence— *failure* to diagnose—actually *caused* the patient's injuries.

The actual trial involved two defendants, the emergency physician *and* the primary care doctor who initially diagnosed bronchitis on September 5th. The autopsy suggests an initially missed septal infarct at the PCP visit and a fatal MI with thrombosis to the LAD on November 6th. We will just focus on the action against the EP; the diagnosis is clear and uncontested. The question here is *if* this was a "diagnose-able" condition when Anna presented at 4:42 AM on the sixth. To answer that question, eight *non-physicians* were chosen; the courts call it a jury ...

II. What Would Greg Do (WWGD)?

Greg Henry, past president of The American College of Emergency Physicians (ACEP), Professor of Emergency Medicine at the University of Michigan, and CEO of Medical Practice Risk Assessment, has been an expert witness in over 2,000 malpractice cases.

Greg opines on evaluation of chest pain, defense and plaintiff strategy, and if he would settle.

> **"If I sit back and state only the pertinent parts of any case, no one will miss this diagnosis— But that's not how patients present."**

Chest pain is still our *biggest* pain. When I first started to do medical legal cases in 1976, misdiagnosis of chest pain accounted for between 35% and 40% of cases. Guess what? In the last three years, chest pain is still about 33% of the cases. The reason is simple. Most people with chest pain don't have something bad. When they do have something bad, it can be deadly.

The public at large is inundated with TV advertisements and dramatic scenarios of chest pain; every layperson can give you the differential diagnosis. The problem is we have a high signal-to-noise ratio. If I sit back and state only the pertinent parts of any case, no one will miss this diagnosis, but that's not how patients present. They have strange stories that go up and down and around. They ascribe their symptoms to factors having nothing to do with their actual disease. Just because you cough doesn't mean it's bronchitis. There's certainly no evidence to suggest that viral bronchitis is made better with a Z-Pack, but don't try telling that to my wife. The complex interaction between scientific medicine and patient satisfaction drives every emergency physician crazy.

What is difficult to avoid in this case is that a 39 year-old woman was awoken from sleep with severe pain between her shoulder blades. This is compounded with the history of a brother who died at age 32 of some medical condition—no matter how you cut it, the brother probably had cardiovascular disease. She smokes 1½ packs per day, is on birth control pills and has chest pain radiating down to her right arm. That is a very difficult scenario to ignore. But I've dissected the facts after knowing the outcome …

As in each case in this book, I'm asked whether I would settle. I make my recommendation while blinded to the outcome. The problem with settlement is that there are huge potential financial loses; this case is not going to settle for a small amount of money. If you tried this case in front of a reasonable jury, you would win 7 out of 10 times. She does have confusing history and improved after leaving the ED.

The defense will have to concentrate on the complexity of the problem, her history of bronchitis and the fact that she felt improved with respiratory treatment. Defense revolves around the fact that 39 year-old women, in general, don't drop dead of heart attacks. The great danger in this case is jury sympathy.

The plaintiff's strategy is simple—heart disease is still as much a common killer of women as it is of men. The fact that she had chest pain running into arms is one of the symptoms taught by the American Heart Association (AHA). As plaintiff, I would bring in posters showing the warning symptoms of heart attack; a simple story and qualified experts could make a substantial impact on the jury.

Would I settle? It's a toss-up. Knowing that we would win this case in 7 out of 10 times, if I could get a settlement for under $200K, I would definitely do it. If not, let's go to trial!

III. The Trial (Monday, September 26, 2005)

➤**Authors' note:** This was a tough trial and a tough case. We all feel for the family and this devoted couple, high school sweethearts who have worked hard and struggled to provide for their family. But who else works in a profession where you can be forced to go to court to defend your actions if there is a poor outcome?

The following is the actual trial transcript. The court's instructions and both opening statements have been significantly shortened. All names have been changed except Mark Jones, who was the actual defense attorney for the case. All other trial testimony is exactly reproduced, but may be shortened and syntax minimally changed to enhance readability. In chapter one, we reproduce the opening statements and in chapter two we focus on the closing statements.

Cast of characters (names changed, except as noted):

The patient: Anna Kamianka
ED physician defendant: Timothy Madison
Plaintiff's attorney: Albert August
Plaintiff's expert witness: Drew Florra (Board certified emergency medicine)
Defense attorney: Mark Jones (actual attorney)

Judge's instructions to jury: Before we hear the opening statements of counsel and begin to take evidence, it will be helpful if you have some preliminary instructions to follow. Later, after you have heard all the evidence, I will give further instructions covering additional [issues of] law. It is the duty of the judge to instruct you in the law and your duty to follow the law.

First of all, it is your exclusive duty to decide all questions of fact submitted to you. In connection with this duty, you must determine the effect and value of the evidence. You must not be influenced in your decision by sympathy, prejudice or passion towards any party, witness or attorney in the case.

The attorneys will have active roles in the trial. They will make opening statements to you, question witnesses and make objections. And finally, they will argue the case as a last step before you hear my final instructions and commence with deliberations. Remember that attorneys are not witnesses. Since it is your duty to decide the case solely on the evidence which you hear in the case, you must not consider as evidence any statement of any attorney made during the trial, [with the exception being] if the attorneys agree to any facts.

The burden of proof is upon the plaintiff to prove the facts necessary to his case by a preponderance of the evidence. Preponderance is the "greater weight of the evidence," that is the evidence that you believe because it outweighs or overbalances in your minds the evidence opposed to it. As jurors, you have the sole and exclusive duty to decide the credibility of witnesses who will testify in the case. As you are all aware, two persons who are witnesses to an incident may often see or hear it differently.

Any fact in this case may be proven by direct or circumstantial evidence. Direct evidence directly proves a fact without having to infer the fact from some other fact. It includes the witnesses who have seen or heard the facts in a case and also includes the exhibits admitted as evidence. Circumstantial evidence, on the other hand, is the proof of facts from direct evidence from which you may reasonably infer a fact in question. For example, if the question in a case is whether Johnny ate a piece of cherry pie, *direct evidence* is a witness who says she saw Johnny put a piece of pie in his mouth and eat it. *Circumstantial evidence* is a witness who testifies that she arrived in the kitchen to see Johnny standing there with an empty pie tin and cherry pie on his face.

So with those definitions … Mr. August, [for the plaintiff], are you prepared with your opening statement?

Opening statement, plaintiff's attorney, Mr. August: Good morning ladies and gentlemen. May it please the court? This is our chance to give you an overview. Please relax. I wouldn't be surprised if you're a little nervous. I'm a little nervous. I know Mike (her husband) is a little nervous. I think it's appropriate we're all a little nervous.

This is a very, very important matter. It involves the destruction of a life and the destruction of a family because of the negligence of two different doctors at two different times. And as the evidence unfolds in this case, you will see that this was truly a preventable tragedy.

Anna Kamianka was a working housewife and mother of three sons. Her contribution to the family was immeasurable. She was the center of the family. She was the glue that held them together. She was the motivating force that got things done. The family relied on her.

Dr. Madison [the ED physician] latched onto the prior diagnosis of bronchitis and in the end, that's exactly what he came up with as a conclusion for what was wrong with her. You will not find anything in this record to even suggest that he asked about family history. He didn't know. He didn't ask. If he had, she would have told him. Why is that important? Well, you got chest pain. You have radiation. The possibility of it being cardiac is clearly there. Chest pressure, chest tightness, suspicious for cardiac problems, but he didn't ask. Had he asked, he would have discovered that she had 5 risk factors for cardiac disease. Dr Madison didn't even take an EKG. No enzymes. No cardiac workup. Sent home with a prescription for an antibiotic. She was flashing red lights about a heart problem, and no tests were done.

Anna didn't have to suffer a heart attack. She didn't have to die. I can't speak for you, but I have seen several TV commercials telling people that if they have chest pain, get to an ER. That's just what Anna did on November 6th. The problem is that Anna did what she was supposed to do. These two doctors did not. And, unfortunately Anna is not here today as a result. And that's what I said at the onset, Ladies and Gentlemen, that this was truly a preventable tragedy.

Opening statement, defense attorney, Mr. Jones: Good morning, folks. I represent Dr. Timothy Madison. We're not going to be discussing Dr. Madison's personal and family life like we will Mrs. Kamianka's, so in a sense you won't get the same sense for him as a person, but you will get a very clear picture of Dr. Madison as a physician. You will hear from him twice in this case, first when he is called by Mr. August for cross-examination and again later in the case when I call him to testify in his own defense. You will learn that he is an intelligent, conscientious, and thorough physician. He's board certified in emergency medicine. He has seen thousands and thousands of patients.

Among those thousands of patients, it is not unusual that several times a day he will see somebody with chest pain and somebody with respiratory problems like bronchitis. These are not unusual problems for patients in an emergency department. And it is not unusual that a doctor orders an EKG, not just for chest pain, but for any number of complaints.

You will see records of Dr. Madison's dictated note; a thorough history, exam and what he thought was going on with the patient. He [documents] that she was having pain in her back with a cough. Oh, that hurts. Had the cough bad enough to throw up. She strained herself. Oh, man that hurts here; it's radiating down my right arm.

So what's this case all about? [Mrs. Kamianka] has a cough—she's coughing up yellow sputum. Dr. Madison pushed on her chest and it was sore—that's what we call reproducible pain. The first thing you [the jury] will have to decide is whether Dr. Madison deviated from the accepted standard of care. We believe he did act appropriately. We are confident that when you have [looked at the evidence] you will walk back into this courtroom and give Dr. Madison his defense verdict.

➤**Authors' note:** So now the allegations are better defined. It is indisputable that she had chest pain, but the doctor is relying on his history and evaluation and thinks she has an infectious cause. How will he defend himself on the stand? How would you defend yourself on the stand? Let's see …

Cross-examination of defendant ED physician, Dr. Timothy Madison, by plaintiff's attorney Mr. August:

Q. Mr. August (plaintiff's counsel): Would you agree with me that potential cardiac symptoms include back pain, chest pain, vomiting, and arm pain?

A. Dr. Timothy Madison (defendant): They are potential symptoms, that's correct.

Q. Now, when you are interested in trying to determine if a patient has myocardial ischemia, what do you do?

A. Initially I would try and elicit a history. I would look at notes and vital signs that the nurse has taken. And then I would examine the patient and make a determination if further testing needs to be done.

Q. Well, I was talking about a patient where you suspected cardiac ischemia, all right?

A. Yes.

Q. So it is true that after the history and physical is taken in a patient with potential cardiac ischemia, you would order an EKG?

A. That is a possibility.

Q. And you would probably order blood work, cardiac enzymes?

A. That's a possibility also.

Q. Part of what you're doing when you're talking to the patient and getting this history is also to assess risk factors, right?

A. In relation presenting with cardiac symptoms?

Q. Right, yes.

A. That's correct.

➤**Authors' note:** The defendant cannot really answer any other way to these questions, but what he wants to say is, "I did *not* think this patient had cardiac ischemia. So, *of course* I didn't get an EKG." This part of the trial is not damning, just a few statements of fact. It is also by the plaintiff's attorney and there will be plenty of time for Dr. Madison to defend himself when he is called back to the stand by his defense attorney.

The ECG is a simple test, inexpensive, noninvasive and could almost certainly have diagnosed the MI. There are false positives; for example, a chronically flipped T wave without an old ECG for comparison could prompt an unnecessary admission, but a STEMI is very specific. Does that mean all chest-pain patients require an ECG? Absolutely not.

However, if a patient has chest pain, the nidus is to prove that the pain is not from ischemia, just as a young woman with pelvic pain and a positive pregnancy test has an ectopic until proven otherwise. An *alternative explanation* for her symptoms, such as a productive cough suggesting bronchitis, goes a long way toward excluding ACS/MI. But just as important as proving a likely diagnosis is excluding the more life-threatening diagnoses per our mantra, "Think Worst First."

The doctor continues with a plausible explanation of deciding not to order an ECG. It seems reasonable and well thought out. It seems like something many of us would do. But how does he answer the questions in front of a lay-jury? Pretty well, I think. But stay tuned for the plaintiff's expert opine on the utility of an ECG.

Continued cross-examination of defendant ED physician, Dr. Madison, by plaintiff's attorney, Mr. August:

Q. So what about Mrs. Kamianka's presentation makes it OK *not* to do an EKG?

A. You're saying that with this presentation I'm obliged to rule out a cardiac origin. I'm saying that is not the case. There's no evidence that the patient had ischemic cardiac disease. The presentation was one of bronchitis and an infectious upper respiratory disease; and as such I'm not obliged to rule out a cardiac origin.

Q. What does a patient need to have as a minimum to get an EKG when they come to the ER with chest pain, if you're the one covering the ER?

A. Well, that patient certainly wouldn't present with a productive cough so [severe] she is throwing up with resulting chest pain.

➤**Authors' note:** What does a guy have to do to get a drink around here?

Q. Can a patient who comes in with a productive cough that's coughing hard, coughing enough to vomit, can that patient still have a heart attack?

A. All things are possible.

Q. Can they still have a heart attack when their complaints include chest pain?

A. Yes, they can.

Q. And that's pretty important to rule out if you have a test that's easily accessible to you in the emergency room, isn't it?

A. To order that test, you need to have an indication.

Q. Truth is, doctor, you never even considered a cardiac cause of Mrs. Kamianka's chest pain complaints, did you?

A. It was in the differential but as I got further history and physical exam, it went further and further down the list.

➤**Authors' note:** Do lawyers know about *diagnosis momentum*? You betcha!

Q. Doctor, isn't it true that once Mrs. Kamianka mentioned the fact that she had been to her family doctor and had a diagnosis of bronchitis some weeks before that you presumed the same diagnosis and operated accordingly?

A. No, absolutely not. I based my treatment upon my interview with the patient. Upon the history that I obtained, upon my physical exam and the treatment of the patient in the emergency department. I do not base my treatments and evaluations upon another physician.

➢**Authors' note:** How about controversial observations such as the fact that women with cardiac symptoms present atypically? Is this even true? (Read commentary by Amal Mattu and Emilie Cobert at the end of the chapter).

Q. A person can have an MI and still have pain between the shoulder blades?
A. Yes, they can.

Q. You talk about it as an atypical presentation of heart disease, is that what you said?
A. That's exactly what I said.

Q. You are aware of the fact that women more often present with atypical symptoms than men, right?
A. Yes, women can.

Q. Was it the cervical spine scoliosis that caused you to think this was not cardiac in origin?
A. No. It was part of the entire workup. That, in and of itself, did not prevent me from getting an ECG. What you're doing is taking each finding specifically and singling it out, and I'm saying I took all those *in context* and as such did not order an ECG.

➢**Authors' note:** Well done. We all understand what he means. How does the plaintiff's attorney wrap this up for the jury? The end of the questioning is always interesting; it is an attempt to leave a lasting impression. The following three questions can only be answered in one way. They have nothing to do with the medical decision-making or the quality of care rendered, but they really don't make the physician look too good. It is a clever approach since the attorney knows before he even starts how the doctor will answer—he knows the glove will fit. See how he inserts the word "doctor" into the last question; my guess is that it wasn't said in the respectful way ... more like a dig ...

Q. You don't have any reason to disagree with the coroner about the cause of death, do you?
A. No, I don't.

Q. [Was there any] evidence of bronchitis on autopsy?
A. No.

Q. As of November 2002, *Doctor*, is it true and do you agree that cardiovascular disease was the number one killer of women in the United States?
A. Yes, I believe that it was.

MR. AUGUST: Thank you very much.

THE COURT: Doctor, you may step down. Ladies and gentlemen, we're going to take our morning break. Break for about 25 minutes. You can go downstairs and have a cup of coffee. Please don't discuss this case among yourselves or with anyone else. Don't form or express any opinions until you have heard all the evidence. All rise for the jury.

➤**Authors' note:** Remember that part about the ECG? The following is the plaintiff's expert's testimony. I will tell you this—I know this guy. He teaches nationally. And he doesn't come across as a medical "whore," he comes across as having a responsible thought process ... if a bit judgmental ... Mr. August cuts right to the chase:

Direct examination of plaintiff's expert witness, Drew Florra, MD, FACEP (board certified emergency medicine physician) by plaintiff's attorney, Mr. August:

Q. Based on your training and experience as well as your review of the materials in this case, do you have an opinion as to whether Dr. Madison violated the standard of care in his treatment of Mrs. Kamianka on the morning of November 6th, 2002?

A. Yes.

Q. Are these opinions based upon reasonable medical probability?

A. They certainly are. All the opinions are more likely than not, at the very least. The opinion is that the standard of care—in other words, what a reasonably prudent physician would do under similar circumstances, was not upheld. That was not done.

Q. What is the basis of that opinion?

A. You can make it complicated or simple. I think simple is best. This was not an exceptional case in any way. This was a 39 year-old woman who came to the ED with chest pain about 5 in the morning and it's described many times in the chart. It's true it included some words like sharp, front and back, but also was described as pain between the shoulder blades, radiation down the arm, and also midsternal chest pressure. When a 39 year-old person comes in with those complaints, in our society, an EKG is mandatory. It's not a judgment. It's not a thought. It's mandatory. And that wasn't done.

The tragic thing is 10 or 12 hours later the patient died of coronary disease. It is virtually certain that if a simple EKG, which costs almost nothing, they charge about $40 for it but the actual cost is nothing, and it's non-invasive ... almost certainly would have been abnormal and would have saved her life.

Q. I want to back up a step here, Doctor. You said it's mandatory, it's required—it's not a matter of judgment. There has been testimony in this case that the physician has judgment when it comes to deciding what tests to order when a patient presents to the ER with various complaints. Why do you say in this instance there is no room for judgment?

A. I think that's a fair question because, you know, it's not like in emergency medicine most things are cut and dry. It's actually hard to think of things that are, but this is one. The fact is that this isn't a *rare* disease, this is *coronary* disease. Half the people in this room are going to die of it. Every single person has a relative or a friend that has died of a heart attack. We are in this business to find this disease. Amazingly enough, we have a pretty good test that's non-invasive, and it's pretty cheap: it's an EKG.

And it's just very clear that when people come in even without chest pain, [for example with] some of the other symptoms like nausea or vomiting, but certainly with midsternal pressure and radiation down the arm, in our society most lay people would know that—you have to do an EKG. Since it's such a common and lethal disease, that it is simply required. It doesn't matter if you think the person has bronchitis or is crazy, whatever you think, you still have to do the EKG.

Q. Does it matter what the potential risk is for the underlying condition when making the determination that an EKG has got to be done?

A. I think I see what you mean. Let's say, for example, a good careful physician honestly believed that the person was ten times as likely to have bronchitis as to have a heart attack. But you had a simple test that could rule out a heart attack with some good probability, or certainly could rule it in. Obviously, you would have to do it because if you miss the bronchitis, so what? It really doesn't matter. It's not even clear the treatment of bronchitis makes much difference. But when we're talking about ACS, that's one of about 5 conditions in emergency medicine that we are not allowed to miss. We only get one shot at it. So even when we have a very low suspicion, we have to go ahead and do the test to rule it out.

➤**Authors' note:** Ok, ok, good arguments. Still, in the middle of cold and flu season? Did these arguments sway the jury?

IV. The Verdict

Judge's instructions to jury (shortened): Good morning ladies and gentlemen. Welcome back. The evidence portion of the trial has now concluded. As I indicated, you're going to hear the instructions of law and the arguments of counsel this morning.

By agreement of the parties, instead of hearing closing arguments first, you're going to hear the instructions of law from me.

In determining whether an issue has been proven by a preponderance of the evidence, you should consider all of the evidence, regardless of who produced it. If the weight of the evidence is equally balanced, or if you are unable to determine which side of an issue has the preponderance, the party who has the burden of proof has not established such issue. Specifically, the plaintiff alleges that Dr. Madison as a treating emergency medicine specialist was negligent in failing to work Anna Kamianka up for a potential cardiac problem.

The issues for you to decide are the following. Number 1, has the plaintiff proven that the defendant was negligent in one or more of the respective claims against him? Number 2, if your answer to this first question is yes, was such negligence a proximate cause of the injuries and damages sustained, including death of the decedent?

➤**Authors' note:** The judge goes on to define how the jury is to make their decision. Read closely, since this will be important later:

Additional judge's instructions to the jury: Although some other physician might have used a different method of diagnosis, treatment or procedure than that used by Dr. Madison, this will not by itself prove that Dr. Madison was negligent. The mere fact that Dr. Madison used an alternative method of diagnosis, treatment or procedure is not by itself proof of negligence. You are to decide whether the diagnosis, treatment, or procedure used by Dr. Madison was reasonable in accordance with the standard of care required of a physician in his field of practice.

Plaintiff's attorney, Mr. August: Objection! To preserve the record, your honor, I would like to renew the plaintiff's objections to the charge or the absence of certain charges. First of all, the plaintiff objects to the inclusion of a charge on "different methods" because we believe the evidence in this case does not support the giving of that charge.

The Court (Judge): Okay, right, well, your objection is noted.

➤**Authors' note:** Well, it all seems reasonable to me ... but I'm no judge. The following is the jury verdict:

The Court: My bailiff has informed me you have reached a verdict
Jury Foreman: Yes.
The Court: Will the foreman please hand the verdict forms over?
(Tendered)
The Court: All right. Has the plaintiff, Mike Kamianka, proven by a preponderance of the evidence that defendant, Timothy Madison, was negligent? (Reads.) The answer is "no." This is signed by seven jurors.

Summary: The jury found in favor of the doctor 7–1 (and against Kamianka).

V. The Appeal (March 1, 2007)

➤**Authors' note:** But this was not the end of the story ... The actual patient encounter occurred on November 6, 2002, and after an extensive legal process and a huge sigh of relief, the doctor is absolved. Now, almost five years after the initial patient visit, the doctor is informed the jury's decision has been appealed. Ugghh!

The following is the plaintiff's allegation for appeal and the defense argument against appeal.

Plaintiff: The trial court erred in instructing the jury, over plaintiff's objection, that there were "different methods" of diagnosing the plaintiff's decedent's medical condition when there was no evidence that more than one method is acceptable to diagnose coronary artery disease." Kamianka argues that the trial court should not have given the "different methods" jury instruction, because the expert testimony established that the only acceptable method of definitively diagnosing coronary artery disease is a cardiac work-up. Kamianka contends that this instruction misled the jury in a matter substantially affecting Kamianka's rights.

Defense: Dr. Madison argues that the instruction was proper because the trial testimony established that acceptable alternative methods of diagnosis existed for Mrs. Kamianka's condition, i.e., chest pain associated with a cough.

Appeals Court impression: Although this instruction has been found appropriate under the facts of certain cases, it is concerning that *different methods for diagnosis, treatment and procedure* are all encompassed under this one instruction rather than parsed out. However, where the issue involved is whether the physician negligently failed to diagnose a particular disease from the observed symptoms, the instruction is misleading to the jury. In such a case, the instruction implies that even where multiple conditions may exist (bronchitis or coronary artery disease), as long as the physician followed a method for diagnosing one of the potential conditions, the doctor may be absolved of negligence. The question here is not whether the physician followed an accepted method for diagnosing bronchitis, but rather, whether the physician failed to recognize that the observed symptoms indicated the presence of heart disease.

Accordingly, we conclude that the trial court erred. The issue is not whether the doctors chose between two recognized methods of diagnosis, but whether they negligently failed to recognize that Mrs. Kamianka's symptoms required that they perform a cardiac work-up to rule out coronary artery disease. Chest pain and coughing were the symptoms, not the diagnosis. Kamianka's assignment of error is sustained.

Judgment: Reversed and remanded. It is ordered that appellant [plaintiff] recover from appellee [defendant] costs herein taxed. The court finds there were reasonable grounds for this appeal.

Authors' note: Wow! How about going through years of depositions and a long trial which rules in your favor, only to have the defense verdict overruled two years later on what seems like a technicality?

VI. The Twist

It is surprising what happens next: instead of proceeding to a new trial, the defense decides to settle. Settle? After winning? How much did they get? Below is an interview with the actual defense attorney, Mark Jones, who reveals their reasoning.

VII. Guest Interview—The Legal Analysis: Mark Jones, JD

- Roetzel & Andress, LPA, Cleveland Ohio
- Mr. Jones was the actual defense attorney in this case

Authors: *We are doctors, trained to use our clinical judgment and not "cookbook" patients. How did you respond to the plaintiff expert's allegations that an ECG always needs to be done?*
MJ: Plaintiff focused on the complaint of chest pain and made the valid point that chest pain from coronary ischemia in women can deviate dramatically from the "classic presentation," placing the ED physician on notice that an ECG is always required. The defense focused on the primary presenting complaint being a severe cough, with *associated* chest pain. The defense argued that:

1. A presenting complaint of chest pain is so common in the ED and can arise from any number of causes, that it would be unreasonable for the standard of care to demand ECGs for all chest pain presentations.
2. All chest pain is not the same, and medical judgment informed by experience and the particulars of the presentation establishes the standard of care
3. It was reasonable for the ED physician to conclude from the totality of the presentation that the likelihood of coronary ischemia was very low and the likelihood of severe bronchitis was quite high.

Authors: *Before the initial trial, did you consider settling? How confident were you that a defense verdict would prevail?*

MJ: Yes, settlement was considered. Significant efforts to settle were undertaken prior to trial, but the demand remained too high. Plaintiff had a well-respected expert and much of the medical literature was supportive of his argument. Prior to the start of trial, it was felt that a defense verdict was a 50–50 proposition. As trial proceeded I became more confident of a defense verdict.

Authors: *Were you surprised with the jury's verdict?*
MJ: No. A jury is capable of coming to any result, and sometimes I am elated by the verdict, sometimes disappointed. Although I am often surprised by events during the trial of a case, I am never surprised by a jury verdict. In this case, it seemed the strident testimony of plaintiff's expert turned the jury off to his testimony; this was not his demeanor at his deposition some months earlier. I was pleasantly surprised by my client's testimony at trial; although he had never been a witness and was very anxious, he presented himself to the jury as confident, competent and thorough. It was this combination of plaintiff expert's poor presentation and the defendant's very good presentation that carried the day.

Authors: *Why did you lose the appeal?*
MJ: Plaintiff appealed on an issue regarding the instructions of law given to the jury. Although it was unlikely that the one instruction faulted had any impact on deliberations, it was not an instruction supported by the evidence presented at trial. The appellate court found error in giving the instruction and sent the case back for trial on all issues.

Authors: *If you won once, why did you think you couldn't win again?*
MJ: The defense felt that in re-trying the case, plaintiff's counsel would adjust his presentation and avoid problems the defense took advantage of in the first trial, and therefore the likelihood of a defense verdict would still be a 50–50 proposition. At trial I was able to take advantage of some inexperience on the part of plaintiff's expert witnesses, an advantage I would lose at a retrial. The doctor was also exhausted by the whole process and wanted to end it.

Authors: What was the settlement amount?
MJ: In settlement negotiations the demand became very reasonable (though I can't reveal the exact amount).

VIII. Medical Discussion—Evaluation of Chest Pain

Guest authors:

Emilie Cobert, MD, MPH
Department of Emergency Medicine
University of Maryland Medical Center
Baltimore, Maryland

Amal Mattu, MD, FAAEM, FACEP
Professor and Residency Director
Department of Emergency Medicine
University of Maryland School of Medicine
Baltimore, Maryland

From the beginning of emergency medicine training, we are taught a simple concept: "rule out the worst first." It is perfectly acceptable for other specialists to create differential diagnoses starting with the most *common* causes of chief complaints, but in emergency medicine we must always work backwards, considering the most *deadly* diagnoses first. That disparity is most important when caring for patients with chest pain. Though GERD, bronchitis and chest wall strain may be the most common causes, acute coronary syndrome (ACS), aortic dissection and pulmonary embolism are the most deadly. When other physicians hear hoofbeats they think of horses, but emergency physicians think of lions and tigers and bears, then work backwards toward the benign diagnoses.

Using that mind-set, let's evaluate this case. An adult patient presented to the ED with several chief complaints, including "back pain, chest pain, vomiting, and arm pain." The triage note then listed once again back pain ("between shoulder blades") with radiation down the right arm, and described the character of the chest pain as being midsternal chest pressure. The treating physician listed "chest pain, coughing, and vomiting." When considering some of the "lions and tigers and bears" that could account for this set of complaints, one must certainly consider cardiac (ACS, pericarditis/pericardial tamponade), vascular (aortic dissection) and pulmonary (pulmonary embolism) causes. The history and physical examination are then critical in deciding if any of the deadly diagnoses can be reasonably ruled out or if further testing is necessary.

In this case, there were two main diagnostic failures which threw the physician off the track. First, the physician found "horses" in the benign diagnosis of bronchitis; the productive cough and recent history of bronchitis diagnosis led him to a premature closure of the investigative process. It is important to remember the presence of a benign condition does not exclude a concomitant deadly condition.

The second major mistake stemmed from the first, an inadequate evaluation of the patient. When evaluating chest pain, we like to use the mnemonic OLDCAAAR to ensure an adequate history:

- O – Onset
- L – Location
- D – Duration
- C – Character
- A – Alleviating/aggravating factors
- A – Associated symptoms (dyspnea, diaphoresis, nausea/vomiting)
- A – Activity at onset
- R – Radiation

In this case, there is only a partial description of Mrs. Kamianka's symptoms, in particular, her chest pain. Furthermore, the physician did not fully address the back pain or arm pain that was in the initial triage assessment. Were the back and arm pains related to or radiations of the chest pain? Was there a recent trauma? Was the chest pain in any way exertional? Was this cough characteristic of her previous episodes of URI/bronchitis? Had a more-detailed history been documented, it possibly would have prompted further testing.

There's no question that the presentation was not "classic;" instead it was "atypical," a term not clearly defined in the literature. Physicians know classic ischemic chest pain well: chest pressure worse with exertion, with radiation of pain down the left arm, and associated anxiety[1] and sometimes nausea, vomiting and diaphoresis. The logical extrapolation is that without the above complaints, the presentation is considered atypical.[2] Two subgroups are commonly recognized as being high risk for having atypical presentations when ACS is present: the elderly and diabetics. However, in recent years we've found that women are also a high-risk group.

Cardiovascular disease is now the leading cause of death for women in the United States.[3] While it's true that women with ACS tend to present most often with chest pain,[4,5] atypical presentations tend to be more common in women than in men. Frequent "atypical" presentations in women include jaw/neck pain, mid-back/posterior shoulder pain, right arm pain, fatigue, nausea, vomiting and indigestion.[6,7] One study demonstrated a statistically-significant greater prevalence of women's AMI presenting with *cough*,[8] as occurred in this case. The takeaway point here is *not* that every woman presenting with fatigue or cough needs cardiac enzymes and a stress test, but rather that these complaints do not rule out the deadly diagnosis.

One of the interesting issues brought up by the plaintiff's expert was electrocardiography. Would an electrocardiogram (ECG) have been the key to clinch a diagnosis of ACS on September 5th when she visited her PCP or on November 6th when she presented to the ED? Not necessarily. An initial ECG has a sensitivity for AMI of up to 60%[9] and as many as 10% of AMI patients may never demonstrate significant ST segment changes or T wave abnormalities.[10] Many emergency physicians would interpret this data as saying that an ECG would have had a 60–90% chance of making a cardiac diagnosis—for this reason, there is generally a low threshold for obtaining ECGs in patients where the diagnosis could be ACS/MI.

The plaintiff's attorney pointed out that cardiac risk factors should have been elicited. However, recent literature has demonstrated that cardiac risk factors actually play very little role in predicting the likelihood of ACS.[11,12] Instead, risk factors are most useful in predicting long-term risk. Nevertheless, it seems that a jury would be easily impressed with her risk factors: heavy smoker, hypertension and family history of early cardiac death.

When all is said and done, who has the better argument?

- In favor of the plaintiff: Here's a 39 year-old woman with multiple cardiac risk factors, presenting with midsternal chest pressure radiating to the right arm and vomiting. The physician focused on her cough instead of doing what a good emergency physician is supposed to do—rule out the life threats! He did a lackluster history, didn't pay attention to the clues the nursing notes were giving him and didn't even do a cheap, simple test that would have saved her life. He took the easy way out by clinging to a benign diagnosis and now Anna Kamianka is dead!

- In favor of the defendant: This patient's presentation was *entirely* consistent with a non-cardiac type of presentation … so much so that even an ECG was not indicated. As the chart shows, she had a cough productive of yellow sputum, post-tussive vomiting with back pain and sharp chest pain directly related to the cough. She improved after treatment—show me the literature that indicates that ACS presents with a productive cough and wheezing that resolves with aerosols! We know that ECGs are usually non-diagnostic, so if you are going to argue that this patient needed an ECG, you must also be arguing that this patient needed an admission and full work-up. And that means that everyone showing up in the ED with a chest cold must be admitted!

This is a tough call. In fact we, the authors (Emilie and Amal), ourselves disagree on which side has the stronger argument, but we agree that the case could go either way based on the likability and believability of the expert witnesses and defendant. We also agree that a couple of extra minutes spent on the HPI would have likely prevented this lawsuit, even if not the patient's outcome.

Emergency physicians would be prudent to follow a few simple rules when making a benign diagnosis:

1. A strong case must be made in the chart for the benign diagnosis.
2. A thorough history (especially HPI) and physical examination should be documented, which reflects consideration of the deadly possibilities.
3. Any chart discrepancies must be addressed.
4. Any "red flag terms/phrases" (e.g., "midsternal pressure" and "radiation down the arm") must be addressed.

Without this, the best physicians can do is to cross their fingers when the summons and complaint are received.

IX. Authors' Summary

What can we learn from this bizarre case? Since completing this chapter, I have had several weeks of ED shifts … all in Ohio … all in November. The fact is that bronchitis is a dime a dozen—and who has bronchitis without *any* chest pain?

- When a patient has URI symptoms and chest pain, inquire about exertional pain or associated dyspnea or diaphoresis. If that had been done in this case, the doctor would have learned a fact we have not yet discussed: Though it may sound indelicate, it was brought up at trial that Anna and her husband had "relations" the night of her MI, and the exertion caused chest pain.

- Though multiple-complaint patients are time-consuming and often frustrating, each complaint still needs to be specifically addressed no matter how obvious the diagnosis, no matter how much static on the language line, no matter how long they have had fibromyalgia …
- Not to sound too much like a broken record, but "read the nurse's notes, read the nurse's notes, read the nurse's notes …"
- When the findings on evaluation do not mesh with the chief complaints, explain your thought process in a progress note. If the note is not convincing even to *you*, go back to the bedside, confirm the history and ensure life-threatening diagnoses are not occurring.
- Have a low threshold for performing an ECG in patients with chest pain.

It turns out the key to almost all these cases is decidedly low tech—with diagnostic uncertainty, we need a *great* history.

References

1. Silverman ME. William Heberden and some account of a disorder of the breast. Clin Cardiol 1987; 10:211-3.
2. Jones ID, Slovis CM. Emergency department evaluation of the chest pain patient. Emerg Med Clin N Am 2001; 19:269–82.
3. Zbierajewski-Eischeid SJ, Loeb SJ. Myocardial infarction in women: promoting symptom recognition, early diagnosis, and risk assessment. Dimens Crit Care Nurs 2009;28:1-6; quiz 7-8.
4. Patel H, Rosengren A, Ekman I. Symptoms in acute coronary syndromes: does sex make a difference? Am Heart J 2004;148:27-33.
5. Kudenchuk PJ, Maynard C, Martin JS, et al. Comparison of presentation, treatment, and outcome of acute myocardial infarction in men versus women (the Myocardial Infarction Triage and Intervention Registry). Am J Cardiol 1996;78:9-14.
6. D'Antono B, Dupuis G, Fleet R, et al. Sex differences in chest pain and prediction of exercise-induced ischemia. Can J Cardiol 2003;19:515-22.
7. DeVon HA, Zerwic JJ. Symptoms of acute coronary syndromes: are there gender differences? A review of the literature. Heart Lung 2002; 235-45.
8. Goldberg R, Goff D, Cooper L, et al. Age and sex differences in presentation of symptoms among patients with acute coronary disease: the REACT trial. Rapid Early Action for Coronary Treatment. Coron Artery Dis 2000; 11:399-407.
9. Fesmire FM, Percy RF, Wears RL, et al. Initial Q wave and non-Q wave myocardial infarction. Ann Emerg Med 1989; 18:741-6.
10. Brady WJ, Morris F. Electrocardiographic abnormalities encountered in acute myocardial infarction. J Accid Emerg Med 2000; 17:40-5.
11. Han JH, Lindsell CJ, Storrow AB, et al. The role of cardiac risk factor burden in diagnosing acute coronary syndromes in the emergency department setting. Ann Emerg Med 2007; 49(2):145–52, 152 e141.
12. Body R, McDowell G, Carley S, et al. Do risk factors for chronic coronary heart disease help diagnose acute myocardial infarction in the emergency department? Resuscitation 2008; 79:41-5.

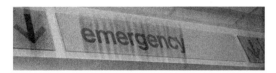

CASE 2

A 42 YEAR-OLD FIREMAN WITH SHOULDER PAIN: WHEN A LIFELINE BECOMES A NOOSE

Primary case author Michael Weinstock

PART 1—MEDICAL

I. The Patient's Story 39

II. The Doctor's Version (the ED Chart) 40

III. The Errors 41

    a. Risk Management/Patient Safety Issues #1–4 41

        Back to the Future 43

    b. Risk Management/Patient Safety Issues #5–6 44

IV. The Bounceback 44

PART 2—LEGAL

I. The Accusation/Cause of Action 47

II. Deposition/Trial Testimony 47

III. What Would Greg Do (WWGD)? 59

IV. The Verdict 61

V. The Appeal 62

VI. Legal Analysis —Jennifer L'Hommedieu Stankus, MD, JD (Interview) 63

VII. Medical Discussion—David Andrew Talan, MD 66

VIII. Authors' Summary 69

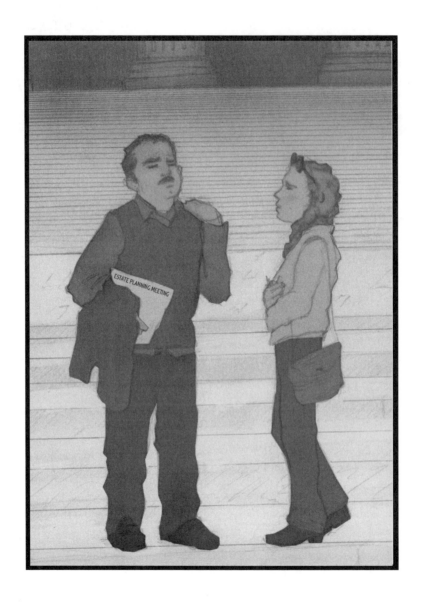

A 42 YEAR-OLD FIREMAN WITH SHOULDER PAIN:
WHEN A LIFELINE BECOMES A NOOSE

This patient was initially seen by a Physician Assistant who performed a history and physical, made a diagnosis, spoke with the primary care physician, and still asked the physician to see the patient. The physician re-examined the patient and documented a thorough note.

Deep thoughts:

1. *We are taught early in our careers that abdominal pain out of proportion to exam equals mesenteric ischemia. How about pain out of proportion to our diagnosis?*
2. *In addition to the HPI, what other historical information is important to obtain?*
3. *Does a referral from an urgent care or primary care physician obligate the ED doctor to perform certain tests?*
4. *How does a plaintiff's attorney use damages to garner sympathy from a jury?*

PART 1—MEDICAL

I. The Patient's Story

David Lykins is a loving father of three boys and devoted husband to Jill, currently 15 weeks pregnant with their 4th. His career started as a firefighter and paramedic, working his way up to Battalion Chief. David likes to spend as much time as possible with his family—Jill brings the boys to the firehouse every few days, and he spends several hours with them. His friend remembers, "To the kids, the firehouse was a big playground … he kept them running."

Co-worker John Bennett described David's approach as Battalion Chief: "He was very strict with us, but it was because he was concerned about our safety. You could tell he really cared. He was almost like a father, even though he was younger than [me]."

The following story of a squad run demonstrates David's decication to his job. On February 24, 1999, a 911 call dispatched the team to the scene of a worker with his leg caught in an auger, "wrapped around like a piece of spaghetti." Though this was a new situation, David took charge and directed everyone, including officers of his own rank. During the 45 minutes that it took to extricate the worker, the worker said, "David talked to me, as I was laying there, waiting to get untrapped. [He] asked me how many kids I had and what my name was and, you know, tried to keep me conscious… After my accident I was in the hospital and Mr. Lykins came after a run and just checked on me to see how I was doing. I was lucky to be alive."

In the beginning of March, 2000, David begins to have problems of his own. He has severe left shoulder pain and presents to the Emergency Department at Shady Valley Hospital.

II. The Doctor's Version (the following is the actual documentation of the provider)

Chief complaint per triage RN (March 2, 2000 at 10:30AM): c/o left shoulder pain … (see below) Arrives via wheel chair (WC).

| ARRIVAL/TRIAGE TIME: 1030 | ARRIVAL VIA: ☐ Ambulatory ☒ WC ☐ Emergency Medical Service | Immobilized ☐ Yes |
| CHIEF COMPLAINT: c/o left shoulder pm … sew … … … Symptoms |
| INITIAL ASSESSMENT: retox'd … nppfied, afternoon. PAV: … |

Chief complaint (physician assistant, Ed Heller) at 10:45: This is a 42-year-old male who is a fire fighter for Fairtown. He says he was lifting patients yesterday. He complains of left shoulder pain. He says he is unable to move his left arm. He has had no trauma as far as a fall. He has done only lifting. He never had anything like this before. Review of systems is otherwise negative. There is no chest pain, shortness of breath, diarrhea or constipation. No dysuria. No numbness or tingling of the extremities. No peripheral edema.

PAST MEDICAL HISTORY:
Allergies: NKDA
Meds: None
PMH: He has a history of abdominal pain two weeks ago. CT scan was done. He does not know the results or what they were looking for. He is vomiting here possibly due to the pain.
SH: Unremarkable
FH: Unremarkable

Date: 3/2/00

```
VITAL SIGNS
Time    Temp(F)   Pulse   Resp   Syst   Diast
10:30    97.8      111     18     102     67
```

PHYSICAL EXAMINATION: The patient is alert and oriented. He is somewhat inappropriate as far as pain in relation to complaint and history. He refuses to move his arm. He is in an extreme amount of pain when I try to move his arm or touch him whether on his arm or on his clavicle. He has good grip. He is able to extend and flex his elbow and pronate and supinate. He has good distal light touch sensation, pulses and capillary refill.

TESTING (10:55): Left shoulder and clavicle XR: No fracture of shoulder or clavicle

EMERGENCY DEPARTMENT COURSE:
11:05 – Demerol 50mg, Phenergan 25mg IM
12:25 – Phenergan 25mg IM
12:50 – Repeat vitals: Pulse 102, Resp 16, BP 102/65

PROGRESS NOTE (PA Ed Heller): I talked with Dr. Oster [the primary care doctor] who says the patient tends to sometimes overreact to his health care needs, and it does not surprise him that the gentleman will not move his arm and that his physical examination is not in proportion with his complaint and history.

DIAGNOSIS (12:57): Left shoulder pain/strain

DISPOSITION: Rx: Vicodin. Left arm in a sling with instructions to rest with no lifting. Apply ice and return to ED if worse. Soft diet. Dr. Oster will see him in the next two to three days.

ATTENDING NOTE (actual documentation from ED attending physician, Dr. Timothy Vaughn)**:** This is an attending note to accompany the dictation by the PA: He is a healthy male firefighter. He apparently has had some left shoulder pain after lifting patients over the last couple of days. It is very painful with range of motion and any palpation. He has no abdominal pain, chest pain or shortness of breath. Apparently, these symptoms started roughly at the same time. He has had no fever. He has had no skin breaks to that shoulder. He is very uncomfortable with any movement of his shoulder. On palpation, there is no erythema or swelling. His left upper extremity neurovascular examination is intact. The x-rays are normal. The patient is vomiting, and I do not have a good clue as to the cause of this, other than the pain from his shoulder. We have given him Phenergan on two occasions with some improvement. This looks to be more musculoskeletal, and certainly, I see no evidence of any referred pain. This is very joint specific. There is nothing on his examination or in his history that makes me think this is a septic joint.

Ed Heller, PA
Timothy Vaughn, DO

III. The Errors—Risk Management/Patient Safety Issues

➤**Authors' note:** This seems like a straightforward shoulder strain, pain with motion and palpation. But is this the whole story?

Risk management/patient safety issue #1:

Error: Not reading nursing notes.

Discussion: Can you decipher the hieroglyphics recorded by the nurse? Neither could the doctor. We get "complains of left shoulder pain" (barely). There was no effort to speak with the nurse to discover what was recorded. Her deposition testimony on November 8, 2000 (8 months after the patient presented), finally revealed the answer:

Q. (plaintiff's lawyer): Please read slowly so I can understand

A. (triage nurse): "Complains of left shoulder pain, *chills, fever.*"

Not reading the nurses'/triage notes is a common theme in medical malpractice cases.

✔ **Teaching point:** ALWAYS read the nurses' notes. If not able to be understood, speak with them personally.

Risk management/patient safety issue #2:

Error: History inconsistent with the proposed mechanism.

Discussion: It is recorded that the patient had been lifting—but when? How soon after the lifting did the pain start? It brings to mind one of my favorite anecdotes in the vomiting patient, "I ate at McDonald's last night." OK. So did 30 million other people! If a patient lifts all day, every day and has shoulder pain one of those days, it is important to correlate if the pain started when lifting or at some point after.

This documentation does not build a case for a reliable mechanism. After all, most patients will offer a convenient history, convenient for you and for them. It isn't to intentionally mislead you, it's just what makes sense; patients don't want to be sick and will often offer an excuse to lead you toward the most benign diagnosis. You can choose to accept it without qualification or pursue further history to verify its relevance.

✔ **Teaching point:** Just because most patients with shoulder pain have a strain, doesn't mean they all do.

Risk management/patient safety issue #3:

Error: Too narrow of a differential diagnosis.

Discussion: Could shoulder pain in a 42 year-old man be from a cardiac etiology? Absolutely! Questioning about exertional symptoms, associated symptoms of diaphoresis and dyspnea (which *was* recorded), and cardiac risk factors is advisable. An ECG is a simple and inexpensive screening test.

✔ **Teaching point:** Maintain a high index of suspicion for atypical presentations of life-threatening diagnoses. Everyone is sick until you prove they aren't.

Risk management/patient safety issue #4:

Error: Including conjecture in the note.

Discussion: This point could be argued since it may be important to note that a "patient tends to sometimes overreact to his health care needs," but it does up the ante. We have a 42 year-old Battalion Chief with a new complaint of shoulder pain to the point that he needs to be brought back to his room in a wheelchair. That would be a serious overreaction. Additionally, how does this information factor into the medical decision-making process? Though not overtly stated, we can surmise from the note that for some reason, there was extra concern about this patient; who calls the PCP for a simple shoulder strain? If there was any doubt about the diagnosis before the call, it was laid to rest after learning about his "history" of overreaction.

✔ **Teaching point:** Be careful about including speculative comments in the chart. If you are right, it didn't matter anyway. If you are wrong, such comments will have a profound impact on your defense.

➤**Authors' note:** Ever listen to Paul Harvey? "And now … the rest of story." Well, this case also has a "rest of the story." As it turns out, our patient's pain actually started the day prior, on March 1. This is also part of the "ancient Egyptian writing" recorded by the triage nurse: "symptoms started yesterday afternoon."

March 1, 2000:
- 3:00 PM (one day before ED visit): David and his wife Jill have a meeting with a lawyer to discuss estate-planning matters. As they leave the office, David comments that his shoulder is bothering him.
- 11:00 PM: The pain is stronger and he has a low grade fever. Jill gives him two 800mg ibuprofen.

March 2, 2000:
- 8:00 AM: Jill calls Dr. Oster, the PCP, and finds out David cannot be seen until 11 AM. He is unable to wait that long, so is referred to an urgent care.

Back to the Future—The Urgent Care record per Dr. Benjamin Roth:

- **Triage (9:39AM)** - Complains of intense pain left shoulder which began yesterday
- **History:** Pt works for fire dept, was lifting patients, pain started hours after. Has headache, nausea, vomiting and feels dehydrated. Pt. feels it is not cardiac related but like it's in the muscle. Pt. iced and took ibuprofen. Unable to move shoulder, had fever all night, couldn't sleep secondary to the pain.
- **PE:** Vitals: temp 97.5, pulse 116, resp 16, BP 120/78. Possibly swollen, extremely tender, no redness. ROM is zero. A&O X 3
- **Urgent Care course:** Vomited in clinic X 1
- **Diagnosis:** Severe left shoulder pain, needs septic arthritis ruled out
- Doctor note: Discussed with ER at Shady Valley. Will send him down there for evaluation.

Benjamin Roth, MD

➤**Authors' note:** It is questionable if the ED doctor was aware that the patient was at the urgent care prior to the ED visit; he did note "This is very joint specific" but never specifically mentioned the referral. "There is nothing on his examination or in his history that makes me think this is a septic joint." Was this documented because of the concern of the urgent care doctor, because of a concern of David or Jill, or a concern of the ED doctor or PA? The same diagnosis that troubled the urgent care doctor is mentioned (septic joint), but no other reference is made to the urgent care visit.

When the records were eventually subpoenaed, the hospital was unable to find the urgent care "call-in sheet" or the urgent care record that was sent with the patient. However, the plaintiff's attorney was able to find them both, blowing them up into 4 × 5 foot posters displayed during the trial.

Risk management/patient safety issue #5:

Error: Not speaking with the urgent care doctor.

Discussion: I have sent patients home without the testing recommended by the urgent care, but only after careful consideration and discussion with the patient and the family. For example, a child referred for brain scan after a fall has some radiation risk—with a parental expectation of imaging, they want to be involved in the decision-making process, but usually follow your recommendation to defer scanning.

Was the urgent care doctor's concern reasonable? To summarize, we have a healthy 42 year-old man with severe shoulder pain, fever (possibly masked by the use of ibuprofen at home) and no definitive mechanism suggesting a muscle strain. Searching for another cause of fever would be helpful. Does he have rhinorrhea and cough (typical in March). Further defining what is meant by fever would also be helpful (felt warm or recorded temperature of 100.4° with thermometer). Discovering the timing of an antipyretic can be helpful.

✔ **Teaching point:** When there is a difference of opinion, speaking with the transferring/ referring physician (urgent care or PCP doctor) may allow discovery of important information.

Risk management/patient safety issue #6:

Error: Lost records.

Discussion: Thou shall not kill. Do unto others as you would do unto yourself. Medical records should not be lost. These statements are all so obvious that they don't really justify the ink and parchment that they are printed on, unless somehow, they are not obeyed.

✔ **Teaching point:** A mechanism needs to exist to ensure that the records provided by the referring doctor are available to the treating ED physician.

➤**Authors' note:** As a closing thought, assuming he was aware of the urgent care visit, kudos to the ED physician who did an independent examination, assessment and documentation of the patient. This could have easily been omitted in a patient with a "simple shoulder strain."

IV. The Bounceback

David is discharged from the ED at 12:57 PM, and his wife drives him to the pharmacy to pick up his prescription for Vicodin. On the way, they stop for gas. David vomits, then gets out of the car and urinates on the gas pump. When they arrive at home, David goes to bed. Jill can hear him moaning in pain.

- Midnight – His pain is increasing, and David asks Jill for pain medicine.
- 2:00 AM – He asks for more pain medication.
- 3:30 AM – Jill calls Dr. Oster (PCP). An "on call" doctor returns the call and tells her to go back to the ED if worse or wait until the morning and see Dr. Oster first thing. David says he does

not want to return to the ED because they did not do anything for him when he was there earlier.

- 6:30 AM – David is up and wants to take a bath before going to see Dr. Oster. Jill notices reddening and swelling of David's arm up to the shoulder. It looks like a bruise.
- 8:30 AM – David presents to Dr. Oster's office with the complaint of shoulder pain and nausea. The pain is excruciating. "The patient is hyperventilating and is acutely ill appearing with edema over the left shoulder to the nipple and over the sternum, medially, but no discoloration, warmth or erythema. There is marked pain with motion of shoulder." He is sent immediately to ED.
- Per PCP, "Spoke with ED doctor who accepts the patient."

ED visit #2—March 3, 2000—Almost 22 hours after the initial ED discharge
- 10:15 AM – Temp 91.3, pulse 61, resp 20, BP 93/80. The ED team jumps into action.
- 10:25 AM – David is seen by Dr. Timothy Vaughn (same doctor as yesterday): "Extremely ill-appearing and much worse than when I had seen him yesterday. Skin on chest is ecchymotic and some areas of necrosis and crepitation are noted underneath. We immediately initiated 2 large bore IV's."
- 10:40 AM – Acute change in vitals: pulse increases to 145 and SBP drops to 70→IV fluids and dopamine
- 10:50 AM – Blood cultures taken. Started on Timentin and Clindamycin.
- CBC is normal. Creatinine is 2.5. Elevated LFT's
- **Assessment:** Extremely critical condition with probable multi-system failure, probably from sepsis secondary to some underlying myofascial infection
- Dr. Anderson, general surgeon, is called to the ED to evaluate the patient and observes a discolored, darkened spot about the size of a fifty-cent piece which grows to the size of a softball in a short period of time.
- **ED diagnosis:**
    1. Acute soft tissue infection left side of chest
    2. Septic shock
    3. Multiple organ failure with acute renal and hepatic failure
- 11:30 AM – Taken from the ED to CT scan suite to define extent of the process. Results show necrotizing fasciitis of left anterior chest wall and possibly upper, anterior mediastinum.

HOSPITAL COURSE:
- 12:15 AM – From CT, the patient is immediately taken to surgery. Dr. Anderson performs extensive debridement of the left anterior chest wall. Following the surgery, Anderson was "a little encouraged" because the infection was not more extensive.
- David undergoes a second, "re-look" operation approximately 12 hours later. The infection has not extended beyond the margins of the first operation, no more necrotic tissue is discovered; it appears that the surgery has controlled the infection.
- David is found to have acute inflammation of the gall bladder and further surgery confirms this diagnosis, but also shows right colonic necrosis, which necessitates a right hemicolectomy. This is thought to be from the vasopressors.
- The renal failure worsens, requiring dialysis.

- He suffers extensive necrosis of the digits of both hands and feet.
- Diagnosis of ARDS—he remains on the ventilator.
- David continues a slow, but steady, downward spiral. After a multidisciplinary assessment, it is determined that he does not have a chance of recovering. This is discussed with the family, and comfort measures are taken.
- With his family in attendance, David expires on March 17, exactly 2 weeks after his bounceback visit.

FINAL DIAGNOSIS: Necrotizing myositis, septic shock, ARF, ARDS, multisystem organ failure

PART 2—LEGAL

➤**Authors' note:** How annoying is it when a patient presents from the urgent care with the work-up plan in hand? "The doctor sent me here for an MRI of my knee. ..." Really? On a Sunday? The wrinkle in this case is we don't know if the ED doctor was aware of the Urgent Care visit or the history of fevers. Additionally, the nurse's triage note was illegible. Both these issues were pivotal to the plaintiff's case.

There are two ways to look at this patient. Imagine hearing it presented in one sentence at an M&M conference:

1. *This is a 42-year-old healthy fireman who was lifting patients and presents with shoulder pain, worse with movement. Impression: I see this patient every day. I see this patient ten times a day. I eat this patient for breakfast. ... ibuprofen, pain control, sling, bye bye. ...*
2. *This is a 42 year old healthy fireman who has fever and shoulder pain so severe that the range of motion is zero. He was sent from an urgent care to r/o septic arthritis. Impression: Now I'm not so sure ...*

What happened at the gas station? *La belle indifference:* An apathetic demeanor observed in patients with necrotizing fasciitis/myositis:

"Mr. Jones, we're going to need to amputate your arm."

"OK, doctor—thanks."

Mr. Lykins was obviously in the throes of the disease at the initial ED visit, not even aware that urinating on a gas pump was out of the ordinary. Did the confusion start when he walked out the door of the ED or was it present, but unrecognized, during the initial ED encounter?

I. The Accusation/Cause of Action

Soon after David's death, his wife Jill filed a lawsuit against the initial ED doctor, the physician assistant, Shady Valley Hospital and the primary care doctor. The main allegation was failure to diagnose necrotizing fasciitis/myositis with the subsequent fatal sequelae. The case was not settled, but proceeded to a trial lasting four weeks.

In the first chapter, we included the judge's instructions to the jury and the opening statements. In this chapter, we advance directly to the courtroom drama, an epic struggle between a hard driving plaintiff's attorney who had been friends with the deceased and two of the foremost experts in emergency medicine: Greg Henry and Dave Talan, both experts for the defense at trial. All three have contributed to this chapter. We complete the presentation with the attorneys' closing arguments.

II. The Trial—The following is actual trial testimony, condensed from over 5,000 pages.

Cast of characters (names changed, except where noted):

The patient: David Lykins (actual name)
ED physician-defendant: Timothy Vaughn
Physician assistant: Ed Heller
Primary care physician: Dr. Jerry Oster
Urgent care physician: Benjamin Roth
Plaintiff's attorney: Dwight Brannon (actual attorney)
Defense attorney: Neil Freund (actual attorney)
Defense expert witnesses: Greg Henry and Dave Talan (both board certified emergency medicine, both actual expert witnesses in this case)

Cross-examination of the defendant ED physician, Timothy Vaughn, by plaintiff's attorney, Mr. Brannon:

Q. You never read the triage nurse's note about David Lykins before he was discharged, did you?
A. I—when a physician assistant presents a patient to us, it's my practice to look at the chart. I like to look at vital signs, medications, allergies, and I will glance at the triage note.

Q. You did not read the triage note on David Lykins on March the 2nd, did you?
A. I don't recall, sir.

Q. And when you attempted to read it, you said you weren't able to make out anything but complaint of left shoulder pain, correct?
A. If that is from my deposition, I would have to review that.

Q. Right. I'll let you look at page ten of your deposition. Excuse me just a second while I get it. May I approach the witness, Your Honor?

The Court: Sure.

By Mr. Brannon:

Q. First of all, Dr. Vaughn, is that a true and accurate copy, at least an enlargement, of what you looked at on the date of your deposition?

A. Yes, it is.

Q. When I asked you what the triage nurse had said in her report on March 2nd, you indicated you did not know unless you read the report. Am I correct?

A. I'm sorry. I don't follow your question.

Q. Well, when I said "what did the triage notes tell you about David Lykins on March the 2nd?" what did you tell me?

A. I'd have to look at my deposition, sir.

Q. Did you tell me that you had no independent recollection other than the medical records?

A. I don't understand your question.

Q. Alright. Tell me today, tell the ladies and gentlemen of the jury, what did Nurse Mayo's triage note say about David Lykins, without looking at the report.

A. He had left shoulder pain, fever, chills. He was pale.

Q. Did you know that on March the 2nd when you treated David Lykins?

A. Sir, I'm not sure what I recall about reading that chart.

Q. Would you read your answer [from the deposition] to the ladies and gentlemen?

A. (Reading his own deposition testimony): "The best I can tell is this, there is a complaint of — complaint of left shoulder pain. Then, the next thing I can pick up is symptoms started yesterday afternoon. That's all I can read."

Q. Well, you are not implying that at the time of your deposition in November of 2000, somehow there was some kind of trickery by showing up with copies you couldn't read but you could the original?

A. That's not what I'm implying, sir. You asked if I could read those. I could not read the copies.

➢**Authors' note:** This plaintiff's attorney is sharp! The defendant physician tried to imply that he had read the triage note but was tricked during the trial into admitting that, during his deposition testimony months earlier, he had *not* been able to read the nursing documentation of fever, thereby revealing he was not aware of the complaint of this symptom during the ED evaluation. Ouch!

The plaintiff's attorney next moves to the patient's severe shoulder pain. He tries to establish that the providers did not take Mr. Lykins' pain seriously. Of course, a lot of patients overreact to their pain in the ED. I had a patient tell me once that he has had pain so long he now uses a *logarithmic* pain scale ?! Is it possible to separate those patients who have organic disease from those seeking narcotics? In 1980, Waddell devised a set of physical signs to differentiate patients with the complaint of back pain.[1] Three or more physical signs on exam strongly suggest a non-organic component.

Waddell's signs:

1. Overreaction to the physical exam
2. Widespread superficial tenderness that does not correspond to an anatomical distribution

3. Pain on axial loading of the skull or simultaneous rotation of the shoulders and pelvis

4. Severe limitation on straight leg raise in patients able to sit forward with legs extended

5. Weakness or sensory loss that does not correspond to a nerve root distribution

Was the severity of the pain a factor which should have prompted the doctor to make the diagnosis? The plaintiff's attorney thinks so.

Continuation of cross-examination of defendant ED physician, Dr. Vaughn, by plaintiff's attorney Mr. Brannon:

Q. You saw excruciating pain, did you not?

A. I saw a gentleman with severe left shoulder pain, correct.

Q. Well, let's describe it. Let's describe it. I won't use my word. How did he seem to convey himself in regards to the amount of pain that he was in?

A. He seemed to be in severe pain when the shoulder was moved.

Q. Did he appear to be overreacting?

A. No, sir, I would never make that assessment.

Q. It's in your medical records, isn't it?

A. I did not dictate that. I would never make that assessment of a patient. I've been doing this for nineteen years, and I've never accused anyone of overreacting or faking.

Q. Didn't Dr ... I'm sorry — Mr. Heller (the PA) come to you and say that he had talked to his family physician and that this patient "sometimes tends to overreact to his health care needs"?

A. At the end, sometime after Mr. Lykins had left and I saw Mr. Heller again, he did mention that the telephone conversation had occurred.

Q. Did that help you close the book on your diagnosis here?

A. No, sir.

Q. And, in fact, your diagnosis of shoulder sprain/strain was not correct, was it?

A. At the time, that was the diagnosis that I had arrived at, yes, sir.

Q. Was that the correct diagnosis that you had arrived at?

A. At that time, that was the correct diagnosis.

Q. So, it's your testimony here today that you can state within terms of a reasonable medical probability that David Lykins had no septic process such as necrotizing fasciitis ongoing on March the 2nd of 2000?

A. If that process was occurring, there were there were no external signs that would give us that indication.

Q. Well, is vomiting a sign?

A. Vomiting is a sign, yes, sir.

Q. And past fever is a symptom?

A. That would require some clarification. Many patients present to the emergency department complaining of fever.

Q. That's fair enough. Did you go to him and talk to him and say, now, I've heard that you have had this past fever; can you clarify it for me? Did you do that?

A. Yes, sir, I did.

Q. Did you ask either Jill or David if they had taken a temperature for fever?

A. Yes, I did.

Q. What did they tell you?

A. My -- my response to that is twofold. When I ask a patient if they have had a fever, the first question is, "have you checked it?" If they haven't checked it, I would document no fever. If they have checked it and it is less than a hundred degrees, I would still document no fever. I don't feel that is a clinically significant temperature.

Q. Would you then ask if they have taken any medication for fever?

A. I had reviewed the chart, and there was no medications listed.

Q. Did you ask the patient? Did you ask David Lykins or Jill Lykins if he had taken any medication for the fever?

A. That is asked at triage. I don't specifically ask that question again.

Q. And at least at triage, they didn't report that he had Phenergan that day, did they?

A. That's correct.

Q. That would have been something for you to know?

A. Yes, sir.

Q. But you never asked the patient if he had had any medication, did you?

A. I don't recall if I had asked or not.

Q. Alright. Now, chills and sweats, would that be an important thing to know about?

A. In the face of a fever, yes.

➤**Authors' note:** The patient had taken ibuprofen sometime before the visit, but the exact time is not documented. This is a tricky one, since many patients complain of fever, "My temperature was 98.7 but I normally run at 95 so that's a fever for me." Sometimes, they are wrong. Sometimes, they just want us to take them seriously, and sometimes, they *have* had a fever, which has been reduced by antipyretics.

Mr. Brannon prompted the defendant to admit that not only had he not read the nurse's notes, but that they contained essential information he should have been aware of. Additionally, the nurse's notes were not accurate, lacking any indication that the patient had received the medication Phenergan within the last several hours. The doctor admitted that the nurse's notes were inaccurate and that he did not independently ask about use of other medications, such as ibuprofen, which may have decreased the temperature.

During the trial, Mr. Brannon displayed a 4 × 5 foot poster defining the symptoms of necrotizing fasciitis for the jury. As we follow his questioning, he is going through all of the classic symptoms (fever, chills, severe pain, vomiting) to show the jury that these symptoms were present, but unrecognized, when the patient initially presented. The poster was actually a grease board with symptoms of necrotizing fasciitis and empty boxes next to each symptom. As he went through the testimony, he made a check mark next to each symptom present, but undocumented by the doctor.

On a side note, I thought the stories of 4 × 5 blow up posters were an urban legend meant to colorfully demonstrate a point to doctors in training. I will attest to the fact that this is no fable. I have more than 20 of them from this case still stacked on my back porch.

Q. I'm not saying necessarily, but if you are considering throwing up, isn't it more likely that someone would throw up because they have an infection than because they have a shoulder sprain or strain?
A. Not at all, sir. We see many people with orthopedic injuries with nausea and vomiting.

Q. We? How many have you seen throw up from a shoulder sprain and strain?
A. Again, sir, I —I don't keep—I don't keep numbers. I evaluate everybody individually.

Q. Alright. Now, up here, is this a correct dictation of what you said?
A. I—yes, sir, it is.

Q. Would you read it to the ladies and gentlemen of the jury?
A. The patient is vomiting, and I do not have a good clue as to the cause of this other than the pain from his shoulder.

➤**Authors' note:** The hospital was not able to find either the telephone triage note or the urgent care form. This was brought up repeatedly throughout the trial and was later the "hook" of the plaintiff's closing arguments.

Q. Did you see the Urgent Care form?
A. No, sir, I didn't.

Q. Did you see the phone form?
A. No, sir.

Q. Did you see any indication that Jill had brought David into the emergency room to rule out either septic arthritis or a septic joint? Did you see that?
A. At some point during our interaction, the Lykins' and I had discussed a septic joint. I'm not sure where that had come up. I have it dictated in my note. So, we talked about it.

Q. And they didn't mention that we're here because of the doctor sending us straight down from Urgent Care to rule out a septic joint or arthritis or some kind of infection?
A. Again, sir, I don't recall where that information came from.

Q. So, you don't deny here today in front of the jury that either one of the Lykins or both told you they had come in to have an infection ruled out?
A. That I don't recall.

Q. You've seen Urgent Care forms before, haven't you?
A. Yes, sir.

Q. And you have read them and used them, haven't you?
A. If the patients give them to us, we read them.

Q. And you are saying you never got this?
A. I never saw the Urgent Care form.

Q. Okay. Would you read from the bottom of Dr. Roths' [documentation]?
A. Severe left shoulder pain needs septic arthritis ruled out. Discussed with ER at [Shady Valley]. Will send him down there for evaluation.

Q. What about the phone form?
A. I did not see the phone form.

➤**Authors' note:** The allegation that Mr. Lykins "Tends to sometimes overreact to his health care needs" was another frequent theme.

Direct examination of David Lykins' co-worker, John Bennett, by plaintiff's attorney, Mr. Brannon:

Q. In the years that you worked with him, did you ever see him not do a job because of an injury, a sprain or a strain, or anything like that?
A. No.

Q. Did you ever hear him complain of an injury, sprain or strain?
A. No

Q. Was David Lykins a complainer; "I'm hurt, I'm sore, I'm sick"?
A. Never

Q. How about nausea, anything like that? Was he sick?
A. No.

Q. You knew people that worked with him. What was his reputation for truth and veracity?
A. Everybody trusted him. You knew he meant what he said. He would say what he meant.

Mr. Brannon: Thank you. I have no further questions.

The Court: Thank you. Mr. Freund [defense attorney], cross-examine?

Defense: No questions, your honor.

➤**Authors' note: How did the defense rebut these arguments?** The following are excerpts from two of the 12 defense expert witnesses (the plaintiff called 28 witnesses). Greg Henry is first and David Talan follows.

Direct examination of Greg Henry, expert witness for the defense, by defense attorney, Mr. Freund:

Q. For an emergency room physician, is history important?
A. Yes.

Q. And why?
A. History gives us at least some indication of the disease process which we're looking at.

Q. Okay. And in this particular case, was there any history other than the fact that this gentleman may have hurt his shoulder lifting a heavy object?

A. All we have is about a day and a half history of pain. The only thing we have related to it was lifting. And so at least on a temporal basis, on a time basis, they're related. We have no way of knowing whether those two are actually cause and effect.

Q. As far as the gentleman's physical appearance, his complaint was significant pain in the left shoulder. Is that correct?

A. Well, I don't want to use the term shoulder. It was up here. But it was somewhat broader than that. And that's why when they did his X-ray, they also X-rayed the clavicle, which is your collarbone, running from here to here. So, it was obviously not just a complaint of the shoulder, but of the upper chest area.

Q. OK. Now, as far as the particular patient is concerned, he had been to an urgent care. Is that correct?

A. Yes

Q. And the urgent care physician believed that this individual may have what has been described as a septic joint or septic arthritis of the left shoulder. Is that correct?

A. Right. He didn't have that. He never had that in the course of this process. But that was a thought.

Q. Okay. Now, was that thought considered by Dr. Vaughn (the ED physician) and Mr. Heller (the ED PA) in the emergency room at Shady Valley Hospital on May 2?

Mr. Brannon: Object!

The Court: Overruled.

A. Yeah, by the nature of the write-up, the pertinent positives and negatives included, it was obviously considered because they commented on the temperature and skin coloration that you would see with an acute joint. And the purpose of taking an X-ray is for looking for fluid in the joint, which you would see with an acute septic joint.

Q. Okay. There's been some discussion, doctor, that Dr. Vaughn and Mr. Heller fell below the standard of care when they didn't stick a needle into the left shoulder joint and attempt to aspirate fluid. You're aware of that?

A. Yes.

Q. Okay. Would you tell the ladies and gentlemen whether or not Mr. Heller and Dr. Vaughn fell below the standard of care?

A. Absolutely not! You don't go sticking needles into joints. Joints are sterile areas. You don't go put a needle into areas until you have something palpable. You've got to know where you're going with the needle. So you've got to be able to feel fluid collection, and there was none palpable in this case, nor was there any seen on the X-ray. So, to stick a needle into a joint without a reasonable probability of coming back with fluid would be malpractice.

➤**Authors' note:** What follows are the "even if" arguments. For example, *even if* the doctors knew the urgent care had sent the patient, he still would have been sent home. *Even if* the doctor had deciphered the nurse's note of fever, he still would have been sent home.

These arguments speak to "causation," one of the two points a plaintiff needs to prove (together with standard of care). We know the patient was not correctly diagnosed, and these questions explore "would it have mattered?"

Continued direct examination of Dr. Henry, defense expert, by Mr. Freund, defense attorney:

Q. Okay. Now, you are aware, of course, that Mr. and Mrs. Lykins were sent to Shady Valley Hospital [from an urgent care].

A. Yes.

Q. Alright. I want you to assume that Dr. Vaughn evaluated Mr. Lykins for what was described by Dr. Roth as a septic arthritis or septic joint.

Mr.. Brannon: Object, your Honor.

The Court: I don't know the question yet.

Mr. Brannon: I apologize.

The court: If I could hear the question.

Q. I want you to assume that Mr. Lykins was referred to Shady Valley Hospital to "rule out septic joint" or "septic arthritis." Just assume that as being true. When Dr. Vaughn and Mr. Heller evaluated this patient, is there an indication that they considered whether or not this individual had a septic joint?

Mr. Brannon: Object! Asked and answered.

The Court: Permit it. Overruled!

A. They checked those things which you would have with a septic joint. Again, this gentleman didn't have a septic joint.

Q. The fact that Dr. Roth, who in his workup, thought [he] saw possibly a septic joint, does that mean that these physicians in doing their workup, taking their histories and doing their assessments and their physical examinations should rely on somebody else and their provisional diagnosis?

A. They're obligated to do their own examination and come up with their own diagnosis.

Q. Okay. Now, you are aware, of course, that this individual did present, in addition to pain, with nausea and vomiting and a history of fever. Is that correct?

A. Yes.

Q. Now, when the patient presented at Shady Valley Hospital on March 2 with a history of fever, what would you think about that?

A. You take the temperature and see if they've actually got a fever.

Q. Did they take the temperature and see if he actually had a fever?

A. Yes.

Q. What was his temperature?

A. It was within the normal range.

Q. Alright. Now, are vitals important when you're trying to work a patient up and determine whether or not this patient is really sick?

A. Well, vital signs are an indicator. They're not a perfect indicator. But they are important in what we call the positive. They're not important in the negative.

Q. Okay. Why are they called vitals?

A. From the Latin vitae, meaning from the root is vitae, which we use for life.

Q. Vitals in the emergency room were basically what?

A. They were consistent with somebody in pain. Slight tachycardia. And otherwise they fell within the normal ranges.

➢**Authors' note:** Would a CBC have been helpful, as alleged by the plaintiff?

Q. Alright. Let's assume for a moment that we accept the plaintiff's argument that a blood test should have been done on March 2, and there were clinical indications to do that test. What would a blood test have shown on the 2nd?

A. Well, we know that it [the CBC] was normal when the patient was sick on the 3rd. So, within the realm of reasonable medical probability, it would have been normal the day before as well.

➢**Authors' note:** Did the doctor meet the standard of care?

Q. Okay. Now, doctor, in your examination, you have determined that there was no redness, no swelling, no portal of entry, no marks, no discoloration of the left shoulder. It has been shouted out in this courtroom many, many times that these physicians, Dr. Vaughn and Mr. Heller should have been thinking infection.
Now, what was to lead these physicians to think infection, infection, infection?

Mr. Brannon: Object! He's not stating the facts underlying.

The Court: Overruled!

A. Nothing at this point in time. He looks very similar to other patients who have shoulder pain. I would not be thinking infection at this moment in time.

Q. Do you send all patients out of the emergency room with a diagnosis?

A. I send them out with a clinical impression at that moment in time, because I understand that a diagnosis is sometimes not arrived at with one visit. Now, certain things are easily diagnosed. If you come in with a cut finger, we can pretty much make the diagnosis of laceration. If you come in with vague abdominal pain, in less than 50 percent of cases can we give you a [specific] diagnosis.

Q. As far as discharge, is it appropriate for a physician who has made a diagnosis to ask the patient to come back if the condition worsens? Is that usual or unusual?

A. Standard. The assumption is that we're open 24 hours a day, seven days a week. We'd expect if there's a change, that you come back. That's just the standard discharge line on the chart.

Q. Alright. Based upon your review of the record, from approximately 1:00 o'clock on, until presentation again the next morning, which would be March 3rd, maybe around 10:00, did the patient get worse?

A. Oh, yes, dramatically worse. By the time they got in the next morning with the family practitioner, he was essentially in a pre-shock state.

Q. One final question, then, doctor. As you have reviewed the case and as you have reviewed the depositions of the physicians, do you have an opinion, based upon standards of care and reasonable medical probability and certainty, whether or not these physicians acted reasonably and met the standard of care?

A. Yes, my opinion is this is a very tragic and sad case, and my opinion is they met reasonable standards of care. I'm glad I wasn't the doctor who saw him because we will never know the outcome of the play until the [diagnosis] has actually presented itself.

Mr. Freund: No further questions.

Cross examination of defense expert witness, Dr. Henry, by plaintiff's attorney, Mr. Brannon:

Q. Did you consider Dr. Roth's finding of possibly swelling and Mrs. Lykins' testimony that it looked swollen? [per the Urgent Care doctor's note and the testimony of Jill Lykins, David's wife, which is not reproduced here].

A. I read them both. I've got to depend on two healthcare professionals who saw him at that moment in time. They did not feel it was [swollen].

Q. Well, if they didn't do an adequate exam and Dr. Roth and Mrs. Lykins were correct, you would have a different opinion, wouldn't you?

A. Not from Dr. Roth, because he said "possible." So, I don't know what to do with that. That's not one way or the other. Again, his wife isn't medically trained. So, I would have less credibility in [her impression] than I would people who are medically trained.

Q. If I understand you correctly, March 2nd, when David Lykins came into the emergency room complaining of pain like he had never had before, giving a history of fever and chills, pale, screaming whenever he was touched, throwing up repeatedly, it was your opinion on examination or redirect by Mr. Freund that he wasn't sick. Is that correct?

A. Absolutely not. That's a mischaracterization of the testimony.

Direct examination of Dr. Dave Talan, (ED physician triple boarded in EM, IM and ID) by defense attorney, Mr. Freund:

Q. Would you describe for the ladies and gentlemen of the jury the mortality from necrotizing fasciitis and myositis?

Mr. Brannon: Object!

The Court: Overruled.

A. Both are obvioulsly bad, but the fasciitis, which is the fibrous covering over the muscles, is 30–50%, so that's not very good. But if the muscle is involved, the mortality is in the range of 80%.

Q. Do you have an opinion upon reasonable medical certainty, as to whether the health care providers met the standard of care?

A. Yes. It's my strong opinion that reasonable physicians and physician's assistants would not have made the diagnosis of necrotizing fasciitis or myositis on that date. Their care was consistent with the community standard of care. This is a very, very rare condition that lacked many of the important features that would lead a reasonable physician to make the diagnosis … and that's it in a nutshell.

CLOSING STATEMENTS: The following are the shortened closing arguments from the plaintiff and defense attorneys. Plaintiff goes first, then defense:

Mr. Dwight Brannon (plaintiff's attorney):

What was the prize here? David Lykins wanted three things in his life. One, he wanted to do his very best for mankind. He wanted to be reasonable, responsible and accountable. He wanted security for his family. Worked hard at it. Triple jobs. And still had all that time for his family. Above all, he wanted to be there. He wanted to *be* there. Second, professionally, he wanted to give, he wanted to serve; it was obviously a token of his desire to serve mankind. Third, [serving] his community. This is about the community. Accountability, responsibility: Those aren't hollow terms.

And I ask you in light of the testimony of Dr. Roth [the urgent care physician] who threw him a lifeline, "David, go to the emergency room." And at the emergency room, ladies and gentlemen, the triage nurse didn't meet the standard of care. Then, Mr. Heller didn't meet the standard of care. Then, Dr. Vaughn didn't meet the standard of care. That's the lifeline. And then they called Dr. Oster [the PCP] to close the loop. They closed the loop all right. (Taking a piece of rope from his pocket and tying a large knot.) Instead of giving him a lifeline, they gave him a noose.

This case really needs no convincing. I ask the question what is fair, what is just, what is the standard of care? Ladies and gentlemen, I await your verdict so I can tell the captain that his trip is truly over, his prize is truly won, and that you will post the conscience of this community so that these defendants stop, look, and listen to ordinary people. Because this courtroom is for the victims. This courtroom is for ordinary people. I ask you to realize how important it is and what an important thing [it is] that you do here. I believe that with all my heart. Thank you, ladies and gentlemen.

Mr. Neil Freund (defense attorney):

Court: Mr. Freund, we're ready for the defense close

Mr. Freund: Thanks Judge.

When we selected you folks as jurors, I played a portion of the tape to show you the beautiful family of David and Jill Lykins. I did that for a reason, and I'd like to share that reason with you.

I know from my life's experiences how I react to the death of loved ones. I know how you react to the death of loved ones. And yet, we expect you to come in here and judge us fairly and impartially. We ask that of you. And I know how difficult that is because I have experienced loss. And then we bring you in here and ask you to decide the case on the facts.

I was thinking, okay. Now, how are we going to go about this? And I thought that we would approach it like the doctors approached this case. In fact, what you are doing in this courtroom is making a diagnosis. And how are you going to make that diagnosis? You're going to look at the facts. You are going to render a verdict, which is your diagnosis. And you are going to go about this the very same way that the doctors did when they made their diagnosis in this case.

Common sense and reason. That's how doctors make their decision based upon their medical training. That's how I ask you to make your decision when you go back and talk to each other and deliberate with each other. Common sense and reason. Without hindsight or retrospect. Hindsight is 20/20. Put yourselves in the shoes of the caregivers. And what I mean by "put yourselves in the shoes of the caregivers" is simply, when you're judging my clients, judge them from the information they knew or should have known as the caregivers at that time. Independent of compassion or sympathy.

We have ranges on myositis from 80% fatality to as low as 20%. But you are being asked in this case to take the quantum leap that in this particular case with this particular individual that he would have survived this terrible deadly disease and not only that, but he would have survived it without disability. And you folks, when you are using your common sense, are going to reject that.

We didn't make the history up. Why is that important? Dr. Henry said in the emergency room, it's a snapshot at a particular moment in time. Everybody agrees; all the experts agreed that history was the most important part of the case. Alright. What history was given to Mr. Heller and Dr. Vaughn? He hurt himself lifting. That is the history that Dr. Roth got, and that's the history that we got at Shady Valley Hospital. None of the classic signs of redness, swelling, high temperature or vitals out of whack were present.

I thought I would just highlight some of the testimony that was actually given in this case. When I was asked to represent Dr. Vaughn, Mr. Heller and Shady Valley Hospital, I wanted to find the best experts to review this case. So, I got the literature and found out who wrote more than anybody else. That was Dr. Johns, an infectious disease specialist (name changed, testimony not included here). He's written more, studied it more and seems to know more than anybody else.

Then I thought, but Mr. Heller and Dr. Vaughn are not infectious disease physicians. They specialize in emergency medicine. Then I thought, okay, I wonder if there's anybody out there who is an infectious disease person and an emergency medicine person. That was Dr. Talan, the fellow from UCLA. Did you notice he had sandals on? I couldn't believe it. He's from California; it figures. I was hoping he would stay in the box and not come out!

But anyway, he is one of only two doctors in the United States who is double boarded in emergency medicine and infectious diseases. One of two, and I got him to review the case. He said the case was defensible.

Then, I thought, I need somebody local. So, I went to Ohio State and I had Dr. Hankman (name changed) review the case. Professor, in emergency medicine … the works.

I'm going to do this some more. So, I sent the case to Dr. Henry. Now, Dr. Henry is from Ann Arbor. I wondered what the folks in Ohio will think about a guy from Michigan? I decided that he had the qualifications. Now, his qualifications were a little different, though, because he was boarded in emergency medicine. He also happened to be President of the whole United States of American College of Emergency Physicians, all 22,000 of them. He gave me a favorable review.

Did Mr. Lykins get worse between his discharge from the ER until he returned the next day? Yes. Actually, his condition changed very rapidly over several hours. Now, why does that make a difference? When they were discharged from the hospital at 1:00 o'clock in the early afternoon on the 2nd, they were given the specific instruction to return if the condition got worse. Well, it surely did get worse, and it got worse, according to Mrs. Lykins' own words, about midnight. Okay?

Now, what are we supposed to conclude from going from 1:00 o'clock at the time of the discharge to about 10:00 o'clock the next day until there was a change in condition? Mr. Brannon spent a lot of time talking about the fact that [David Lykins] was a paramedic. Think about that. Here's an individual who, from the testimony of the plaintiff, we're supposed to believe that his eyes were rolling up when he was in our institution on the 2nd. He had every ambulance in Fairtown available to him if he would have chosen to call. But, if we're supposed to believe that his condition was so bad, why didn't he want to go back to the emergency room on the 2nd. It is reasonable to conclude that surgery wasn't indicated on the 2nd?

I had a very good medical professor, a rheumatologist, [who] told me, and it's true, that there are diseases where at one point in time you cannot make the diagnosis and, therefore, you need to see the patient repetitively in order to establish a diagnosis. That's common, very common.

Whether or not you accept the idea that he suffered a strain and that's why the strep A seeded in him or whether you believe that the strep A seeded for some other reason, when you go back and discuss this among yourselves and consider the signs and symptoms, what was there for these doctors and Mr. Heller to diagnose? You will decide that the signs and symptoms were not sufficient to even suspect infection, much less this deadly disease.

Then, take Dr. Anderson [the general surgeon at Shady Valley who took him to surgery on March 3rd] and plug in his testimony that he would not have done surgery on the 2nd. That he would not have cut on what looked to be perfectly viable tissue. You would agree that the earliest time a diagnosis could be made was probably at about 6:30 in the morning [of March 3rd] when he actually had the discoloration, the swelling, and puffiness in his pectoral area.

Probably in hindsight and retrospect, if I had something to do over again in this case, with my client, you know what [that] would be? I would tell Mr. Heller, "Ed, don't use the word 'overreact.' "

When you go back there and you are deciding about whether the doctors and folks at Shady Valley met the standard of care, judge these folks as the facts existed and as the signs and symptoms existed at that time. And if you do, I am convinced that you'll make a decision that's favorable to them. This is not a "send a message to the world" case. I expect that you'll treat Jill Lykins and her family fairly, and we simply ask the same.

So, ladies and gentlemen, it's been a long four weeks. I thank you kindly for your attention. I hope I haven't bored you too much, and I look forward to your verdict. Thank you very much.

III. What Would Greg Do (WWGD)?

Greg Henry, past president of The American College of Emergency Physicians (ACEP), Professor of Emergency Medicine at the University of Michigan, and CEO of Medical Practice Risk Assessment, has been an expert witness in over 2,000 malpractice cases.

Greg presents a unique viewpoint, since he was one of the defense experts in the case. Later in the chapter, another defense exert in the case, Dave Talan, triple boarded in EM, ID, and IM, discusses the evaluation and diagnosis of necrotizing fasciitis/myositis.

"Anyone reading this who thinks they couldn't have missed this case is either an idiot or a liar. This case represents what's wrong with the American system of justice. "

I want to take a slightly different approach to the analysis of this case. I know the outcome. I was a part of it. I was the expert witness for the defense.

This case represents what's wrong with the American system of justice. No one likes what happened. A good guy and a great father, an all-around credit to the community, died. Is anyone happy about this? No! But there is nothing that the doctor can do about it, and blame should not be cast for simply experiencing a horrible outcome.

There is something fundamentally wrong with the system where we cannot take care of a family without having to criminalize a physician. Dwight Brannon is a great attorney. He is smart. He is articulate, and I have great respect for his skills. Our interaction in this case was an epic struggle. The problem is, the system shouldn't work this way. I wasn't happy about knowing that if I did my job well, a family would not be compensated. But the final analysis was: this wasn't malpractice. Malpractice is not about him being a good guy or a bad guy. If he was Simon Legree, he still deserves medical care which comports with the standard of care. To find a villain in this case is to be going at it from the wrong direction. Dr. Talan and I are friends. He is brilliant on the stand. But again, the issue is not the presentational skills of Dr. Talan or myself. The issue is: did the physician act in such a way as to comport with the standard of care?

Anyone reading this who thinks he/she couldn't have missed this case is either an idiot or a liar. This is a young man. He was lifting. He has pain from the lifting. Pain can cause nausea and vomiting. He had tender muscles. To think that this man, a non-drug shooter, with no history of any major illness, should have a necrosis on a chest wall is almost beyond belief.

I first saw a case like this in the hospital as a freshman medical student in 1968. You can do the math on that, but that's a lot of years to see cases, and I have never seen another. To think that I would walk in and make this diagnosis is crazy. Secondly, it is astounding that the wife would take him home and on the way he would become encephalopathic, pee on a gas pump, and would not be immediately brought back. I think this strongly influenced the jury.

By the time this patient returned, he was a dead man walking. All the king's horses and all the king's men were not going to solve this problem. The tragedy of this case is the tragedy of America. We have fallen. We are now a country that is more concerned with process then with product. Why anyone believes we need lawyers and insurance companies to handle basic humanitarian needs is beyond me. It is an embarrassment to the society at large that this type of process occurs.

IV. The Verdict

As reported by The Dayton Daily news, March 29–30, 2002 (combined articles, minimally edited and shortened). Note: Doctors' names have been changed to remain consistent within chapter. Written by Rob Modic:

DAYTON—An urgent-care doctor threw a "lifeline" to a Fairtown firefighter who had a deadly infection, but Shady Valley hospital and its staff turned it into a "noose" that killed the man, the lawyer for the firefighter's widow told a jury Thursday.

After 2½ hours of deliberations, a jury found for Shady Valley Hospital, an emergency room doctor, his assistant and a Fairtown doctor sued by the widow of a firefighter who died of a massive infection.

Mrs. Lykins later saw that a physician assistant, Ed Heller, had recorded that he had called Oster [the primary care physician] on March 2, 2000, who said Lykins "Tends to sometimes overreact to his health care needs." Oster denied he had said "overreact" and Heller said he mistakenly used the word. Plaintiff's attorney Dwight Brannon contended the remark caused the emergency room doctor and staff to doubt Lykins' claims of pain. But defense attorney Neil Freund countered that the conversation took place after doctors decided to discharge Lykins.

The eight-member Montgomery County Common Pleas jury, which needed at least six jurors to reach a verdict, gave six votes for the emergency room physician, Dr. Timothy A. Vaughn and his assistant, Heller. Four alternate jurors, who sat through the entire four-week trial, said they split 2–2.

Defense attorney Freund offered his condolences to Jill Lykins and claimed the victory that upheld the treatment David Lykins received as meeting the medical standards for care. "On behalf of Dr. Timothy Vaughn, Ed Heller and Shady Valley Hospital, we are grateful and thankful to the jury for their verdict," Freund said. "We believe the doctors associated with Shady Valley Hospital and all of the hospital staff give quality care within this community, and we are thankful that the jury agreed with us. This was a tragic case in which a fine family was devastated with a terrible disease, and we feel for the family and especially for Mrs. Jill Lykins and her children." Lykins' attorney, Brannon, said afterward that the case would be appealed.

Why did the defense win? The following are results of a *jury perception study* (conducted after the trial)

- Demographics:
  - 53% female
  - Age range: Young adult to sixties
  - Education: 20% with bachelor's or graduate degrees
- Facts supporting David Lykins (plaintiff):
  - The ED staff didn't take the situation seriously.
  - Vomiting should have indicated that David was suffering from more than a strained shoulder.

- o ER staff did not communicate with each other in an efficient manner; they ignored the urgent care form, the telephone referral form and the triage nurse's notes.
- o The fact that David was a paramedic should have factored into the diagnostic equation and led to a more proactive approach and recognition that he would not be exaggerating his condition.
- Facts supporting Shady Valley Hospital and defendants
  - o Mr. Lykins should have gone right back to hospital when he woke up instead of taking a bath (loss of valuable time).
  - o Necrotizing fasciitis is an extremely rare condition with limited window of diagnostic opportunity, and it would not be fair to hold the staff responsible for failing to diagnose it.

Thoughts of the actual attorneys:

Plaintiff's attorney, Mr. Dwight Brannon:

- "Biggest case I ever lost—Was out-experted—I shouldn't have lost it."
- "I have tried six cases of necrotizing faciitis. This was my first [loss]. I have won all the others. I would like an opportunity to re-try this case."
- Note: Per Mr. Brannon, the unrecovered plaintiff expenses for the preparation and conduct of the trial were approximately $250,000.

Defense attorney, Mr. Neil Freund:

- "We got killed during the case, absolutely mauled by the newspapers."
- "According to Dr. Talan, expert witness for the defense: 9/10 or 10/10 ED physicians would have missed this diagnosis."

➤**Authors' note:** When I initially contacted Mr. Brannon, he told me he wanted a chance to re-try this case, and he got his wish. At the 2010 Essentials of Emergency Medicine conference in San Francisco, CA, a mock trial was held with several participants from the original trial, including Dwight Brannon as the plaintiff's attorney and Dave Talan as the defense expert. With Mel Herbert as the judge, Billy Mallon as the plaintiff's expert, and Scott Weingart as the volunteer physician defendant, the four week trial unfolded over the course of an hour. A true jury of his peers, composed of six emergency medicine physicians, one physician assistant and a nurse practitioner ruled again for the defendant, 6–2.

… but back to the original trial. This was not the end of the story.

V. The Appeal: The court's decision was appealed. The following is a brief summary of the 19-page appeals decision:

From our review of the record, we conclude that any errors committed by the trial court were harmless. We further conclude that the record does not support the claim of improper conduct on the part of the defendants, defense counsel, or the defense witnesses.

There is competent, credible evidence to suggest that David's diagnosis of strain/sprain on March 2 was reasonable and that the proper diagnosis could not be made until the following day, when the signs of discoloration and swelling appeared.

We have found no evidence in the record to demonstrate any relationship between the failure to retain [the urgent care] records and the treatment of David Lykins. In other words, the timing of the diagnosis and David's death were not caused by the hospital's failure to keep those forms. It is clear from the record that Heller and Vaughn ruled out septic arthritis in David's shoulder, as requested by the urgent-care physician. It is further undisputed that David did not have septic arthritis of the shoulder.

All of Lykins' assignments of error having been overruled, we affirm the judgment of the trial court. Judgment affirmed.

VI. Guest Interview—The Legal Analysis: Jennifer L'Hommedieu Stankus, MD, JD

- Former medical malpractice defense attorney and military magistrate
- Long-standing member of ACEP'S Medical-Legal Committee and Ethics Committee
- Contributing writer for ACEP News
- Adjunct professor at Regis University
- Most importantly, a senior emergency medicine resident at the University of New Mexico

Note: We will hear from her again in Case 9.

Authors: *You started out as a police officer then went to law school. Did it turn out to be what you expected?*
JS: When I started out as a medical malpractice defense attorney, straight out of law school, I believed the law was black and white; if there was no clear negligence, there could be no verdict for a plaintiff. As a hospital attorney, it was my job to determine the standard of care, and subsequently who should win and lose. If I found the standard of care was breached, with resultant harm, I felt obligated to reach a settlement that would adequately, but not excessively, compensate the patient for the harm suffered, and the patient would thank me for my efforts. I could not have been more wrong on every front.

These cases are about the money at stake, not about determining if negligence occurred or not. The average cost of bringing a case to trial is $100,000, usually paid out of pocket by the plaintiff's attorney. This is a huge risk. This impacts the award to the patient, as the attorney's contingency fees are subtracted from the settlement or judgment. Even with large awards, the patient is not compensated as much as one would expect. Standard of care is not always easy to determine; it is difficult for people to look only at a snapshot in time and remain objective. Even experts disagree, particularly in emotionally-charged cases such as this.

Authors: *Let's cut right to the chase, does the fact that the patient died increase the chance of a verdict for the plaintiff?*
JS: The worse the outcome, the better the plaintiff's chances. This case is horrific. The patient was a previously healthy, productive member of the community who was a loving father and husband. He went from a state of health to death in a matter of days. How can that be? How is it that a physician trained in emergency medicine could not see such an aggressive disease process? How could the patient be discharged with abnormal vital signs and told he had a mere shoulder strain, and within minutes of leaving become so encephalopathic that he urinated on a gas pump?

These are the questions that will go through the minds of the jurors. They are the questions that may go through the minds of other physicians. It is very difficult to get past the emotion of this vibrant firefighter's death and focus on the information available at the initial ED encounter. Even if necrotizing fasciitis was in the differential diagnosis, would it have changed the outcome? Dr. Talan argues no (below). Further, there was no physical sign of this disease, since it was likely deep in the muscle, not at the level of the skin. Labs may or may not have been useful. In hindsight, placing the patient in observation may have revealed the disease process, but with his symptoms at the time, this admission would not qualify at my hospital.

There have been many instances where juries render a verdict for the plaintiff, even where they believe that a physician was not negligent, merely because they wanted the patient or his or her family to have some compensation for their terrible loss ... and this was a terrible, terrible loss.

Authors: *What were the biggest risk management mistakes at the initial visit?*
JS: Some have already been discussed, including knowledge of the referring physician's concerns, not inquiring when the triage note could not be read, inaccurate medication history from the nurse and discharge home with abnormal vital signs.

Two points deserve special mention. First, when things don't add up and the ED work-up is exhausted, strict instructions for return should be clearly communicated to the patient. The patient and family must feel comfortable about returning, and these discussions should be clearly and thoroughly documented in the medical record. I found it amazing that the patient's wife did not feel comfortable immediately returning to the ER, despite watching her husband urinate on a gas pump and vomit on the way home. That was a big change.

Second, never, ever, make a judgment about a patient or another provider in the medical record—ever. Not only is it unprofessional, but it is usually inaccurate. It makes the provider look uncaring, which fosters an assumption that the patient is not getting the best care. It is the "frequent flyers," chronic pain patients, drunks and "over-exaggerators" who are the most challenging because they need to be objectively examined every visit.

Authors: *Did the involvement of a mid-level provider (MLP) increase the risk of a bad outcome?*
JS: I don't think so in this case. But, anytime there is communication between providers about patients, particularly with an unclear diagnosis, there is a strong risk of framing or anchoring bias. Here, the MLP presented the patient as having a shoulder strain. The patient himself related his symptoms to lifting on the previous day. He did not tie in the fevers and chills.

In cases such as this, biases are difficult to escape. But again, where things do not add up, take a step back and try to think of what else could be going on. Ask the history questions again. Physical exam was not useful here in terms of making this diagnosis, except to the extent that there was zero range of motion and extreme tenderness to palpation, but that wasn't until the following day. Still, pain out of proportion in a successful fireman is a bit unusual and probably deserves a second look (thus the second provider).

It is OK to tell a patient that you do not yet have a good explanation for what is going on and that is not unusual in many disease processes. Here, the patient's wife testified that the ED didn't do anything for her husband's condition, and she didn't feel that would change if she returned. Perhaps framing the aftercare instructions differently would have allowed her to feel more comfortable about returning.

Authors: *Who is legally more responsible, the doctor or MLP?*
JS: This depends upon state law. In some states, the MLP is acting under the physician's license, almost like a resident. In others, the MLP may practice independently. In this case it is a moot point, because the physician went and did his own exam and is therefore equally, if not more, responsible. The responsibility rests on the person with the highest level of training, who had direct involvement in the case.

Authors: *Are you surprised by the jury's decision in this case?*
JS: Absolutely. Even where the standard of care seems clear, one is not guaranteed a certain result. I agree with Dr. Henry that anyone could have missed this case, and that at the time of presentation, proper care was given.

Yet, there were so many things that a jury could have latched onto. The first was the sympathy factor, since this was a shocking, sudden, horrific loss. The second was the judgment about the patient in the medical record. It gave the impression that the patient was not taken seriously and raises the question whether or not the outcome could have been better with a more thorough and thoughtful evaluation; would the physician have gotten more labs such as a CBC, sed rate, CK, or CRP? How about a chest CT? Juries love to latch onto anything that will allow them to help a sympathetic cause. The images of the patient urinating on a gas pump and vomiting right after leaving the hospital are powerful.

Authors: *How would you approach the plaintiff and defense strategies?*
JS: In terms of winning this case, the plaintiff should not have focused so heavily on the recommendation from the urgent care physician because that wasn't the diagnosis anyway. He should have focused on what else it could have been, given that things didn't add up. He could have emphasized what other diagnostic imaging could have been ordered to find the diagnosis. I would have hammered [the point] that this patient's significant signs of disease were discounted, as evidenced by the fact that within minutes of discharge he was not able to function normally. Was there really such a big change within minutes? I would argue that the patient and family must have been made to feel that their problem was insignificant because they chose not to go back to the emergency department, even despite these significant changes.

To win a case, there should be clear and convincing negligence. Here, that wasn't the case. Further, there has to be harm caused by a delay in diagnosis. One of two leading experts in infectious disease testified that this process was such that the patient would not have survived, regardless of the time of diagnosis. We are governed by a legal system in which physicians are afraid of being sued, even when they have met the standard of care or when the standard of care is not completely clear. Dr. Henry said, "This case represents what's wrong with the American system of justice." I agree.

VII. Medical Discussion—Diagnosis and Management of Necrotizing Fasciitis and Myositis

Guest author: David Andrew Talan, MD, FACEP, FIDSA
Professor of Medicine, UCLA School of Medicine
Chair, Department of Emergency Medicine, Olive View-UCLA Medical Center
Faculty, Division of Infectious Diseases, Olive View-UCLA Medical Center

Dr. Talan serves on the editorial boards of the *Annals of Emergency Medicine, Emergency Medicine News* and *Pediatric Emergency Care* and is a reviewer for *Clinical Infectious Diseases, JAMA* and *The Medical Letter*. Dr. Talan has written and researched extensively on infectious diseases. He is triple boarded in emergency medicine, infectious diseases and internal medicine.

I review cases both for plaintiffs and defense. I have opined and testified for both sides, although my opinions often do not support the case of the referring attorney. My academic niche is the intersection of emergency care and infectious diseases. I am primarily an emergency physician, but occasionally practice as an infectious diseases consultant, and as such, I am frequently asked to review medical-legal infectious disease cases that involve emergency department care.

This case is more than an intellectual exercise for me since I was actually a defense expert and testified at the trial. I felt that the care provided met with the applicable standard of care and that, even had the diagnosis of necrotizing myositis been suspected at the first emergency department visit, it was unlikely that Mr. Lykins would have survived.

In order to address the issue of negligence, one has to consider both the epidemiology and presentation of patients with necrotizing skin and soft tissue infections. Severe pain is a typical finding and was certainly present in this case. However, pain is an ubiquitous and non-specific symptom, and patients themselves frequently misdirect physicians by ascribing more logical explanations for it than a rare and otherwise occult infection.

As we witnessed in this case, Mr. Lykins, who certainly was well experienced in demanding physical activity and his body's response, consistently related his symptoms to mechanical lifting. Even later, when his infection was suspected, he pointed to a lifting injury. The emergency staff demonstrated diligence in contacting Mr. Lykins' primary care physician, and they certainly could not be blamed for his offering that Mr. Lykins sometimes "overreacts."

Certainly cynicism about a patient's complaint of pain is a common trap in evaluating parenteral drug abusers who are at risk for necrotizing fasciitis. In the absence of more specific findings of a skin and soft tissue infection, these explanations for the cause of Mr. Lykins' pain made diagnosis much more challenging.

A skin and soft tissue infection is suspected when there is a mechanism to acquire an infection and is accompanied by supportive findings. The lack of a predisposing factor, such as a wound, needle use, chronic lymphedema, vascular insufficiency or diabetes, was a compelling factor to direct the diagnosis away from infection.

The examinations recorded also were consistent in their description of the absence of redness, warmth, and swelling, the more specific hallmarks of infection. There were no signs of crepitance or soft tissue gas on X-ray, no other skin findings sometimes seen in necrotizing syndromes, such as hemorrhagic blebs and darkly discolored skin, and no evidence of compartment syndrome. Vomiting was present, but it is a non-specific symptom and one that would more commonly accompany severe pain due to a musculoskeletal injury than be one of only a few other symptoms of an occult infection.

The urgent care physician suspected a septic joint at the visit preceding the emergency department evaluation, and limitation of range of motion was present. However, as documented on examination and implied by the extent of the X-rays ordered, the area of tenderness extended well beyond the joint, and there were no local inflammatory findings.

Certainly, an emergency physician is not obligated to pursue a diagnosis made by a previous provider if he or she does not observe findings to support that diagnosis, particularly when this would require an invasive diagnostic procedure (i.e., arthrocentesis). In retrospect, we know that had the joint been tapped, it would have been negative anyway.

Knowledge of the patient's history of fever was a major issue in this case. I am not critical of the emergency department staff for not calling the urgent care physician since no reasonable expectation existed that he would be able to provide any information that would not be directly available from the patient and his wife. The emergency department nurse should record her notes legibly, and good practice dictates that a PA or doctor should read the nursing notes.

While it is natural in light of the subsequent tragic consequences of this case to be critical of the inconsistency among provider notes, ultimately providers have to independently confirm a patient's history. The emergency department attending physician specifically documented in his contemporaneous charting that Mr. Lykins "has not had fever" and that the patient was afebrile during his stay, and the physician clearly considered the diagnosis of a septic joint. Unless one concludes that the attending fabricated this history, in the absence of other findings to suggest infection, I think that his evaluation and diagnosis were reasonable.

Of note, an admitting physician later recorded that Mr. Lykins had a fever a few days before, which may have explained the apparent inconsistency of the histories and helped explain the pathogenesis of the disease. Mr. Lykins was ultimately diagnosed with Group A streptococcus necrotizing myositis. This was a bacteremic infection that may have very well started out as a streptococcal pharyngitis, perhaps accompanied by fever, which then localized to an area of damaged tissue. Perhaps, this was due to the injury of the left shoulder Mr. Lykins described. Why some patients with terrible infections do not mount fever, even many hours after taking antipyretics, is one of the cruel ironies of human biology and a circumstance that can lead to delayed diagnosis, one that is generally over-represented in medical malpractice cases.

It was suggested that a complete blood count should have been sent for analysis, perhaps triggered by a history of fever, and its results would have led to an earlier diagnosis. Whereas this is possible, I think it's unlikely. Mr. Lykins' total white blood cell count would have likely been elevated, consistent with infection but also consistent with severe pain from a rotator-cuff tear. Similarly, the proportion of neutrophils could have been non-specifically elevated. The lab at this hospital did not report immature neutrophils, so that information would not have been available. The white blood cell count could also have been normal, since it was normal the next day despite progression of the infection.

A laboratory-based scoring system has been developed for the diagnosis of necrotizing fasciitis, called the Laboratory Risk Indicator for Necrotizing Fasciitis.[2] It consists of the following components: elevated white blood cell count, creatinine, C-reactive protein, glucose, decreased hemoglobin and decreased serum sodium. These components were largely derived from patients with clinically-obvious necrotizing infections and uncomplicated cellulitis, and therefore it is unclear if this index would be helpful at an earlier stage of disease in patients like Mr. Lykins, without local signs of a skin and soft tissue infection. The only diagnostic test that would have been of value is inspection of the deep tissue in the operating room—good luck getting a surgeon to take a patient without any local findings.

The treatment of a necrotizing skin and soft tissue infection is immediate surgical debridement or amputation of all non-viable tissue, antimicrobials and hemodynamic support. In this case the etiologic pathogen was Group A streptococcus, an organism that is susceptible to many antibiotics, including penicillin. Both clinical and experimental data support the adjunctive use of antibiotics that inhibit protein translation at the ribosome, such as clindamycin and linezolid, in order to block toxin production and kill organisms that are metabolically active but at stationary growth. Controversy exists around the efficacy of intravenous immunoglobulin (IVIG).

The reason that infectious diseases are among the most common diagnoses leading to malpractice suits is that they are potentially curable, provided that the diagnosis is suspected early enough. In this case had a surgeon been willing to take Mr. Lykins to the operating room to explore his shoulder area for evidence of necrotizing fasciitis on the evening of the first emergency department visit, it is likely that this diagnosis would have been confirmed about 24 hours earlier than it was. Logically, this would have increased Mr. Lykins' odds of surviving the infection.

However, his chance of survival would have to meet the legal standard of more likely than not (i.e., 51%), in order to be sufficient to support causation. No studies exist in which patients with suspected life-threatening infections were randomized to immediate or delayed therapy and then followed for their outcome. Therefore, causation is largely expert opinion based on:

- Known outcomes of the disease
- The health of the host
- The condition of the host and extent of the infection at the time of the possible earlier diagnosis
- The virulence and susceptibility of the infecting organism(s)
- The time difference between the possible earlier and actual treatment

In this case, the overall mortality associated with necrotizing fasciitis is about 30%.[3] Prognosis is worse in patients with advanced age and co-morbidities and if shock is present. In this sense, causation would be supported since Mr. Lykins was in good health and, at the time of the first emergency department visit, he was hemodynamically stable. However, the deeper the infection, the worse the prognosis, and when it substantially involves the muscle, (necrotizing *myositis*), the mortality is much higher—one review suggests it is uniformly fatal.[4]

In addition, since debridement is the cornerstone of treatment, outcome also is greatly affected by the site of infection and the potential for tissue to be safely removed. In the case of truncal infections, as occurred here, options for amputation are limited. Since Mr. Lykins localized his symptoms to the shoulder and upper chest, even had he been diagnosed earlier, there was a very good chance he would not have survived.

VIII. Authors' Summary

What can we take away from this tragic case?

- Progress notes: Two were done and well done. There was a lot of data from which to defend this case. Of course, it's better if it doesn't even go to trial in the first place …
- Always read the nurse's notes. A history of fever without alternative explanation may have prompted consideration of this disease entity.
- Be careful about using conjecture in the chart. Even the defense attorney told the jury that use of the word "overreact" was unfortunate. Think of it this way: if the patient actually is overreacting, it doesn't help you. And if the patient actually has something bad, it *definitely* hurts you.
- Ensure protocols exist so records are not inappropriately discarded. Pen your initials, date and time on the records before scanning into the chart.
- Discuss diagnostic uncertainty with the patient and the family so they know exactly when and why to return.

References

1. Waddell G, McCulloch JA, Kummel E, et al. Non-organic physical signs in low back pain. Spine 1980;5:117–25.
2. Wong CH, Khin LW, Heng KS, et al. The LRINEC (Laboratory Risk Indicator for Necrotizing Fasciitis) score: a tool for distinguishing necrotizing fasciitis from other soft tissue infections. Crit Care Med 2004 Jul;32(7):1535–41.
3. Stevens DL. Invasive Group A streptococcus infections. Stevens DL. Clin Infect Dis 1992 Jan;14(1):2–11.
4. Yoder EL, Mendez J, Khatib R. Spontaneous gangrenous myositis induced by Streptococcus pyogenes: case report and review of the literature. Rev Infect Dis 1987;9[2]:382–5.

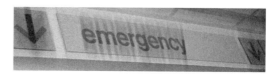

CASE 3

A 15 YEAR-OLD GIRL WITH HEADACHE: A GRANDMOTHER'S 9/11 STORY

Primary case author Michael Weinstock

PART 1—MEDICAL

    I. The Patient's Story 73

    II. The Doctor's Version (the ED Chart) 74

    III. The Errors—Risk Management/Patient Safety Issues 75

    IV. The Bounceback 78

PART 2—LEGAL

    I. The Accusation/Cause of Action 79

    II. What Would Greg Do (WWGD)? 79

    III. Deposition/Trial 81

    IV. Legal Analysis—William Bonezzi, Esq. (Interview) 88

    V. The Verdict 89

    VI. Guest Interview—Plaintiff's Expert Witness: Dr. Leslie Neuman 89

    VII. The Appeal (Continued Interview of William Bonezzi. Esq.) 90

    VIII. Medical Discussion—Jonathan Edlow, MD 90

    IX. Authors' Summary 93

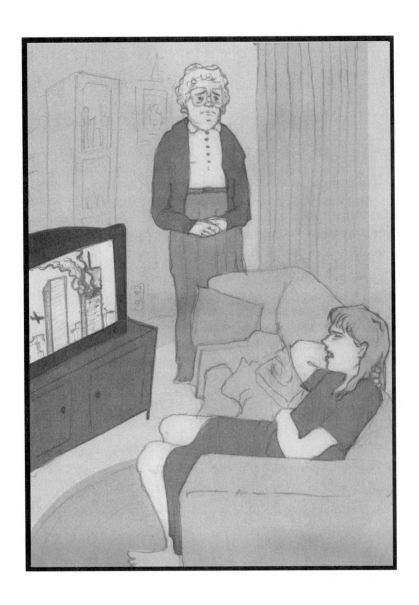

A 15 YEAR-OLD GIRL WITH HEADACHE: A GRANDMOTHER'S 9/11 STORY

America has had many defining moments throughout the years. For many, we remember exactly where we were and what we were doing. On the morning of September 11th, 2001, I was working an 8 AM–4 PM shift in the Emergency Department. The day started slow. After I had seen a few patients, I checked the news on the computer; the report just before 9 AM was that a small commuter plane had crashed into one of the buildings of the World Trade Center. Soon, we knew the whole story.

Deep thoughts:

1. *Which historical factors are most important in the evaluation of headache?*
2. *Should we evaluate similar complaints differently when the patient presents per EMS?*
3. *How does the evaluation of headache differ in the pediatric population?*
4. *What role should "associated symptoms" play in the evaluation of a "chief complaint?"*

PART 1—MEDICAL

I. The Patient's Story

Peggy is a 15 year-old high school student, usually to bed by 7:30 so she can be up at 5AM for school. She does not smoke or drink. She is one of three sisters, but is separated from her siblings and her parents; the other two sisters live with their father, and her mother lives in Phoenix, Arizona.

Peggy's home situation is unique; she lives with her grandmother, an engaged and caring person, founder of the Give the Children a Chance organization and host of *Gospel Dimensions* on WXYZ-FM. One of five grandchildren, Peggy has had some emotional issues, twice "cutting" herself, one time placing multiple parallel incisions on the left forearm and another time eight on the left shin.

On the afternoon of September 11, 2001, only hours after United 93 hits the ground in Stonycreek, Pennsylvania, Peggy begins to cough and develops a headache. Her grandmother tries to get her into the car to take her to the doctor, but is unable—at 2:15 PM Peggy's grandmother dials 911.

At 2:20, the paramedics arrive to find Peggy sitting on the couch. They record: "Patient had a sudden onset of neck and head pain this am after coughing. Denies dizziness, nausea, vomiting, numbness/tingling of extremities. ABC intact. Is able to move her neck."

They transport and arrive in the ED at 14:43.

II. The Doctor's Version (the following is the actual documentation of the provider)

Date: September 11, 2001 at 14:53
Chief complaint: Headache
Nurse's note: Pt. c/o coughing and neck and head pains c/o stiff neck. Ears plugged – some nausea and vomiting of thin liquids. Pain scale 5/10

HISTORY OF PRESENT ILLNESS (Per physician assistant, Ms. Kelly McKinney): Patient complains of throbbing frontal headache(s) for a few hours prior to arrival. No n/v, blurred vision, photophobia, numbness, fever. Patient denies it is the worst headache ever. No trauma. Stated it started after a coughing spell. The condition has remained unchanged since onset. There has been no reported treatment prior to arrival.

REVIEW OF SYSTEMS: Unless otherwise stated in this report or unable to obtain because of the patient's clinical or mental status as evidenced by the medical record, the patient's positive and negative responses for constitutional, psych, eyes, ENT, cardiovascular, respiratory, gastro-intestinal, neurological, genitourinary, musculoskeletal, integument systems and systems related to the current problem—are either stated in the preceding or were not pertinent or were negative for the symptoms and/or complaints related to the presenting medical problem.

PAST MEDICAL HISTORY:
  Allergies: NKDA
  Meds: None
  PMH: Asthma
  Soc Hx: Nonsmoker

The History of Present Illness, Review of Systems, and Past and Social History are complete to the best the patient or the patient's representative was capable of reporting or could not be obtained because of the patient's clinical or mental status as evidenced by the medical record.

EXAM:

VITAL SIGNS						
Time	Temp(F)	Rt.	Pulse	Resp	Syst	Diast
15:00	97.8	TM	70	20	174	94

CONSTITUTIONAL: Alert and well developed
MENTAL STATUS/PSYCHIATRIC: Age-appropriately oriented to time, place, 3rd person. Affect appropriate for age.
HEAD: Without temporal or scalp tenderness, masses, or lesions.
EYES: PERRL, EOMI: No discharge or conjunctival injection.
EARS: TMs without perforation, injection, or bulging. External canals clear without exudate.
NOSE: Normal mucosa and septum.
THROAT: Pharynx: without injection, exudate, or tonsillar hypertrophy. Airway patent.
FACE: No tenderness or swelling.
NECK: Supple. No tenderness. No lymphadenopathy.

LUNGS: Clear to auscultation and breath sounds equal.

HEART: RRR, nl heart sounds, without pathological murmurs, ectopy, gallops, or rubs.

NEUROLOGICAL: Cranial and cerebellar functions normal. Motor functions intact.

ED COURSE:

16:00 – Ibuprofen 600mg PO. Soft collar neck. Ice pack

DIAGNOSIS: Headache

DISPOSITION (16:39): Patient was discharged home by the ED physician. Return in 2–3 days if no better. Condition upon discharge _____ [undocumented]. Rx for ibuprofen 600mg TID. Return to ER if symptoms change.

Kelly McKinney, PA-C
Bruce Hanninger, DO

III. The Errors—Risk Management/Patient Safety Issues

➤**Authors' note:** There is a Bob Dylan line that comes to mind, "I can't help it if you might think I'm odd, if I say I'm not loving you for what you are, but what you're not." The documentation on this chart is quite good … as it reads. But is there more to this story?

Risk management/patient safety issue #1:

Error: Poorly defined onset of headache.

Discussion: When a patient presents with headache, fever, rash and confusion, my neighbor can make the diagnosis. The trick with headache is to find the life-threatening diagnosis lurking around the corner. Arguably the most important historical element in a headache patient is the onset.

Answers to the "onset question" can vary widely. Often, a patient will say the onset is sudden only to mean that it started over a period of a few hours. That may be "sudden" in relation to the time span of their life, but certainly not our definition of sudden; reaching maximum intensity in less than one minute.

✔**Teaching point:** Every headache patient needs to have a clearly defined documentation of *onset*.

Risk management/patient safety issue #2:

Error: Inaccurate documentation.

Discussion: One of the most important aspects of the documentation is the general appearance of the patient. It is our Malcolm Gladwell's "Blink" moment. It is our gestalt as we walk into the room; "sick or not sick?" The appearance is documented here, but in a very general and nonspecific manner: "Alert and well developed. Age-appropriately oriented to time, place, 3rd person. Affect appropriate for age." To me, it sounds like it came from a computer pick-list.

Consider this exchange during the deposition of the plaintiff's expert witness William Biggs by the plaintiff's attorney, Louis Latiff:

Q. When a patient presents in severe pain, do they always provide 100% accurate information?
A. Sometimes a patient in severe pain is unable to give a history until you've treated their pain and have them feeling better.

Q. Is it fair to say that Mrs. Rainey's (the grandmother) version of her interaction with Dr. Hanninger and Ms. McKinney (PA-C) is not entirely consistent with the [documentation provided]?
A. Yes.

Q. Is it fair to say that Mrs. Rainey's version describes Peggy as having severe pain and at some point screaming?
A. Yes, sobbing.

Q. That's not noted anywhere in the physician's report, is it?
A. That's correct.

Another interesting fact was unearthed during the trial; Peggy was examined while in the wheelchair. Her pain was so severe she was not able to even get on the cart.

✔ **Teaching point:** One of the most important parts of the documentation is describing if the patient appears sick or well.

Risk management/patient safety issue #3:

Error: Contradiction between the triage note and the doctor's note.

Discussion: The triage note not only mentions vomiting, but describes the material Peggy vomited as "thin liquids." The specific nature of the description makes it believable, compared to the doctor's note which stated in the first ROS notation: "no nausea/vomiting." If there is a discrepancy between the triage note and the doctor's note, the more credible of the two wins, unless the physician addresses the discrepancy and declares the former inaccurate based on the findings.

✔ **Teaching point:** Just because your initials trump the nurse's initials doesn't mean your documentation automatically trumps theirs. Corny as it sounds, the providers should care for patients as a team.

Risk management/patient safety issue #4:

Error: No exploration of associated symptoms of vomiting and neck pain.

Discussion: The primary complaint recorded by the nurse was headache, but there were other symptoms mentioned in the triage note, which were not explored further. Could the patient have had primary neck pain which then radiated up into the head, perhaps from a carotid or vertebral artery dissection? How about meningitis? She was coughing. Could pneumonia have been present? PE? Spontaneous pneumothorax?

✔ **Teaching point:** One complaint per customer doesn't fly in Emergency Medicine. When there is more than one complaint, they all need to be explored (remember Case 1?)

Risk management/patient safety issue #5:

Error: No progress note.

Discussion: This is challenging, but no less necessary, in a busy community ED. Who has the time to write a progress note on every patient? Additionally, when ankle inversion is the mechanism and the X-ray is negative, it is easy to intuit from the chart why the physician arrived at the diagnosis of "sprain." But there are some patients who leave the ED with *diagnostic uncertainty*; Peggy was one.

The diagnosis recorded by the doctor was the same as the chief complaint, which is fine. But clearly, the exact cause of the headache was not defined. Writing a progress note will often force the physician to think through the decision-making process and differential diagnosis, often prompting them to re-check and re-examine the patient. If the progress note does not even convince *you*, it will definitely not convince a jury!

✔ **Teaching point:** Write a progress note on all high-risk patients.

Risk management/patient safety issue #6:

Error: Reassurance because this is not the "worst headache of her life."

Discussion: I had a neurosurgeon see one of my patients in the ED a few years ago, commenting to me later that the patient didn't have a headache with a "thunderclap" onset. Really? Get your head out of the textbook into the reality of ED headache presentations. What patient ever uses that terminology? If we sent home all chest pain patients not pointing to an elephant sitting on their chest, we would spend more time in court than at the bedside!

I personally never use the phrase "worst headache of life" and discourage the nurses from documenting it unless it is an unsolicited comment from the patient. After all, the first headache in your life is also the worst headache in your life (by definition). Besides, who would ever answer "no" to this question, particularly when the "questioner" is holding a syringe of Dilaudid and Phenergan?

What's most important is the onset and whether or not the patient's headache is unusual in any way. Reporting that the headache is the "worst of my life" is just one of many ways patients can relay to us that this headache is something unusual, unlike anything they have ever previously experienced. So, what makes a headache "unusual" enough to raise concern is the onset, intensity, new location, onset with exertion and certain associated signs or symptoms, such as syncope or neck pain, to name just a few.

Another curious note in regard to our patient; here is a 15 year-old girl, who does not suffer from frequent headaches, being transported to the ED on 9/11 by squad because her grandmother couldn't even get her into the car. Here is a girl in such severe pain that she is examined in a wheelchair. Here is a girl screaming and sobbing in pain. And I ask this—how could this *not* be the worst headache of her life?

✔ **Teaching point:** Use caution when using catchphrases. Don't expect patients to conform to a textbook description of their symptoms.

Risk management/patient safety issue #7:

Error: Gobbledygook! No. Not a medical term. But, nonetheless, I said "Gobbledygook!"

Discussion: Definition: *unintelligible language, especially jargon or bureaucratese.* We can trace its origins back to Maury Maverick, a man whose last name became synonymous with a politician who refuses to conform to the party line. (Though "mavericks" *can* change …) The term "gobbledygook" first appeared in print in the *New York Times Magazine* on May 21, 1944, being inspired by the turkey, "always gobbledy gobbling and strutting with ludicrous pomposity."

So, let me again reproduce the documentation from Peggy's chart: *"Unless otherwise stated in this report or unable to obtain because of the patient's clinical or mental status as evidenced by the medical record, the patients positive and negative responses for constitutional, psych, eyes, ENT, cardiovascular, respiratory, gastrointestinal, neurological, genitourinary, musculoskeletal, integument systems and systems related to the current problem—are either stated in the preceding or were not pertinent or were negative for the symptoms and/or complaints related to the presenting medical problem."* If anyone knows what this means, please write. If anyone thinks this protects you from a legal standpoint, please don't!

✔ **Teaching point:** Sometimes gobbledygook is just gobbledygook.

➤**Authors' note: Summary/question:** When there is a poor outcome, does it help to have documented, "Patient denies it is the worst headache ever?"

IV. The Bounceback

September 15, 2001—(PCP visit—four days after initial ED visit) Peggy goes to see her primary care physician. Her complaint is neck pain. He takes a history and examines the patient, prescribes flexeril for her neck pain and sends her home to return if worse. It is unclear whether the doctor knows she had recently been to the ED with a headache.

October 7, 2001—The country wakes to the following headline: U.S. Strikes Afghanistan
In a press conference, President George W. Bush said the United States and its allies launched an attack Sunday night on targets in Afghanistan to retaliate for the September 11 attacks on New York and Washington.

The battle is now joined on many fronts," Mr. Bush said. U.S. and British forces have taken "targeted actions" against Mr. bin Laden's terrorist network and against the military command of the Taliban militia.

October 8, 2001—Peggy is not up for school. At 5:10 AM her grandmother goes to her room to see if she is awake and finds her unresponsive. The paramedics are called. There is no attempt at resuscitation. Peggy is pronounced dead.

October 9, 2001—As published in *The Abdicator* (compilation of two articles): **Teen dies at home**—Peggy Rainey, a 15-year-old South Kruesdale Avenue girl who had been hospitalized recently, died this morning at home and the County coroner's office removed her body, police said. They do not suspect foul play. The girl's grandmother found her unresponsive and not breathing at 5 AM. The coroner will determine the cause of death.

AUTOPSY (October 9, 2001):

- Intracerebral hemorrhage due to ruptured berry aneurysm of proximal left posterior communicating cerebral artery
- Acute "jet lesion" blood channel into left frontal lobe and left lateral ventricle with 30ml left lateral ventricle hemorrhage
- No gross evidence of thrombosis or chronic hemorrhage of aneurysm. No hemosiderin staining around site of aneurysm
- Acute pulmonary congestion and edema
- No alcohol, drugs, carbon monoxide or growth from blood cultures
- Mid and distal left forearm have multiple linear parallel incisional-type scars, some of which appear to be paired injuries. Inner mid left shin has 8 parallel linear incisional-type scars

PART 2—LEGAL

I. The Accusation/Cause of Action

Plaintiff originally filed her complaint in September of 2002.

- Plaintiff alleges that Peggy's pain and suffering and her death could have been prevented had the healthcare providers met their respective standards of care and detected or diagnosed Peggy's aneurysm.
- Had this aneurysm been detected, plaintiff claims that Peggy could have had life-saving surgery to clip the aneurysm.
- Peggy's death was proximately caused by the defendants' negligence in failing to detect, diagnose, and treat her aneurysm.

II. What Would Greg Do (WWGD)?

Greg Henry, past president of The American College of Emergency Physicians (ACEP), Professor of Emergency Medicine at the University of Michigan, and CEO of Medical Practice Risk Assessment, has been an expert witness in over 2,000 malpractice cases.

Greg discusses evaluation of headaches, trial strategy, and if he would have settled.

"Even the largest plaintiff's whore in the world cannot testify that every headache needs to be worked up for a subarachnoid hemorrhage"

This is a patient that I have seen hundreds of times. Headache is one of the most common complaints in the emergency department. Peggy had a sudden onset of neck pain after coughing, but the majority of these patients will have nothing.

This patient was seen unfortunately during the time of the World Trade Center attack. If you don't believe things like that can distract physicians, you don't understand human physiology; all of a sudden our minds are concentrating on something else and now we have a 15 year-old girl whose history and physical examination seem absolutely benign or histrionic.

Parenthetically, I fortunately was not working on that day, but, just like the Kennedy assassination and the landing on the moon, even at my advancing age, I remember distinctly where I was and what I was doing. This will never be a defense for a physician, but it is certainly something we all understand with regard to focus and concentration. It is my general rule never to take personal phone calls, speak to accountants, attorneys or business people while seeing patients. We have enough issues to think about without further cluttering our minds. The smallest distraction might be a problem.

My general thoughts on the case are biased by the nature of the patient herself. I have written on headaches for years. But in the heat of the emergency department, when you have a teenager who has emotional problems, is a known self abuser, and comes in with the headache complaint, there is an innate prejudice against finding physical disease. All of us has had patients with severe psychiatric problems who were later found to have an organic process. There is a point beyond which reasonable suspicion has to be tempered with a statistical probability.

The strategies of the defense are clear; emphasize the rare nature of this disease in a 15 year-old and the standard work up for a headache patient in the ED. Even the largest plaintiff's whore in the world cannot testify that every headache needs to be worked up for a subarachnoid hemorrhage. The plaintiff will talk about the lost opportunity and the fact that subarachnoid hemorrhage is an imminently treatable disease. This is a classic battle of perfection versus standard of care. I would think that a reasonable jury would understand that the work-up of this patient did comport with the standard of care.

This case is imminently defensible simply because you either decide that you're going to work-up every single headache with an MRA and spinal tap or you're going to use some judgment. I don't believe you should take unreasonable chances with the patient's life; by the same token, what constitutes the acceptable "miss rate?" The jury must understand that every adult human being has had a headache. Not every adult has had a major work-up and spinal tap to decide the cause. It would be a mistake for the defense to even mention the 9/11 scenario as having anything to do with a defensive posture in this situation.

The question of settlement in this case is not a difficult one for me. It was not for another 28 days that the disease entity became obvious. The history taken and the physical exam performed seemed logical. The patient was improving. If you don't defend this one on a standard of care basis, what case do you defend? With my insurance hat on, this doctor deserves vigorous defense all the way to verdict.

➤**Authors' note:** Greg Henry gets it out of the gates ... let's go to court!

III. The Depositions/The Trial

Cast of characters (names changed, except where noted):

The patient: Peggy Rainey
ED physician defendant: Bruce Hanninger
ED physician assistant: Kelly McKinney
Plaintiff's attorney: Louis Latiff
Plaintiff's Emergency Medicine expert witness #1: William Biggs
Plaintiff's neurology expert witness #2: Leslie Neuman
Defense attorney: Bill Bonezzi (actual attorney)
Defense Emergency Medicine expert witness: Edward Eubank
Forensic pathologist for defense: Harry Manning

Direct examination of plaintiff's expert witness Dr. William Biggs, board certified emergency physician, by plaintiff's attorney Louis Latiff.

➤**Authors' note:** The witness alleges that the history taken was incomplete and that if it had been adequate, the doctor would have been alerted of sentinel headache/bleed. His allegations are cleverly rebuffed later by the defense attorney.)

Q. Is the history taken adequate for an emergency room physician?
A. No.

Q. Why not?
A. First, the history of the present illness is totally inadequate. It does not meet the standards [for a patient] who presents with a headache. The review of systems is inadequate and inconsistent with other data. The physical exam records the blood pressure one time, and it's a crisis blood pressure. This is never addressed or repeated. One big deficiency is this record does not record a differential diagnosis, which is ... which is a major feature of every encounter. And the discharge condition isn't given. There's no re-evaluation. There's nothing about response to treatment. It's an inadequate record.

Q. What is the nature of the history of present illness that you have cause for concern for?
A. The standard for history of present illness that every medical student is taught early in their training is that there are seven items that have to be addressed, and these items aren't addressed, and if they had been addressed, I think the outcome would be different. These items are the location of the pain. That is addressed. The character, throbbing. That is addressed. The onset and the time course. Is it sudden onset? That's a major thing that isn't addressed. The mitigating factors or precipitating factors, we know from the run sheet that this was precipitated by coughing, and that isn't addressed [by the doctor]. So, you know, by not addressing these important elements, the consideration of the cause of her headache was not there.

➤**Authors' note:** Wow, this guy is tough! I'm glad he wasn't my attending when I was a med student … or maybe if he had been, I would be a better doctor. … He does have some good points, but would any of this have changed the outcome? Are the standards for a medical student the same as an ED attending? Does this equate to improved patient care? Whereas the onset is certainly important, would mitigating factors or location have made a difference in the evaluation? His answer about the HPI almost sounds like a rant, like he is responding to faculty in his institution or maybe a rogue student. Look what happens later. The defense's "cross" cleverly forces him to admit that many of these deficiencies actually *were* addressed.

Cross-examination of plaintiff's expert witness Dr. Biggs by defense attorney Bill Bonezzi:

Q. You indicated that the history and physical were deficient because not all of the items were obtained that should have been, those seven items that you talked about?
A. Yes.

Q. Well, he found out about the location of the pain, did he not?
A. Yes.

Q. He found out about the character of the pain?
A. That's true.

Q. He found out about the onset or the time course of the pain? "Patient complains of throbbing frontal headaches for a few hours prior to arrival."
A. Yes.

Q. Now, I note that on the history of present illness portion of the record, there is a statement there that says "Stated it started after a coughing spell."
A. Okay, I'm sorry. So that was addressed. I'm sorry.

Q. He also found out …
A. The time of onset, yes, but not the suddenness or its relationship to the cough.

Q. Well, was there suddenness?
A. He doesn't say. He does say it started after the coughing spell.

Q. Well, we just read what the grandmother said (not reproduced here), and her deposition said, "I don't think the neck and the head pain was brought on by the coughing." So, I guess what I'm looking at is, you know, there's nothing here or in the grandmother's testimony that would suggest that there was a sudden onset of headache, was there?
A. It's in the EMS note: "Patient had a sudden onset of neck and head pain this AM after coughing."

Q. Well, do you know whether or not the sudden onset of head and neck pain was brought on by the coughing? We don't know, do we?
A. Right. We don't know with an absolute degree of certainty, but putting the whole thing together, it all fits. And it's my opinion, and I hold this to a reasonable degree of certainty, that the sentinel bleed was brought on by the coughing and/or the hypertension.

Q. … are you aware that Dr. Harry Manning (the forensic pathologist) disagrees that there was a sentinel bleed?
A. No.

➤**Authors' note:** What? What? *Not* a sentinel bleed? How is defense ever going to go *there*? Ever heard of hemosiderin? Yeah, I have too—23 years ago in medical school.

Continued cross-examination of EM expert witness Dr. Biggs by defense attorney Bill Bonezzi:

Q. You're aware of what hemosiderin is, right?
A. Yes.

Q. Okay. And are you aware of whether or not, if there is a subarachnoid bleed, that if the brain is examined in an autopsy, there'll be evidence of hemosiderin?
A. Actually, I never thought about it. I don't know. I don't know the answer to that.

Q. Fair enough. Did you review..
A. I practice in the emergency department.

Q. Did you review the deposition of Dr. Harry Manning, who is a forensic pathologist?
A. No.

➤**Authors' note:** This guy is getting paid *how much*? Well, likely more for an hour on the stand than you made the last three shifts arguing with drunks at 3 AM and he didn't even *read* the path report? Really?

Deposition (direct) of defense expert witness Dr. Harry Manning (forensic pathologist) by defense attorney Bill Bonezzi:

Q. Did you reach any conclusions concerning Miss Rainey's cause of death?
A. Yes. The cause of death was a ruptured aneurysm.

Q. To what extent was the history important in determining the cause of death?
A. It had very, very, very little relevance.

Q. What factors did you take into account in coming to a decision on that?
A. The autopsy report and the microscopic slides. There was no evidence of thrombosis or clotting of the aneurysm. There was no evidence of chronic hemorrhage or evidence of a previous hemorrhage. There was no hemosiderin staining anywhere around the site of the aneurysm. There's no evidence that she suffered a previous bleed anytime more than four or five hours before she died.

Q. And you reached that conclusion based upon what factors?
A. The autopsy report findings call it an "acute jet lesion." There's no evidence of thrombosis and no evidence of hemosiderin.

Q. When you reached this conclusion, were you aware that Peggy Rainey had gone to the St. Steven's emergency room on September 11, 2001—and complained of a severe headache?
A. Yes.

Q. You are able to eliminate any consideration as to whether this history suggested that there may have been some earlier problem with this aneurysm that occurred prior to October 8th, 2001?
A. Although she may have had a headache and nausea and vomiting four weeks earlier, there is no evidence in the autopsy that she'd had a previous bleed. There is absolutely no evidence in the autopsy of anything being older than a couple of hours, and I concur with the pathologist who did the report and the coroner who signed it off.

> **Authors' note:** So there was no staining with hemosiderin, and therefore, she didn't experience a sentinel bleed. Maybe an enlarging aneurysm or other type of headache, but not a bleed. Even if a CT and LP had been done on September 11, he contended it would have been negative and not changed the outcome. The defense attorney further uses Dr. Manning's testimony to focus on the extremely rare occurrence of this diagnosis:

Q. How common is it for a 15-year-old to have an aneurysm of the nature that Peggy Rainey did?
A. Rare

Q. How rare?
A. Very rare

Q. How many cases?
A. Out of about 6,000 autopsies, I think I remember personally seeing two.

> **Authors' note:** The whole crux of the plaintiff's allegation is that if a CT and LP had been done, the sentinel bleed would be confirmed and the aueurysm would have been diagnosed and clipped. The following is this allegation played out by Dr. Biggs (plaintiff's ED expert witness) and then by Dr. Leslie Neuman, a neurologist also hired by the plaintiff as an expert witness:

Direct examination of plaintiff's EM expert witness Dr. Biggs by plaintiff's attorney Louis Latiff:

Q. Should Dr. Hanninger have ordered a CT scan?
A. Yes.

Q. What would the CT scan have shown?
A. The CT scan has a 95 percent sensitivity to see a subarachnoid hemorrhage.

Q What if the CT scan hadn't shown it?
A. If the CT scan does not show a subarachnoid hemorrhage and it's a high-suspicion case, then the standard of care is to perform a lumbar puncture, which is sensitive to detect virtually 100% of subarachnoid hemorrhages.

Q. Is it your opinion, Doctor, that Dr. Hanninger's failure to order a CT scan for Peggy Rainey was beneath the standard of care?
A Yes.

Q. Is it also your opinion, Doctor, that Dr. Hanninger's failure to order a lumbar puncture was beneath the standard of care?
A. Yes. I know that the risk for someone who has a sentinel bleed, the risk of a re-bleed within three weeks is 50 percent, and the risk of death from a re-bleed is about another 50 percent. For the first month after a sentinel bleed, the risk of a re-bleed is about 1 to 2 percent each day, and neurosurgical interventions greatly reduce this risk. And I would say to a reasonable degree of medical certainty, looking at the whole time course and all the data … That's my opinion. Is it absolute? No, nothing in medicine is ever absolute. But it's more likely than not, in my opinion.

> **Authors' note:** Another of the plaintiff's expert witnesses was Leslie Neuman, a neurologist. He gives testimony, but it seems that his standards are of a neurologist, not of an ED physician.

Direct examination of plaintiff's expert witness Dr. Leslie Neuman (neurologist) by plaintiff's attorneyLouis Latiff:

Q. You have many patients who come into your office with neck pain and a headache, do you CT scan [all of] them?
A. Do you want the real answer?

Q. I do.
A. Yes. Every patient that I see that has a headache gets a CAT scan.

Q. Is there any difference in the standard of care and treatment between neurologists and emergency room physicians?
A. I don't think so. I do not—I don't believe so. I mean, there are certain things that transcend certain specialties, where there is a lot of crossover. In this case, I think an emergency room physician [and] a neurologist, those front-line specialties could evaluate this type of situation.

Q. Was the standard of care met in the emergency room on September 11, 2001?
A. I believe it was not met.

Q. What is the basis of your opinion?
A. … the many issues we talked about, unusual headache, first time severe headache unusual enough to warrant transport to an emergency room, headache onset with coughing, some nausea and vomiting, complaints of neck stiffness, high blood pressure, all of those factors together …

Authors' note: Well, how about the high blood pressure? It was checked once and was 174/94, certainly high for a 15 year-old girl (who probably usually runs 90/60), but not unexpected for someone in severe pain. A recheck might have been nice since the elevated BP was brought up more than once by the plaintiff as a risk of SAH. Her blood pressure was elevated on 9/11, but did she have a diagnosis of hypertension?

Additional considerations are whether or not the hypertension was a physiologic response to an acute CNS event? It is a well-known phenomena that acute stroke results in a hypertensive responsive to preserve cerebral perfusion pressure. If the claim is made that the hypertension is due to severity of pain (you see where I'm headed with this), how can we claim this wasn't an unusual headache, based on the intensity alone?

Continued cross-examination of plaintiff's expert Dr. Biggs by defense attorney Bill Bonezzi:

Q. You have a concern with the blood pressure?
A. This was another big "red flag." She had a blood pressure of 174/95. This is a 16 year-old girl with no record of hypertension who comes in with this high blood pressure. Hypertension is a major risk factor for severe headaches. Those readings are equivalent to a middle-aged man coming in with a blood pressure of 250/150. We see strokes in adolescents with blood pressures of 150, 160, 174. That's a serious red flag flapping in the breeze that something's wrong here.

Q. (By Mr. Bonezzi): [tries to interrupt]: Dr. Biggs …

A. Hypertension is a risk factor for subarachnoid hemorrhage, and acute headache in a 16 year-old with that blood pressure in itself a neurological emergency. The blood pressure was never addressed.

➤**Authors' note:** Ever see the movie "A Few Good Men?" When Tom Cruise has Jack Nicholson (Col. Jessup) up on the stand and decides to go for broke and provoke him into revealing what actually happened with a new recruit who died, with the Nicholson's subsequent, famous line, "You can't handle the truth!" Though the plaintiff's attorney's comparison to an adult BP of 250/150 sounds outlandish to me, I couldn't say for sure if he actually did have data to support that statement. The defense attorney must have been less sure, but decides to go for broke.

Continued cross-examination of plaintiff's expert William Biggs by defense attorney Bill Bonezzi:

Q. Get me the article or give me the study that you're referring to that compares her blood pressure with a male's blood pressure that would be 250/150.

A. I don't have an article that compares that. I'm just telling you that in medical practice, I've been taught this by my professors and so forth, that an adolescent with a blood pressure in that range is serious, particularly an adolescent girl.

Q. You don't have anything to support what you're saying, is that right?

A. Yes, I do. I have 25 years of experience as an emergency physician.

Q. Doctor …

A. I have some fine professors who have taught me that over the years.

Q. Doctor, that doesn't count in a courtroom.

Authors' note: Embarrassing. Ever thought of being an expert witness? The pay is quite good, by the way …

Well, did she have hypertension or transiently-elevated blood pressure? Is the contention that her elevated BP was a cause of the stroke acutely, that she had chronic hypertension setting her up for the aneurysm or more likely that cerebral autoregulation was responding to some CNS insult? She did have a recheck, but not in the ED. It was at the PCP office four days later.

Cross-examination of plaintiff's expert witness Dr. Leslie Neuman (neurologist) by defense attorney Bill Bonezzi:

Q. And, oh, by the way, you are aware that when she went to see her PCP a couple days later, her blood pressure was normal?

A. Right

➤**Authors' note:** We've heard a lot from the plaintiff's folks. How does the defendant rebut this witness? Enter Edward Eubank, Professor of Emergency Medicine. Board certified in emergency medicine, internal medicine, and critical care medicine. He has over 100 original publications, over 50 textbook chapters or invited review articles, and over 100 research abstracts. One of his main contentions is that the primary consideration in a 15 year-old girl with headache, neck pain and vomiting is meningitis.

Cross-examination of defense ED expert Dr. Edward Eubank by plaintiff's attorney Louis Latiff:

Q. [Would it] be unusual for a 15 year-old girl to come into an ER complaining of a severe headache?

A. That isn't the most common age group that comes in with primary headache complaints.

Q. And you're aware that she went to the ER on 9/11, the day that the Twin Towers were struck by the terrorists?

A. I am

Q. Wouldn't you find it even more unusual that a teenager would present herself to the ER complaining of a severe headache if it was simply a common headache where she never presented to the ER with headache?

Defense, Mr. Bonezzi: Objection!

A. No, not necessarily. In fact if anything it could almost be the other way around, that could have induced a stress reaction.

Q. I'd like to give you a hypothetical: A patient's headache was bad enough to present herself to the ER on September 11, 2001. The patient arrives in an ambulance. She was not able to walk as she normally would and was only able to be transported via wheelchair. The patient complains of a headache described as one that is killing her, a stiff neck, nausea and vomiting, the inability to walk and talk. Would your treatment differ in any regard to the treatment given by the ER physician in the file that you reviewed?

A. Well, you're outlining a hypothetical case that has some differences from the documented record in this case. If I picked up that chart [my] number one concern would be meningitis. The number two would be possible meningitis. It would not be subarach-noid hemorrhage. It's very uncommon in 15 year-olds.

Q. And I gather that you would not have ordered a CT scan for this patient?

A. I do not have sufficient information to be able to answer whether a CT scan would be indicated. There are a whole number of additional questions including [questions related to infection, history of headaches, severity of headache] and dependant to the answers to those questions, [I would decide].

Q. Isn't the arrival of someone in an ambulance an indicator that the condition is serious?

A. Yes and no. We have patients that come in by ambulance who are taken off the gurney and sent to the waiting room. Some people use ambulances like taxis. We do a very careful evaluation of a patient that comes in by ambulance, but that doesn't always mean they get put at the top of our priority list.

➤**Authors' note:** Can we causally relate her headache on September 11 to the ruptured aneurysm on October 8?

Q. In your view, you're not convinced that the patient had a sentinel bleed on 9/11?

A. I don't believe we know whether she had a sentinel bleed on September 11th. I'm not a pathologist. I addressed the standard of care in getting a CT scan for working up a possible hemorrhage. Given her symptoms complex, given the course of her subsequent symptoms and how long they went on, I would say there's a very good chance that she did not have a sentinel bleed.

IV. Guest Interview—The Legal Analysis: William Bonezzi, J.D.

- Bonezzi, Switzer, Murphy & Polito, Cleveland, Ohio
- Mr. Bonezzi was the actual defense attorney for the case

Authors: *The doctor was obviously concerned about the patient by asking her if this was the worst headache of her life, but failing to define onset. There were also some discrepancies between the documentation and testimony of the grandmother. How was this rebutted in court?*

WB: The grandmother was cross-examined regarding her recollection of the ED encounter. Her testimony did not comport with the statements she gave to the EMS upon their arrival. The complaints the granddaughter gave to EMS were also contrary to what the grandmother said. The documentation by EMS was important to set the stage regarding what was said to the first responders. I did not argue with the grandmother; instead, I brought out each discrepancy of her testimony vis-à-vis the documents. I knew that was going to be important to the jury, and arguing with someone who was grieving for the loss of her grandchild was inappropriate. The testimony of the PA was very important in supporting what the documents indicated. I ended my questioning with the significance of "the worst headache in your life." I asked what would have been done had the answer been affirmative as opposed to being negative.

Authors: *What were your main arguments to the jury?*

WB: I felt that I had a good standard of care witness, and an even better proximate cause witness. I explained, both in my opening and closing, what a sentinel bleed was, its signs and symptoms and what one would expect to see on autopsy. I also discussed a "jet lesion," the lack of hemosiderin and the fact that it was greater than 21 days from the time the plaintiffs claimed there was a sentinel bleed until the SAH. I indicated that the further out one goes from the original symptoms [of headache] the less likely the original problem was a sentinel bleed. My forensic pathologist was very good at explaining the dynamics of a sentinel bleed, the sequelae of same, and the medical reasoning why the 9/11/01 event was not a sentinel bleed. Plaintiffs did not engage a forensic pathologist and were left only with crossing my expert.

Authors: *Peggy was a "cutter," as described in the autopsy. Were you able to use this as an argument at trial that she was somehow overreacting or not giving accurate story?*

WB: I did not go into the "cutting" because I chose not to retain a psychiatrist to explain its significance. I did not feel that it aided in the defense of the case, which in my estimation needed to be focused on the medicine. Of interest was the fact that the decedent's sisters lived with their father and only Peggy lived with their grandmother. They all lived within the same city. The mother lived in Arizona and rarely came back to visit. Neither the mother nor the father were witnesses in the case.

Authors: *If there is a choice, a standards defense is always preferable, but in this case, causation (hemosiderin) was extremely important. What was your "hang your hat" argument at the trial?*
WB: I will always try to defend a case on both standard of care (SOC) as well as causation. If I do not have a standards defense, I will at times even admit that the SOC was breached. In those circumstances, I literally have to show that the breach of the standard did not cause the injury or death, and concentrate on cause. The more I focus on that, the more the plaintiff's attorney has to follow suit. It is then a trial of medical experts. To proceed with a true cause defense requires a good expert who has the talent to educate and explain to the jury the significance of cause, why the injury or death was not avoidable, and that under the best of circumstances, the outcome would have been the same.

Authors: *When the jury was out, what did you think were your chances of winning?*
WB: I felt very good about the case, but with every case that involves a lot of technical details, I questioned whether I did an adequate job of explaining the medicine and its significance. My physician was very well-prepared, as were my experts. I believed that if my explanations were appropriate, we would win on SOC, but I always felt that the best argument was causation, which this jury never had a chance to decide!

V. The Verdict (2005)—Events:

- On September 13, 2005, Judgment Entry concluded in part that as a neurologist, Dr. Neuman was not qualified to testify as to the standard of care in the emergency department.
- One week into the trial, the family physician, Dr. Hernandez, was dismissed with prejudice.
- The trial continued on into the second week with the defense of Dr. Hanninger (defendant ED physician).

  At the conclusion of the trial, a verdict of 7–1 returned for the defense on Standard of Care. The jury never deliberated on causation.

Summary of verdict: *For* the defendant-physician.

VI. Guest Interview: Dr. Leslie Neuman (named changed)—Neurologist for the plaintiff:

Authors: *What were your main contentions about the evaluation at the ED visit?*
LN: This was not an ER frequent flier. If her headache was bad enough to come to the ER, she should have had a CT scan.

Authors: *Were you surprised with the verdict?*
LN: I thought money would be paid.

VII. The Appeal (September 5, 2006)

Continuation of guest interview: William Bonezzi, Esq., of Bonezzi, Switzer, Murphy & Polito, Cleveland, Ohio. Mr. Bonezzi was the defense attorney for the case.

Authors: *The case was appealed due to the trial judge's determination that the neurologist, Dr. Neuman, was not qualified to testify concerning standard of care in the ED. How did this occur?*

WB: The jury never decided the cause issue because they found 7-1 that the physician met the standard of care (SOC). The appeal was a formality, and the defense verdict was upheld. Originally plaintiffs retained Dr. Neuman as both a SOC expert as well as a cause expert. I was able to demonstrate that Dr. Neuman did not work in an ER, did not know protocols and procedures of an ER, and was not a neurosurgeon. He could not provide testimony relative to what would be done on behalf of Peggy Rainey had a CT scan been ordered and demonstrated a leak. He could not answer whether this "leak" if found would have been "coiled" or removed surgically. As a result, the original Judge was going to rule that his intended testimony would be limited. As a result, plaintiff's counsel dismissed the case with the right to re-file within one year. The case was re-filed, but counsel never retained a neurosurgeon and did not retain a forensic pathologist. As the case progressed, it was apparent that plaintiffs did not have an ER expert. I moved once again to have the case dismissed.

Authors: *Any other thoughts or interesting observations from the trial/ordeal?*

WB: As with any case, preparation was key. I felt that the case was analyzed correctly and the proper experts were retained. The issues were crystallized and testimony was obtained to support the arguments. The most important aspect, however, was the defendant physician's testimony. He had gone over the records thoroughly, he had reviewed his deposition so that he was extremely familiar with it, he was available for many preparation meetings, and he worked with me through the case. I also felt that plaintiff's counsel did not appreciate the nuances of the issue involving hemosiderin, and as a result was not prepared to counter it at trial.

VIII. Medical Discussion—Evaluation of Headache, Diagnosis of SAH

Guest author: Jonathan Edlow, MD, FACEP

Associate Professor of Medicine, Department of Emergency Medicine, Harvard Medical School
Vice Chairman, Department of Emergency Medicine, Beth Israel Deaconess Medical Center

Dr. Edlow is Chair of the June 2008 American College of Emergency Physicians (ACEP) Headache Clinical Policy Task Force.

In addition to clinical duties, Dr. Edlow has authored two books for the general public: *Bull's Eye: Unraveling the Medical Mystery of Lyme Disease,* which was featured on Terri Gross' NPR show *Fresh Air,* and his newest book: *The Deadly Dinner Party and Other Medical Detective Stories.*

I will start out by disclosing that I act as an expert witness on medical malpractice cases, both for plaintiff and defense, and I will further state that diagnosis of subarachnoid hemorrhage (SAH) is a strong academic interest of mine.

With those caveats, let's dissect the case that has just been presented. First, for at least two decades, SAH has been identified as one that emergency medicine physicians have been taught to "never miss." Of course "never" is a lofty goal and, given the variations with which patients can present, the cost of *never* missing a SAH (CT and LP on every headache patient) would be huge. The most common reason for misdiagnosis is not getting a CT scan.[1,2] The notion, as the neurologist testifies, that "every patient with a headache" gets a CT scan is ridiculous. That may or may not be true for a neurologist, but is certainly *not* true (nor should it be) in emergency medicine.

So which patients with headache *do* need a CT?

There is no well-derived and validated decision rule to answer this question. This patient is a 15 year-old girl with a severe headache, without a clear-cut history of a prior headache syndrome, associated with vomiting and that might have started abruptly. There is considerable discussion regarding if it was sudden-onset or not. Although the lawyers can parse out different statements from different individuals, the reality is that the defendant could have obtained this simple fact in about 5–10 seconds of history-taking, and should have. But let's give him the benefit of the doubt on this point.

We still have a young woman who has an unusual, severe headache associated with vomiting; does this patient need a scan? She is neurologically intact with a supple neck. Does the exam help? Unfortunately, there are many serious, treatable neurological diagnoses that can present with a normal exam, including SAH. Meningismus may not develop for 12–24 hours and might not be present at all. So, these are findings that are helpful when present, but useless when not.[3]

Are there any other clues from the case? A blood pressure of 174/94 is important. Whether this number is the same as 250/150 in a male adult is irrelevant. What *is* relevant is that 174/94, in a 15 year-old girl (whose normal pressure is likely closer to 90/60, as the authors point out) is an extraordinarily high value. This blood pressure is a big red flag—but not for the reason that the plaintiff's expert opines. He suggests the patient was hypertensive and therefore at risk for SAH. To me, the significance is that such a high pressure suggests (and only suggests) that something might be going on in the central nervous system. Yes, it could be due to pain, or anxiety. But 174/94? At this level of blood pressure in a 15 year-old, the burden is on the physician to prove that this reading is not significant.

At an absolute minimum, treat the pain and anxiety and re-check the blood pressure. Failure to do this is an error. She had a normal blood pressure four days later in the pediatrician's office, demonstrating that she is not chronically hypertensive. But it does not mean that the pressure was benign, since it could have signified a serious intracranial problem four days prior in the ED and which has subsequently stabilized.

Aneurysms are rare in children; only a few percent of patients with symptomatic aneurysms are children.[4] In one single-institution review, there were only 77 aneurysms found over 27 years.[5] So, I can easily imagine not thinking about a SAH in a 15 year-old with a headache. But SAH is not the only potential cause of this girl's headache. One should have a checklist of "serious" or "cannot miss" diagnoses (things that cause big problems and that are treatable) for every headache patient, at least to consider by history and physical examination. This patient could have hypertensive encephalopathy, meningitis, a non-SAH intracranial bleed (AVM, tumor, vasculopathy), cerebral venous sinus thrombosis, pituitary apoplexy, arterial dissections and other possible diagnoses. All are uncommon, but the bottom line is that this presentation of a severe, unusual headache in the presence of severely elevated blood pressure (which may have developed abruptly) demands an evaluation. Therefore, I would have done a CT followed by an LP if the CT was non-diagnostic. I believe that it was a violation of standard of care not to perform these tests.

That said, would the results have changed the outcome? I don't think so. Regarding proximate cause, the forensic pathologist's testimony is key. If her aneurysm had bled at the time of the first visit, there should have been gross or microscopic signs of the bleeding. Our old friend, hemosiderin, should have been present, and it wasn't. The fact that the plaintiff's expert had not read the pathologist's deposition is astonishing; for an expert not to know the facts of the case is sloppy and irresponsible. Legally, the absence of hemosiderin is the key to the case. The aneurysm had not bled at the time of the first visit; the glove does not fit!

Sentinel headache and sentinel bleed are two different terms that are often used interchangeably, but they actually describe two very different things. A sentinel headache is a severe, unusual headache that precedes a subsequent SAH. A sentinel bleed is an actual bleed that precedes a subsequent SAH. Sentinel bleeds are a subset of sentinel headaches. The vast majority of sentinel headaches are actually bleeds that, in retrospect, were not diagnosed as bleeds at the time (either because the patient never sought medical care or the medical practitioner did not do a work-up). If all sentinel headaches were worked up, the vast majority would be found to actually be bleeds (in other words, a first, clinically mild SAH).

How do we know this? In a pooled analysis of 813 patients with thunderclap headache, normal CT and CSF, 0/813 patients had SAH or sudden death on long-term follow-up. This fact is in part the basis for the ACEP clinical policy on headache that states that patients with thunderclap headache can be safely discharged after a negative CT and LP.[6] However, occasional patients with acute, severe headache will have a cerebral aneurysm that is symptomatic (dissected, clotted or acutely expanded) but not ruptured.[7-10] Despite the number of references, these are the stuff of case reports and should not guide routine care. Some have suggested that CTA should be done to rule out SAH,[11] but I am against this strategy for many reasons too numerous to outline here.[12]

My bottom line with this case: Don't over-think (or under-think, as I think was done here) a case. In patients with unusual, severe headache with vomiting (and extremely high blood pressure that is not otherwise explained), do the CT and LP. If these are negative, you have done a standard work-up, and although you can still be sued if a SAH is missed, it is much more easily defended.

Should she have had an MRI or CTA? This is a matter of judgment.[13, 14] I would not testify against a physician who made a thoughtful decision not to pursue work-up beyond CT and LP. In this particular case, an MRI or CTA would have likely diagnosed the aneurysm, which presumably had acutely expanded, clotted or dissected. The outcome would likely have been far better, but vascular imaging is not standard of care for all patients with thunderclap headache.

In summary, I think that the standard of care was violated, but there was no proximate cause. The pathological evidence shows that she did not bleed at the time of the first ED visit. Therefore, had the standard work-up been done, the CT and the CSF most likely would have been normal, and the outcome would have been the same.

Authors' Summary

Besides hoping this patient never walks (or is transported by ambulance and then wheelchair) into your ED, what can we take away from this tragic tale?

- The initial ED record read well, but during deposition and trial testimony, was revealed to be incomplete. How could her headache have been 5/10 when she was at one point screaming and sobbing in pain?
- There was a discrepancy between the triage note and the physician's note, indicating that the triage note was never read.
- There was at least some diagnostic uncertainty; the presenting symptom was headache and the final diagnosis was headache, indicating that a definitive diagnosis had not been found. This is fine, but in these situations:
  o Discuss this uncertainty with the patient and family so they can become "health care partners" and return if symptoms change, worsen, or persist.
  o Repeat and record your evaluation after some time has passed.
  o Document a progress note to explain why you do not think the most serious causes of the presenting symptom are occurring.
- One technique is to apply what we, the authors, call the "front door-back door" approach:
  o Front door: In-depth exploration of the presenting complaint: onset, duration, exacerbators, etc.
  o Back door: Exploration of top items on the rule-out list: using a headache as an example we need to ask specific questions to rule out SAH (onset), meningitis (fever), mass (weight loss), and others.
- This chapter in no way recommends obtaining CT scans on all HA patients, since in the hands of many experienced EM physicians, this diagnosis may still have been missed. It does argue for an appropriate history, specifically concerning the onset of HA, and an accurate description of the clinical picture.

References

1. Edlow JA, Malek AM, Ogilvy CS. Aneurysmal subarachnoid hemorrhage: update for emergency physicians. J Emerg Med 2008; 34(3):237-51.
2. Kowalski RG, Claassen J, Kreiter KT, et al. Initial misdiagnosis and outcome after subarachnoid hemorrhage. JAMA 2004; 291(7):866-9.
3. Edlow JA, Caplan LR. Avoiding pitfalls in the diagnosis of subarachnoid hemorrhage. N Engl J Med 2000; 342(1):29-36.
4. de Rooij NK, Linn FH, van der Plas JA, et al. Incidence of subarachnoid haemorrhage: a systematic review with emphasis on region, age, gender and time trends. J Neurol Neurosurg Psychiatry 2007; 78(12):1365-72.
5. Hetts SW, Narvid J, Sanai N, et al. Intracranial aneurysms in childhood: 27-year single-institution experience. AJNR Am J Neuroradiol 2009; 30(7):1315-24.
6. Edlow JA, Panagos PD, Godwin SA, et al. Clinical policy: critical issues in the evaluation and management of adult patients presenting to the emergency department with acute headache. Ann Emerg Med 2008;52(4):407-36.
7. Neuman JA, Piepgras DG, Pichelmann MA, et al. Small cerebral aneurysms presenting with symptoms other than rupture. Neurology 2001 Oct 9;57(7):1212-6.
8. McCarron MO, Choudhari KA. Aneurysmal subarachnoid leak with normal CT and CSF spectrophotometry. Neurology 2005; 64(5):923.
9. Raps EC, Rogers JD, Galetta SL, Solomon RA, Lennihan L, Klebanoff LM, et al. The clinical spectrum of unruptured intracranial aneurysms. Arch Neurol 1993 Mar;50(3):265–8.
10. Witham TF, Kaufmann AM. Unruptured cerebral aneurysm producing a thunderclap headache. Am J Emerg Med 2000; 18(1):88-90.
11. McCormack RF, Hutson A. Can computed tomography angiography of the brain replace lumbar puncture in the evaluation of acute-onset headache after a negative noncontrast cranial computed tomography scan? Acad Emerg Med 2010; 17(4):444-51.
12. Edlow JA. What are the unintended consequences of changing the diagnostic paradigm for subarachnoid hemorrhage after brain computed tomography to computed tomographic angiography in place of lumbar puncture? Acad Emerg Med 2010; 17(9):991-5; discussion 6-7.
13. Moussouttas M, Mayer SA. Thunderclap headache with normal CT and lumbar puncture: further investigations are unnecessary: against. Stroke 2008; 39(4):1394-5.
14. Savitz SI, Edlow J. Thunderclap headache with normal CT and lumbar puncture: further investigations are unnecessary: for. Stroke 2008; 39(4):1392-3.

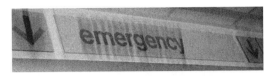

CASE 4

A 36 Year-Old Man with Chest Pain: *The Double Bounceback*

Primary case author Michael Weinstock

PART 1—MEDICAL

I. The Patient's Story 97

II. The Doctor's Version (the ED Chart) 98

III. The Errors—Risk Management/Patient Safety Issues #1–6 99

IV. The Bounceback 101

V. The Errors—Risk Management Patient Safety Issues #7–9 103

VI. Revelation and Final Diagnosis 104

VII. Guest Author— David Sklar, MD 105

PART 2—LEGAL

I. The Accusation/Cause of Action 106

II. What Would Greg Do (WWGD)? 106

III. The Legal Proceedings—Review by the State Medical Board 108

IV. Guest Author—Diane Sixsmith, MD 109

V. Guest Interview—Tim Whiteside, MD 110

VI. The Verdict/Settlement 111

VII. The Press 112

VIII. The Legal Outcome 114

IX. Legal Analysis—Greg Rankin, Esq. (Interview) 114

X. Medical Discussion—Rob Rogers, MD 116

XI. Authors' Summary 118

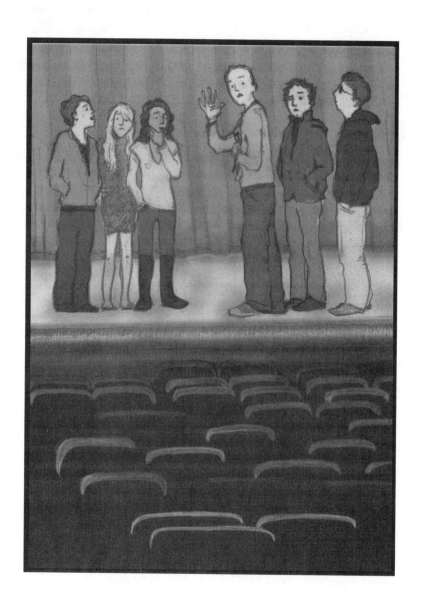

A 36 Year-Old Man with Chest Pain:
The Double Bounceback

Does failure to diagnose a rare condition increase the legal risk if the standard of care is to *miss* the diagnosis? How much credence do we place in normal tests when the history screams otherwise? This case explores one of the most common and most devastating risk management hazards: failure to read the nurses' notes. Because of this case these emergency departments have changed their procedures.

Deep thoughts:

1. *Since we have more training than paramedics and nurses, can we ignore their documentation?*
2. *Is the "double bounceback" more legally troublesome than a single erroneous ED discharge?*
3. *Does a bizarre therapy in the face of a misdiagnosis hurt the physician legally?*
4. *How do we reconcile a patient with anxiety and potentially life-threatening complaints?*

PART 1—MEDICAL

I. The Patient's Story

At the age of 22 Jonathan moves to New York City to pursue his dream of writing a musical. Like most struggling artists, life isn't easy. He spends weekends waiting tables at the Moondance Diner in Soho. He spends weekdays at his keyboard writing songs. His tattered four-story walk up is so tiny, there is a bathtub in the kitchen. Through the years, he has some success writing for Sesame Street and cabarets, but not the big break he has been hoping for.

In the late 80's, he begins work on a new project; he has a vision to create a modern version of "La Boheme." He doesn't merely want to update the opera, but to transform the American musical tradition, appealing to a younger audience raised on MTV, modern film, and changing social values. After two years of hard work, the project is suspended, but he returns to it with a passion after three young friends die of AIDS.

Finally, in1994, he receives a grant to develop his musical at The New York Theater Workshop. He sends his dad a note: "Dear Dad, I quit work. Love, Jon."

In December 1995, dress rehearsals begin. One month later, on Sunday January 21st, he is in the theater for the final week of rehearsals, visualizing his last seven years of hard work. After dinner, at 6:30 to be exact, he is suddenly struck by intense chest pains. He is short of breath and dizzy. He tells a friend, "You'd better call 911, I think I'm having a heart attack," then falls to the floor between the theater's last two rows.

An ambulance rushes him to Cabrini Medical Center. On the way, the paramedics record their diagnosis: "Pleuritic chest pain."

II. The Doctor's Version

Date: Sunday January 21, 1996 at 18:45
Place: Cabrini Medical Center, New York City

Chief complaint (*per nurse* at 18:45): Inspiratory chest pain. Rates pain as 7/10
Chief complaint (*per physician* at 19:00): Epigastric abd. pain

HISTORY OF PRESENT ILLNESS (19:00): Pt. states he ate a turkey sandwich, which didn't taste right. Had dinner and smoked marijuana prior to developing Sx. Hx of ulcers but no hx cardiac disease, no smoking or cardiac risk factors … just finished producing a play… increased stress: Review of systems negative for nausea, vomiting, or diarrhea.

PAST MEDICAL HISTORY:
Allergies: NKDA
Meds: None
PMH: Ulcers, stress
PSH: Negative, non smoker
FH: No family history of heart disease

EXAM (summary):
VITAL SIGNS: Normal
CONSTITUTIONAL: A&O X 3, in no apparent respiratory distress
RESP: Breath sounds clear and equal bilaterally; no wheezes, rhonchi, or rales.
CARD: Regular rate and rhythm, no murmurs, rubs or gallops
ABD: Soft with minimal epigastric tenderness to palpation, no rigidity/rebound/guarding
SKIN: Normal for age and race; warm and dry; no apparent lesions

TESTING: EKG, CXR, blood work are performed but results are not recorded on the chart

ED COURSE:
- Dizzy spell while in the radiology department. Nursing documentation records breathing problems and dizziness while in the ED including the patient saying, "I can't take a breathe." It is unclear from records whether the doctor was informed of this episode.
- "He was pale and clammy," says best friend Jonathan Burkhart, who met him at the hospital. "You've never seen a person breathe as hard as he was breathing."
- Jonathan's friend asks the doctor for an update and is told, "I can't find anything wrong. You'll be out of here in one hour since I want to pump his stomach."

TREATMENT:
- Gastric lavage with NG tube
- 50g activated charcoal per NG
- Torodol 30mg IVP

DIAGNOSIS: Food poisoning

DISPOSITION (22:15): Instructed to eat a bland diet for 24 hours and return to the ED if necessary

Note: The next morning, the radiologist over-reads the CXR as normal.

Michael Meirs, MD

III. The Errors—Risk Management/Patient Safety Issues

➤**Authors' note:** We see patients like this 10 times a day: vomiting, anxious, history of eating a bad turkey sandwich—or do we? This patient provided us with the diagnosis (food poisoning), which is nice, since we can just put it in the bottom box and move on. But wait—which medical school did he attend? No one wants to be sick, and in many cases, patients explain away their symptoms as a benign cause. In this case, there are few historical factors which support the patient's self-diagnosis.

Risk management/patient safety issue #1:

Error: Not reading or acknowledging the nurse's notes.

Discussion: We have all had the medical school experience of presenting a patient's history only to find the attending gets a different history, usually with you feeling nine inches tall. Just because a nurse records a history does not mean the patient needs thousands of dollars of tests: "the worst headache of his life," "child turned blue," "pleuritic chest pain." But it does mean the documentation needs to be acknowledged and either confirmed or refuted by the physician. The options include:

1. Record that you have read the nurse's note and have discussed it with the patient (and/or family), and they deny saying the documented phrase. I usually note that I have confirmed this twice. Two doctors beat one nurse, even if it's just the same doctor asking twice.
2. Seek other ways to confirm which party is getting the most accurate information, such as family members or a squad report. (Note: realize patients may change their story, such as an adolescent who told the triage nurse he was suicidal, but denies it to you since he now realizes he will be "pink slipped").
3. Speak with the nurse to confirm the history documented is actually the history received.

Just as speaking with the nurse is important, valuable information can be discovered from the paramedics. Their observations are particularly valuable in seizure patients, motor vehicle accidents ("When we got there he was completely alert") and with altered-consciousness elderly patients ("Doc, we run on this guy every week, and he is always non-verbal.") In this case, the paramedics found a patient complaining of inspiratory chest pain who had just had a syncopal episode—not a story easily swallowed as food poisoning.

✔ **Teaching point:** Ignore the nurse's documentation at both your patient's and your own peril.

Risk management/patient safety issue #2:

Error: Not digging deeper.

Discussion: A patient with food poisoning would be expected to have more symptoms than mere epigastric abdominal pain (i.e., vomiting or diarrhea). These associated symptoms are not essential for the diagnosis, but without them an alternative explanation should be considered. Was anyone else who had the turkey sandwiches sick? Is there any dizziness or sweating, or at least some nausea? Are there other symptoms (chest pain) which would lead the physician to an alternate diagnosis?

✔ **Teaching point:** When the story is not consistent, return to the bedside and:

1. Confirm the history.
2. Inquire about other important symptoms based on ddx of "can't miss" diagnoses.
3. Re-examine the patient.
4. Ensure disease process is not progressing.
5. Record a progress note.

Risk management/patient safety issue #3:

Error: Performing bizarre therapy.

Discussion: We barely pump stomachs for drug overdose anymore; it is hard to see how it would be helpful to remove a "food-poisoning" toxin already far enough downstream to be causing symptoms. As reported in the *Annals of Emergency Medicine* in 1999, Singer, et al. evaluated 1,171 procedures and reported that NG tube insertion was the most painful.[1] Was the doctor trying to be vengeful or thorough? The old adage, "Doctor, don't just stand there, do something," sometimes needs to be replaced with "Doctor, don't just do something; stand there," particularly when the therapy is unpleasant and ineffective.

✔ **Teaching point:** First, do no harm.

Risk management/patient safety issue #4:

Error: Not addressing documented complaints, i.e., syncope and chest pain.

Discussion:

- Question: "Doctor, have you ever seen a case of ___?"
- Answer: "No, I have never seen a one."
- Question: "Never *seen*, or never *diagnosed*?"

The physician started with a chief complaint of epigastric pain, but after he heard about the bad turkey sandwich, it was all over. The complaints of syncope as documented by the paramedics and chest pain documented by the nurse should throw this differential wide open. Even if the chief complaint was accurately noted to be epigastric pain, there are non-abdominal etiologies that can be responsible for this constellation of symptoms, cardiac ischemia being one of the most serious. An ECG was performed, meaning this diagnosis was considered, but a progress note was not present to explain why the life-threatening diagnosis was not occurring. Additionally, a good history could have easily explored this potentially serious diagnosis with questions about an exertional component, radiation to the shoulder(s) or jaw, associated symptoms of dyspnea or diaphoresis, and of course, risk factors.

✔ **Teaching point:** A diagnosis not considered is a diagnosis not made.

Risk management/patient safety issue #5:

Error: Poor communication between staff and physician.

Discussion: The patient had a dizzy spell while in radiology. (Why was a patient with food poisoning in *radiology*?) There is no evidence this was communicated to the doctor. With the additional history of dizziness and dyspnea, the diagnosis of food poisoning would need to be reconsidered. One of the great advantages of diagnostic testing in the ED is that it prolongs a patient's course, allowing for the disease process to evolve. This seems to have occurred in this case. The doctor was either uninformed about, ignored or chose to not address the change in condition.

✔ **Teaching point:** Empowering staff to communicate with the physician will improve patient care and decrease legal risk.

Risk management/patient safety issue #6:

Error: No repeat abdominal exam.

Discussion: Incorporating a repeat abdominal exam before discharge on all patients with abdominal pain will go a long way in finding the serious/surgical causes. Of all the stomach flus and food poisonings, a few will turn out to be something more serious, perhaps appendicitis or a bowel obstruction. If we see 150,000–200,000 patients in our careers, how many times can we afford to be wrong?

✔ **Teaching point:** Perform a repeat abdominal exam on all patients before discharge.

IV. The Bounceback

Monday, January 22, 1996—Jonathan returns home
- Jonathan is discharged from the hospital at 22:15 Sunday night, and upon wakening Monday morning, he calls the hospital to see if the tests had shown evidence of food poisoning.
- "They couldn't find the results," says Jonathan's friend Eddie, who spent the day nursing him. "But he was told they were sure if there was something wrong he would have been notified."

- The same Monday evening, his roommate Brian returns to their apartment to find Jonathan in bed, short of breath and speaking in a quiet mumble. Brian describes Jonathan's color as "pale and off-greenish." He is only able to eat Jell-O and tapioca pudding. Jonathan asks him to stay and sleep on the living room floor. Brian sets an alarm and wakes up every couple of hours.

Tuesday, January 23, 1996
- When Jonathan wakes up, his symptoms have improved, but come evening, his chest pains have again become intense.
- His roomate Brian calls Cabrini and a hospital attendant says the hospital is unable to get access to the records from Larson's previous visit, so he takes Jonathan by cab to St. Vincent's Hospital and Medical Center, which is closer than Cabrini.

ED VISIT #2: ST. VINCENT'S HOSPITAL AND MEDICAL CENTER

Date: Tuesday, January 23, 1996 at 23:00
Place: St. Vincent's Hospital and Medical Center, New York City

CHIEF COMPLAINT: Chest pain

Triage (23:00) – The nurse triages patient as "urgent" and records chief complaint of right-sided "inspiratory chest pain" for 4 hours. "The patient thinks his pain may be from heartburn."

HISTORY OF PRESENT ILLNESS (00:40): Pt. complains of fever and right sided, inspiratory chest pain which is a tightness, which he rates as 7/10. Pt. complains of "not feeling right." Pt. denies malaise, cough, diaphoresis, myalgia, N/V/D

EXAM:
 VITAL SIGNS: Temperature 100.4 degrees, elevated heart rate of 100, respiratory rate elevated to 22, wide difference between systolic and diastolic blood pressure
 CONSTITUTIONAL: Alert and oriented
 LUNGS: Clear to auscultation bilaterally
 CARD: Regular rate and rhythm without m/r/g
 ABD: Soft and nontender without r/r/g

TESTING: CXR and EKG—Both read as normal by ED physician

ED COURSE: Vital signs not repeated.

DIAGNOSIS: Viral syndrome with instructions to follow with his own physician. Condition: Improved

Paul Votapek, MD

> ➤**Authors' note:** A friend later describes Jonathan's appearance in the ED. "He was slumped over in a chair with his head in his hands, just completely out of it, white as a ghost, sweating and pissed off." He remembers Jonathan saying, "I just don't know what it is. I feel like shit, but they can't find anything, and I just don't feel right."

V. The Errors—Risk Management/Patient Safety Issues—ED Visit #2

➤**Authors' note:** You can call a bounceback annoying, or be thankful for a second chance to "get it right." Often, the ED return patient is irritating to the staff; "That headache lady with the sunglasses is back *again*." In this case, it is hard to know if the physician was even aware that the patient had been seen several days earlier.

Risk management/patient safety issue #7:

Error: Diagnosis momentum.

Discussion: In 2002, Croskerry described "bias" in medicine, later popularized in *How Doctors Think*, a best-selling book by Jerome Groopman. Croskerry termed "diagnosis momentum" to describe a physician who gets locked into a diagnosis too early in the evaluation and is unable to escape[2]—sort of like the Eagles' song "Hotel California" where " ... you can check out anytime you want, but you can, never leave."

✔ **Teaching point:** The biggest impediment to a correct diagnosis is often a previous diagnosis.

Risk management/patient safety issue #8:

Error: Not repeating vital signs.

Discussion: This is becoming a recurring theme. Elevated heart rate not rechecked in a patient who is "white as a ghost," diaphoretic and has his "head in his hands" is never a good sign. A re-evaluation and progress note are in order.

✔ **Teaching point:** Address abnormal vital signs and test results.

Risk management/patient safety issue #9:

Error: Not recognizing a bounceback patient as high risk.

Discussion: A bounceback patient is high risk and has a higher chance of misdiagnosis, and a higher likelihood of needing admission.[3] Here is a suggested approach to the bounceback patient:

1. Thank the patient for returning
2. *Sit down* when taking history
3. Perform a complete evaluation with each visit—do not be misled by *diagnosis momentum*
4. Specifically ask the *main reason* for the return visit
5. After history is taken, summarize to the patient what was just told to you
6. Ensure all documented complaints are evaluated
7. Review the documentation from the *previous visit* looking for:
   - Symptoms that were not evaluated
   - Abnormal findings not addressed
   - Accuracy of initial diagnosis
   - Appropriateness of treatment
8. Document a progress note explaining the medical decision-making process

9. Address concerns with family members

10. Provide after-care instructions which are action and time-specific.

✔ **Teaching point:** Though often seemingly annoying, treat the bounceback patient gently.

VI. The Revelation and Outcome

The writer we have been discussing is Jonathan Larson, author of the musical *Rent*, one of the longest-running shows on Broadway, closing recently after a run of 12 years.

Wednesday, January 24, 1996—ED Discharge to Home

- In the early hours of Wednesday morning, during a cab ride home from St. Vincent's, Jonathan complains of continued pain and tightness in his chest saying, "Nothing has changed."
- In the morning, the radiologist over-reads the CXR: "Heart size upper limit of normal."
- Later, a cardiologist reads the EKG, writing "question lateral MI." There is no follow-up with the patient.
- Larson calls his father and tells him he has chest and lower back pain and a low-grade fever.
- Around 7:30 PM Wednesday night Jonathan arrives at the theatre for a preview with 200 invited guests. His musical receives a standing ovation, but Jonathan is noticeably different. "He was moving slowly and didn't speak loudly," the director noted. "Jonathan was usually an exuberant guy, and he was behaving gently."
- He meets with a New York Times reporter around midnight who says the music is tremendous and would change the direction of musical theater. Jonathan says he needed to respond in some way to celebrate the lives of his friends who have died young. "It's not how many years you live, but how you fill the time you spend here," Jonathan said, prophetically in hindsight, about the meaning of his play. He leaves the theater in a cab, planning to meet with the director in the morning. He arrives home at 12:30 AM.

Thursday, January 25, 1996

- At 3:40 AM, Jonathan's roommate Brian returns home to find a gas flame burning under a scorched tea kettle and Jonathan lying on the floor. Brian opens his shirt and begins chest compressions, yelling, "Wake up! Wake up, Jon!" The police arrived shortly after and pronounce him dead. It is the day before opening night.

Friday, January 26, 1996

- **Autopsy:**
  1. Cystic medial degeneration of the aorta, likely from undiagnosed Marfan's syndrome
  2. Twelve-inch aortic dissection from base of aorta 1½ cm superior to the aortic valve to the bifurcation of the common iliac arteries
  3. Hemopericardium and cardiac tamponade with 700cc blood in pericardial sac

RENT **Preview**—Later that night, the curtain rises on the first preview. The rock opera's opening night ended with no applause. The audience, cast, and crew sat completely silent until an unidentified voice said, "Thank you, Jonathan Larson." Within a few months *RENT* moves to Broadway, where it wins the Pulitzer Prize, four Tony Awards, six Drama Desk awards and three Obie awards.

VII. Guest Author: David Sklar, MD, FACEP

- Professor of Emergency Medicine, University of New Mexico School of Medicine
- Associate Dean & Designated Institutional Officer, Graduate Medical Education
- Author of *Unanticipated Death After Discharge Home From the Emergency Department*, Annals of Emergency Medicine, June 2007

When patients present with classic symptoms, most physicians will make the diagnosis. Few will miss pulmonary embolism in patients with chest pain, shortness of breath and hemoptysis. Patients with searing chest pain radiating to the back will be evaluated for aortic dissection. It is with the atypical presentation of a relatively rare condition where the expert clinician may make a difference. Experienced physicians may recognize more extensive patterns of disease and have better access to these patterns stored in their memory. They have seen myocardial infarctions that presented without chest pain and the pulmonary embolism that presented without shortness of breath. They are able to identify subtle clues that suggest a patient has a serious condition and not a benign process.

Diagnostic accuracy for self-limited problems is not very important since they resolve without treatment. It is a tragedy to misidentify a patient with a life-threatening problem and discharge that patient home. Unfortunately, discharge of emergency department patients who subsequently, unexpectedly die of conditions related to the emergency department visit are distressingly common.[4]

In a study we performed at the University of New Mexico, over a period of 10 years, 58 emergency department patients died unexpectedly within seven days after discharge of a condition related to their initial emergency department visit, of which 35 had a possible error.[4] Possible errors led to nine patient deaths within seven days of their emergency department visit, per 100,000 discharges. Atypical presentation such as that of Jonathan's occurred in 54% of our error cases. Abnormal vital signs occurred in 83%.

It may not always be possible to identify an atypical presentation, but we need to recognize abnormal vital signs. We should seek an explanation and re-check them prior to discharge since they may be the earliest clue that a physiologic process is amiss or suggest that the patient's problem, even if undiagnosed, could be life-threatening. In Jonathan's case, tachycardia, though a non-specific finding, in conjunction with near syncope and chest pain, might have suggested a reduced cardiac output and prompted additional investigations.

There were other clues; the diagnosis of food poisoning in the absence of diarrhea or vomiting was unlikely. Syncope in the theater and the later sensation of dizziness and shortness of breath while at radiology were not adequately explained. The passing of the NG tube to pump the stomach has no support in the medical literature and, though not dangerous, was unnecessary and suggestive of poor diagnostic reasoning. The second visit provided more clues—abnormal vitals, history of syncope, unexplained chest pain, abnormal EKG, any of which might have suggested a serious condition requiring additional testing, examination or history.

Because of the atypical presentations of aortic dissection, it is not likely the diagnosis would have become apparent to most physicians by history or physical exam alone. However, the risk of seriousness might have been recognized and might have led to more work-up. Through careful attention to abnormal vital signs, clinicians can become alerted to the evaluation of serious, atypical presentations and be prompted to seek other clues to the diagnosis.

We cannot all be expert diagnosticians, but we can utilize all the tools of experts to guide us when confronted with difficult cases, such as the tragic death of Jonathan.

PART 2—LEGAL

I. The Accusation/Cause of Action

- Family sues with an initial demand of $250 million, estimating revenues from *RENT*, in a negligence lawsuit against both hospitals.
- A report on *PrimeTime Live* raises serious questions and results in an investigation by the New York State Health Commissioner, Dr. Barbara DeBuono. The investigative process includes extensive review of the ED visits, 29 interviews, plus the advice of eight physicians, including three with expertise in emergency medicine and five board-certified radiologists.

[As quoted]: "Mr. Larson's condition was misdiagnosed at both hospitals," said State Health Commissioner Dr. Barbara DeBuono. "We do have concerns about the appropriateness and medical soundness of the treatment Mr. Larson received in their emergency rooms." (Note: one of the emergency physicians and the medical director of ED #1, Cabrini, shed light on the process later in this chapter.)

II. What Would Greg Do (WWGD)?

Greg Henry, past president of The American College of Emergency Physicians (ACEP), Professor of Emergency Medicine at the University of Michigan, and CEO of Medical Practice Risk Assessment, has been an expert witness in over 2,000 malpractice cases.

Greg discusses care of the double bounceback patient, defense of the case and how a State Board review differs from a standard negligence lawsuit.

> **"[In the ED] we have oceans of mediocrity surrounded by moments of terror and regret"**

I have to confess having knowledge of the case. Not only do I have know of this case, but everybody in the country knows of this case—we also know of the similarly tragic deaths of John Ritter and Richard Holbrooke.

This admitted, the principal problem with this book is clear—we present cases which are *something*. Most of the things that we see in the emergency department are *nothing*. In truth, we have oceans of mediocrity surrounded by moments of terror and regret. In my 140,000 patient experiences, I don't ever remember seeing a young man of this age with Marfan's syndrome and an aortic dissection. It is easy to forget the rarity of this disease. There are only 3,000 to 4,000 thoracic aortic dissections in the United States each year, which means the average emergency physician might see one, even in a busy institution, every seven or eight years. Do the math.

Goethe said, "We see only what we know." When "what we know" is a diagnosis, we try and make the history and physical fit that diagnosis. The presenting complaints of this patient are syncope and chest pain, but we dress it up with everything else: "I ate a bad turkey sandwich." To ascribe causation to the turkey sandwich is to spell disaster. If the standard of care is what actually happens, in this disease it is to have missed it on the first one or two presentations. The diagnosis is always eventually made—unfortunately when it occurs post-mortem, it doesn't count for much.

Paramedics' and nurses' comments are equivalent to the physicians' in a courtroom: these people are viewed as healthcare professionals that have both training and experience and a right to put their opinions on paper. The expectation of the public is that the physician will have accounted for the pre-hospital and triage notes when formulating a diagnosis. Ignore Allied Professional notes at your peril!

The concept of the "double bounceback" always needs to be sung as an emergency medicine anthem. If they are in for the second time, take a really good look; if they are in for the *third* time, admit. It doesn't really matter why they returned—if they have been back three times and the diagnosis is confusing, the problem is not resolved. In this particular case, the initial evaluation and bizarre therapy probably didn't do much to establish the physician's credibility, but they also didn't do much to harm him intellectually or legally.

Patient safety issues begin and end with diagnosis momentum. We get channeled as we see patients. When you see the patient for the second visit, listen to that little voice that says, "Something here isn't right." An even greater attribute is to look at a previously - assigned diagnosis and question its basis. There is no substitute for actually putting fresh eyes on a case. I'm aware of at least two insurance companies who request that return visits are seen by different eyes and unbiased neurons.

The defense in this case will be obvious:
- We are talking about rare disease
- The patient believes he has a cause for his symptoms that seems plausible to the emergency physician
- The vast majority of patients who present with such vague symptoms have no easily discernable medical problem

That doesn't mean we have a right to miss everything, but on the same basis we can't work up everyone for everything.

A decision to settle or try this case is more based on sensationalism than science. A famous person has died; the reasons for such a death may be secondary to the emotional appeal to a jury. For the family to sue for $250 million is ridiculous. The family had no reasonable expectation that they would receive all of that money. On that basis the federal government ought to attach a suit asking for the taxes they would receive if this sum had been paid out to the decedent. There is definitely harm to the defense from the sensationalism and this would force me, as the representative of the insurance company, to seriously consider a reasonable settlement.

It is important to point out that families often don't just want money but may need some form of recognition or plan for quality improvement. I have settled cases in which part of the settlement was attaching a plaque in a room in the ED dedicated to the family member who they lost. I have seen cases where a family wants the physician to listen to their story of grief as a part of their settlement agreement. It is the wise attorney who takes all of these things into consideration when deciding on the resolution.

As was noted, this case was turned over to a State Board for review. State Board reviews are much different than standard negligence lawsuits. It depends on the state, but I have seen Boards with unbelievable power and act without constraint; the state of New York is notorious. I have personally been involved in the defense of physicians who have been taken before the New York State Board of Medicine; the investigation is begun with a presumption of guilt. They have any amazing ability to find physicians who believe very bizarre things about the standard of care, but physicians are just people—there are variances on how we work-up disease.

Appearances before State Boards should put a tingle down the spine as they have a political agenda to show they are acting in the interests of the citizens of the state. The actual facts are almost never of importance. What they need are pelts from the hides of physicians to nail to the wall. It is clearly the uninformed and uninitiated who would go to such a meeting without proper counsel.

(Note: Upon writing, Greg did know the outcome of this case—this case was presented initially as an EM RAP bounceback presentation in January 2009.)

III. Review by the State Medical Board

The cast of characters:

The hospitals: Cabrini and St. Vincent's
The family
The State Medical Board of New York
37 physicians and witnesses interviewed under the watchful eye of the press

IV. Guest Author: Diane Sixsmith, MD, MPH, FACEP

Chairman, Department Emergency Medicine, New York Hospital Queens
Assistant Professor of Emergency Medicine, Weill Medical College of Cornell University
Expert witness for the NY Office of Professional Misconduct (OPMC) in the case of Jonathan Larson

The death of Jonathan Larson was a front-page item in all the local newspapers. The analogy to his own musical was too great to ignore. A later feature article in the New York Times was even titled "A Composer's Death Echoes in His Musical." The tabloids emphasized the fact that Jonathan had visited not one, but two New York City EDs in the days before his death; every ED director's worst nightmare.

Faced with the media attention, the Office of Professional Medical Conduct (OPMC) of New York State felt compelled to investigate whether the care met accepted standards. The Office is the working arm of the New York State Board of Professional Medical Conduct, one of 70 state medical and osteopathic boards in the U.S. and its territories. In New York, the Board is composed of hundreds of physicians in all the recognized specialties who are appointed to a voluntary three-year term by the governor. Another hundred or so members are laypeople.

While the OPMC investigates complaints about physicians, physician assistants and specialist assistants and monitors practitioners who have been placed on probation, it refers its findings for final decision to the State Board. Such decisions usually involve the medical license, but also may deal with substance abuse treatment, medical or psychiatric evaluation and practice monitoring.

In New York, physicians come to the attention of the OPMC through a variety of channels besides high-profile media cases. Malpractice claims, individual patient or family complaints, and referrals by other physicians or hospitals are all funneled through the OPMC and then reviewed for significance. If a particular incident or complaint appears to have merit, a medical investigator and a physician employed by the OPMC assemble the relevant medical records and interview the relevant parties, including the physician under investigation. They may also ask to see individual physician peer review or credentialing files, looking for other evidence of problematic conduct or care. The findings are then sent to an outside reviewer of the physician's own specialty.

I was the outside reviewer in Jonathan Larson's case. My job as a reviewer was to determine whether there were deviations from the accepted standard of care and whether these constituted negligence or gross negligence, incompetence or gross incompetence. My opinions were summarized in a written report, which was then used by the Office to determine whether the physicians should be charged and brought to a hearing before the Board. The main purpose of the hearing would be to determine whether the physicians should be allowed to continue to practice medicine, since the overarching mission of the State Board is to ensure public safety.

I reviewed the medical records from both EDs and the transcripts of interviews that had been taken with all the providers involved. A segment of *PrimeTime Live* had an interview with a cardiologist who opined that Jonathan's X-ray clearly showed aortic abnormalities, so I had his case blindly and anonymously reviewed by cardiologists, radiologists and ED physicians at my own hospital in an attempt to bring some objectivity to my review. To each of my colleagues, I presented the information in the ED record regarding history, vital signs and physical findings and then asked them to review the X-rays and EKGs and come to a tentative diagnosis and disposition. They were all surprised at the final diagnosis. None of them considered the chest X-ray significantly abnormal, and none of them considered the diagnosis of aortic dissection.

I was considerably bothered about the fact that in the first ED, Jonathan had an NG tube placed and was given activated charcoal, and I expressed this in my report. While I felt that this was not something that the majority of physicians would have done, we give other physicians considerable latitude in administering therapies that they believe may have efficacy.

I suspected that a better history could have been elicited at both EDs. The one essential aspect of the history that may have changed the outcome, the "bounceback," appeared not to have been known by the second ED providers. Was the failure to impart knowledge of the previous visit Jonathan's or the ED staff's failure to record it? I also was concerned that the dizzy spell while in the radiology suite at visit #1 was not more fully evaluated. But in the end, I felt that "there but for the grace of God go I" or any of my colleagues. In adhering to the information as it appeared in the records, without giving in to my own unproved suspicions about cursory histories or incomplete examinations, I concluded that on neither visit did Jonathan appear to have any red flags that warranted further work-up or criteria that justified further observation or admission.

Per the guidelines of the OPMC, incompetence is defined as acting without sufficient knowledge or skill; negligence is failing to provide the care that a reasonably competent ED physician or the majority of ED physicians faced with similar circumstances would provide. Since I felt that most physicians would have ended up doing a similar work-up and then discharging Jonathan, I concluded that there was no negligence or incompetence. Moreover, I felt that aortic dissection was a diagnosis that almost no one would have included on his or her differential diagnosis list.

➢**Authors' note:** If you had to choose, which is preferable, a State Board review or a standard, run of the mill grilling in the courtroom? Neither? We agree!

V. Guest Interview: Tim Whiteside, MD

One of the physicians interviewed, as well as named in the lawsuit, was Tim Whiteside, a very capable physician, double boarded in EM/IM. He was the ED Director at Cabrini in 1996. He currently heads performance improvement at Hawaii Emergency Physicians Associates.

Dr. Whiteside was the ED director at Cabrini Medical Center (ED visit #1)

Authors: *Did you see the patient at the initial visit?*
TW: No. I first learned about the patient from the Nurse Manager the next day. The nurses were concerned that a patient diagnosed with food poisoning was treated with lavage and charcoal since they had never seen that before. I reviewed the case and discussed this with the physician and was still a little unclear about the reasoning.

Authors: *What did the ED doctor say about the case?*
TW: His impression was that the patient would be better in 24 hours. He did not specifically address the chest pain with the patient. He was really focused on this being GI-based.

Authors: *The CXR was over-read the next day. Was there a discrepancy?*
TW: There was no discrepancy in the CXR report from radiology.

VI. The Verdict/Settlement—Per the State Medical Board
(Obtained under the Freedom of Information Act)

June 9, 1997: Whereas the New York State Department of Health has conducted surveys and inspections of [Cabrini Medical Center and] St. Vincent's Hospital and Medical Center and has found alleged violations of Article 28 of the Public Health Law and Title 10 (Health) of the Official Compilation of Codes, Rules and Regulations of the State of New York and Whereas the parties wish to resolve this matter by means of settlement instead of an adversarial administrative hearing;

NOW, THEREFORE, IT IS STIPULATED AND AGREED AS FOLLOWS:

1.   The matter relating to alleged violation of Article 28 of the Public Health Law and 10 NYCRR, as set forth in the Statement of Deficiencies, dated December 10, 1996 is settled and discontinued with prejudice upon the terms and conditions set forth in this Stipulation and Order.

2.   The Respondent, for the purpose of resolving this administrative matter only, admits the existence of substantial evidence of violations of Title 10 (Health) of the Official Compilation of Codes, Rules and Regulations of the State of New York, as set forth herein, as follows:

A. Cabrini Medical Center (ED #1):

1. ED doctor did not fully evaluate the chief complaint of chest pain. No information was presented that considered or eliminated the possible causes of chest pain.
2. There is no evidence the physician interpreted the CXR or CBC prior to ED discharge, contrary to established emergency room procedures.

3. The diagnosis of food poisoning was not supported by patient symptoms or complaints except for possible epigastric tenderness and description of turkey sandwich with a bad taste. Use of NG tube was inappropriate and unnecessary.

4. No repeat vital signs despite nursing documentation of breathing problems and dizziness.

5. **Summary:** Not correctly diagnosed and incorrectly treated.

6. **Penalty:**
   - Issued statement of deficiency and fine of $10,000.
   - Required plan of correction which would relate to the care of all patients. The plan must be generic in nature, aimed at preventing such deficiencies in the future. It must include intended completion dates and mechanisms established to assure ongoing compliance.

B. St. Vincent's Hospital (ED #2):

1. Vital signs including pulse were abnormal and were not repeated, as required by hospital's own protocol.

2. Patient was triaged as "urgent" but not evaluated by a physician for 1 hour and 40 minutes after triage, not consistent with written triage procedures mandating evaluation within one hour.

3. With exception of fever, diagnosis of viral syndrome was not supported by Mr. Larson's condition or presenting symptoms. There was no malaise, cough, diaphoresis, myalgia, nausea, vomiting, nor diarrhea.

4. **Summary:** Not correctly diagnosed and incorrectly treated.

5. **Penalty:**
   - Issued statement of deficiency and fine of $6,000.
   - The respondent shall develop, submit and implement an acceptable plan of correction within time frames acceptable to and subject to the department's monitoring.
   - The respondent shall submit quarterly progress reports to the Department on each of the components of this Stipulation and Order for a one-year period commencing with the effective date of this Stipulation and Order with assessment of effectiveness.

VII. The Press

State Faults Hospitals for "Rent" Tragedy—NY Daily News
by Joe Nicholson and Anne E. Kornblut—December 13, 1996 (shortened)

The author of the hit musical "Rent" was twice misdiagnosed and sent home from hospitals to die, just days before he was about to unveil the work that brought him international acclaim, state health officials said yesterday. As the main artery from his heart was about to burst, Jonathan Larson went to two of the city's most prestigious hospitals with excruciating chest pains, dizziness and shortness of breath. But doctors told him he had food poisoning or a viral syndrome and sent Larson, 35, home, where he died of an aortic aneurysm on his kitchen floor.

Larson's health problems were "not correctly diagnosed and inappropriately treated" at Cabrini Medical Center and St. Vincent's Medical Center, investigators said. The hospitals were hit with unusual fines totaling $16,000 after the state's four-month probe, and doctors at both hospitals were referred for investigation by the state's Office of Professional Medical Conduct.

"A number of deficiencies exist between the department's report and the medical facts in this case," said a statement from St. Vincent's Medical Center. "Our exhaustive review indicates that Mr. Larson's evaluation at St. Vincent's was medically thorough and appropriate."[State health commissioner] Dr. DeBuono conceded that diagnosing the aortic aneurysm "would pose a challenge to the best clinician," particularly because of Larson's young age and lack of history.

The musical, a modern version of "La Boheme" depicting life on the lower East Side, played to sellout performances at the New York Theater Workshop before it moved to Broadway's Nederlander Theater, where it won prestigious Tony and New York Drama Critics' Circle awards. Three months after Larson's death, "Rent" won the 1996 Pulitzer Prize.

On Anniversary of a Son's Death, Contracts and Awards Are Small Comfort
The New York Times—by Rachel L. Swarns—January 26, 1997 (shortened)

Allan Larson buries his grief in the stacks of paper towering precariously on his desk, in the pages of the book about and in the cards and letters from fans overwhelmed by his son's creation, the hit musical "Rent." And sometimes at night, in the hazy place between wakefulness and sleep, he finds himself believing that his son is still alive, that the telephone will ring and that Jonathan Larson, the curly-haired, ebullient playwright and composer, will be on the line, humming the riff of a newly penned song.

"I have my moments, when I still can't believe, because it shouldn't be," said Mr. Larson in an interview yesterday, on the one-year anniversary of his son's death. "But you wake up and it's the same nightmare," said Mr. Larson, who flew to New York from New Mexico with his wife, Nanette, to spend the day with the cast of the musical. "This year has been a roller-coaster ride from hell, and it continues to this day."

Last night, about 100 friends and relatives commemorated his death. Gathered on the stage of the Nederlander Theater, where the show is performed, they sang the anthem, "Seasons of Love." The actors in "Rent," a contemporary American version of the Puccini opera "La Boheme," have had to get used to working without him. But some say they still feel his presence. "Every time there's an empty seat in the theater, we like to think that Jonathan's there," said Anthony Rapp, the actor who plays the character Mark.

Yesterday, before the stage gathering, the actors shared their memories of the young playwright, who grew up in White Plains pounding on the family piano. "His big eyes, his smile, his laugh, his big ears, his curly hair, the way he always looked like he was up to some mischief, that's what I remember," said Daphne Rubin-Vega, who plays the role of Mimi in the musical. "A year ago today, we just sat there on the stage, huddled together," she said. "We spoke. We cried. And today we want to be together."

Mr. Larson's father, who scattered some of his son's ashes on Broadway, said he could think of no better place to spend the day than with the actors. "You want to be with family," he said. "They're family now."

VIII. The Legal Outcome

The suit was settled for an undisclosed amount. Part of the money is currently used to fund educational efforts by the National Marfan Foundation.

IX. Guest Interview—The Legal Analysis: Greg Rankin, JD

- Managing partner at Lane, Alton & Horst in Columbus, Ohio
- Over 30 years of medical practice defense
- Recognized in 2009 edition of The Best Lawyers in America in the specialty of medical malpractice

Authors: *What is the difference between defending a case against an allegation from a patient and from a State Medical Board?*
GR: There are many differences between *civil litigation,* in which a patient is suing a physician for negligence, and an *administrative proceeding,* in which a state medical board is taking action against a physician's license. One of the main differences is the stakes involved:

- In a civil malpractice action, the consequence to the physician is an award to the plaintiff of money damages, which are typically covered by professional liability insurance. There are, of course, exceptions to this when the amount sought and/or recovered by the patient against the physician exceeds the physician's policy limits, in which the physician's personal assets are subject to garnishment. In a malpractice action, the rules of evidence govern. They typically preclude a plaintiff from introducing evidence of prior acts and/or findings of negligence on the part of the physician.

- In an action filed by a state medical board, the potential is for the physician to lose his license to practice medicine, either temporarily or permanently. Typically, there is no monetary sanction against the physician. In a state medical board proceeding, prior claims against the physician can be introduced.

Authors: *Is the first or second ED physician at greatest legal risk?*
GR: With respect to the conduct of the first ED doctor, there are a number of factors which could have made his case more defensible. First, had he reviewed (and noted in the chart), the EMT/nursing note, this likely would have sent him down a path different from food poisoning. The physician should have noted that he had reviewed these records, as well as the diagnostics studies and blood work. The physician should have set forth his thought processes and/or a differential diagnosis to reflect that he had considered other etiologies besides food poisoning. Finally, there is no mention of the patient's condition at the time of discharge.

The second ED doctor did err by failing to note that this was a "bounceback." This information should have been elicited in the history, either by the nurse or the physician. Bounceback patients should be assessed at higher risk for this reason and should trigger an even more detailed and thorough assessment than usual.

Because Mr. Larson died from an undiagnosed condition does not mean that the physicians are automatically liable for the death. Aortic dissection is an extremely rare condition, which places it further down the differential. Though the first physician also missed the diagnosis, that physician may have less exposure at trial since the second physician should have been able to build upon the initial failed diagnosis and continued symptomatology of the patient. The second ED physician had the "last clear chance" to arrive at the correct diagnosis and commence treatment at a time that likely would have saved the patient's life.

Authors: *What factors play into the decision to settle or go to trial?*
GR: A settlement is arrived at by looking at the following considerations:

- What are the chances of a defense verdict?
- Is this case defensible on the standard of care or proximate cause?
- If there is a plaintiff's verdict, what is the likely and maximum monetary exposure?
- What medical expenses were incurred by the plaintiff?
- What are the lost wages or lost earning capacity of the patient?
- What are the non-economic damages to the plaintiff, i.e., pain and suffering, emotional distress, mental anguish?

Other less predictable factors include:

- The venue where the case will be tried
- Whether the jurors are generally considered to be conservative or liberal
- Are there aggravating circumstances in the underlying case, such as gross negligence on the part of the defendant or an attempt to modify or dispose of records?
- Will there likely be adverse publicity surrounding this case?
- Are there significant sympathy factors favoring the plaintiff, such as the death of children?

Authors: *Would you have settled this case or gone to trial?*
GR: I would have attempted to settle this case for a reasonable sum. However, the plaintiff's demand of $250 million is far beyond the scope of potential jury verdict range. It appears that the plaintiffs were more focused on extracting a "pound of flesh," rather than a reasonable settlement figure. Sometimes we are forced to try cases that are going to lose because the plaintiffs are unwilling to accept a reasonable sum as a settlement.

Authors: *When a case is settled, is the doctor still entered in the National Practitioner Data Bank?*
GR: All cases which are settled on behalf of the physician are reported to the National Practitioner Databank regardless of the amount. The physician does have the opportunity to submit his own statement explaining the circumstances under which the case was resolved. Cases are typically subject to a confidentiality clause so as to prohibit either side from discussing the terms of the settlement publicly. This is done to encourage settlement and to prevent situations where a settlement will be used to cause embarrassment or harassment to a physician.

➤**Authors' note:** This settlement was also subject to a confidentility clause; we spoke with the Larson family attorny who was helpful and supportive, but would not reveal specifics of the settlement.

X. Diagnosis and Management of Aortic Dissection

Guest author: Rob Rogers, MD FACEP, FAAEM, FACP

Associate Professor of Emergency Medicine
Department of Emergency Medicine, The University of Maryland School of Medicine
Director of Undergraduate Medical Education
Baltimore, Maryland

Presentation of Aortic Dissection

The classic presentation of aortic dissection entails an elderly patient with acute onset and "tearing" or "ripping" chest pain that radiates to the interscapular area. This is fine for those of us studying for the recertification boards in emergency medicine, but what about the patients we see day in and day out? How do these patients really present? Luckily, there are quite a few patients with a classic presentation which lends itself to a speedy diagnosis, but what about the rest? The central issue is that acute aortic dissection can present in many different ways, many subtle and atypical.

Much of what I know about the varied presentations comes from my medicolegal work, both for the defense and plaintiff. One of the most interesting aspects of acute aortic dissection is that some patients present with signs and symptoms that are not ascribable to the disease, often presenting in cardiac arrest. The clinical bottom line is this: Chest pain that radiates to the back or abdomen should in many cases be worked-up to exclude this lethal disease.

What about Jonathan's case? Why the disease was never considered.

You can speculate about why the diagnosis was missed in Jonathan's case, but I'll share with you some of my thoughts. First, he was young. For some odd reason many clinicians assume that young patients can't be sick. The second reason relates to a phenomenon that we see all too often in emergency medicine: labeling patients with diagnoses that don't fit the clinical picture. How does food poisoning explain chest and abdominal pain? Jonathan reportedly had no nausea, vomiting, or diarrhea. When is the last time you saw a patient with "food poisoning" without these symptoms?

Red flags on Jonathan's first and second visits

The plaintiff's attorney's strategy is based on knowing the final diagnosis and looking backwards to pluck out potential red flags. It's not that easy moving forward with a patient in the ED. We don't have a definitive diagnosis, but we have the responsibility to formulate a differential diagnosis and come up with a preliminary diagnosis. One red flag in Jonathan's care was unexplained chest and abdominal pain. I have studied Jonathan's case for years, and I still cannot definitively say that the EP should have made the diagnosis. Perhaps if someone had put together the chest and abdominal pain—but that is a stretch. Also, consider the pleuritic nature of the chest pain on the initial visit. At that time, a ventilation-perfusion scan would have been the diagnostic test of choice to exclude pulmonary embolism, and if done, would not have diagnosed the dissection. Today, he would have had a CT scan to evaluate for PE which would likely have diagnosed the acute aortic tear by shear luck. That has happened to me a few times …

The other red flag, and one of the biggest, is that he "bounced back" to the emergency department. Patients who come back with the same complaint or have any deterioration in their status are giving us a "second chance." Jonathan came back for a second ED visit with severe chest pain and was diagnosed with a viral syndrome. If you really think about it, how many patients have you seen with a viral syndrome who complain of severe chest pain? Was this an opportunity to explore other diagnoses? Probably.

How often is CXR normal (as it was with Jonathan)?

A study by von Kodolitsch showed that the chest X-ray is approximately 67% sensitive for diagnosis and is insensitive in excluding the disease.[5] If this is your strategy, I suggest changing it. I have personally seen at least five cases of acute aortic dissection where the initial chest X-ray was completely normal.

How do we diagnose aortic dissection without irradiating everyone?

It is my opinion that you in fact cannot exclude the disease without a CT scan. Several years ago I was a believer that d-dimer was going to be the test that would allow us to exclude the disease, but the d-dimer literature is not that good.[6-9] The sensitivity has a wide range, but is not adequate to exclude this life-threatening process. Bottom line: You can't rule out the disease without a CT scan. Of course, taking a detailed history on chest pain patients aids us in risk stratifying who needs the CT in the first place.

Pearls

- Emergency physicians should always attempt to explain a patient's symptoms; if the diagnosis does not fit, then consider additional history or further diagnostic studies.
- A very common element in missed aortic dissection malpractice lawsuits is combined symptoms "above and below the diaphragm" (e.g., chest and abdominal pain, chest and severe leg pain, chest and back pain).
- A good risk management strategy is to ensure your chart reflects consideration of dissection by documenting equal pulses and absence of a diastolic murmur, or recording a progress note.
- Chest pain and neurologic symptoms should lower your threshold to rule out aortic dissection.

The Bottom Line

Acute aortic dissection isn't that common, and it can be impossible to diagnose even under the best of circumstances. My answer is simply to be thorough in the evaluation of patients with chest pain, considering the possible life-threatening possibilities no matter the age of the patient. Ensuring the chart reflects the medical decision-making process will go a long way in protecting the physician in court.

XI. Authors' Summary

Mr. Larson had pain described by friends as severe, with associated shortness of breath and two near-syncopal episodes. In retrospect, in a patient with probable Marfan's syndrome, these symptoms fit neatly into a picture of aortic dissection. But it is easy to see how this unusual diagnosis could have been missed, especially if it wasn't in the physician's differential.

Like many of our patients, Jonathan Larson did not want to have a serious diagnosis, telling the first physician about a bad turkey sandwich and the second that he thought he had heartburn. Both physicians were led astray. But both missed opportunities to make the diagnosis, including reading the nurses' and paramedics' notes, getting additional history from his friends in the ED, reassessing Jonathan after he deteriorated during his initial ED visit with a near syncopal episode, and having time and action-specific follow-up in a patient who is discharged with diagnostic uncertainty.

The second visit was more troubling because he was now a bounceback patient, putting him at higher risk of having a serious underlying problem. Jonathan also had another serious risk for misdiagnosis: a previous diagnosis. His tachycardia was not recognized or reassessed. His CXR was possibly misread, and over-reliance was certainly placed on testing above clinical findings. The ECG was abnormal with an unrecorded impression.

Jonathan's father, Allan Larson, summed up the feelings of any parent who survives his child: "Parents should never have to cry for their lost children."

Thanks to:

- Allan Larson, Jonathan's father, who supported this work and clarified details of Jonathan's life during the course of several telephone calls
- Jonathan Martin, Director of Education at the National Marfan Foundation
- Sora Newman, from National Public Radio, for focusing the commentary
- The State of New York Department of Health

References

1. Singer AJ, Richman PB, Kowalska A, et al. Comparison of patient and practitioner assessments of pain from commonly performed emergency department procedures. Annals Emerg Med 1999;33:652-8.
2. Croskerry P. Achieving quality in clinical decision making: Cognitive strategies and detection of Bias. Acad Emerg Med 2002; 9:1184-204.
3. Martin-Gill C, Reiser RC. Risk factors for 72-hour admission to the ED. Am J Emerg Med 2004;22:448-53.

4. Sklar DP, Crandall CS, Loeliger E, et al. Unanticipated death after discharge home from the emergency department. Annals Emerg Med 2007;49:735-45.
5. Kodolitsch Y, Nienaber CA, Dieckmann C, et al. Chest radiography for the diagnosis of acute aortic syndrome. Am J Med 2004;116:73-7.
6. Sutherland A, Escano J, Coon TP, D-dimer as the sole screening test for acute aortic dissection: a review of the literature. Ann Emerg Med 2008;52:339-43.
7. Sodeck G, Domanovits H, Schillinger M, et al. D-dimer in ruling out acuteaortic dissection: a systematic review and prospective cohort study. Eur Heart J 2007;28:3067-75.
8. Sbarouni, E., Georgiadou P, Marathias A, et al. D-dimer and BNP levels ih acute aortic dissection. Internat J Cardiol 2007;122:170-2.
9. Ohlmann P, Faure A, Morel O, et al. Diagnostic and prognostic value of circulating d-dimers in patients with acute aortic dissection. Crit Care Med 2006;34:1358-64.

Additional reading

- Elefteriades JA, Barrett PW, Kopf GS, et al. Litigation in nontraumatic aortic diseases: a tempest in the malpractice maelstrom. Cardiology 2008; 109:263.
- Juang D, Braverman AC, Eagle K. Aortic dissection. Circulation 2008; 118:e507-e510.

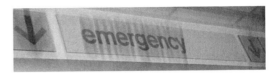

CASE 5

A 38 YEAR-OLD WOMAN WITH ABDOMINAL PAIN: CT OUT OF PROPORTION TO EXAMINATION

Primary case author Kevin Klauer

PART 1—MEDICAL

   I. The Patient's Story 123

   II. The Doctor's Version (the ED Chart) 123

   III. The Errors—Risk Management/Patient Safety Issues 125

   IV. The Bounceback 127

   V. The Outpatient Visit 128

   VI. The Third Visit 128

   VII. The Final Diagnoses 129

PART 2—LEGAL

   I. The Accusation/Cause of Action 129

   II. The Depositions 129

   III. What Would Greg Do (WWGD)? 130

   IV. The Outcome—Settlement vs. Trial? 131

   V. Guest Interview—Gillian Schmitz, MD 132

   VI. Medical Discussion—Peter Rosen, MD (Interview) 135

   VII. Legal Analysis—Karl Schedler, JD 137

   VIII. Authors' Summary 139

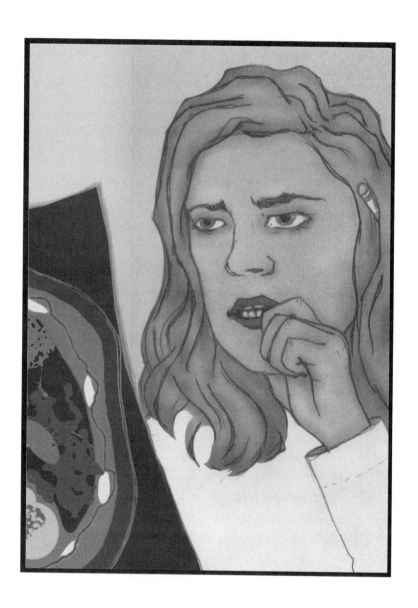

A 38 YEAR-OLD WOMAN WITH ABDOMINAL PAIN: *CT OUT OF PROPORTION TO EXAMINATION*

Abdominal pain is a complex diagnosis with many potential etiologies, some serious and many not. Per the Centers of Disease Control, September 8, 2010, abdominal pain presentations have increased by 31.8% over the last eight years, equating to almost two million more visits per year (seems most come to my ED at 3 AM). The use of advanced imaging has increased from 19.9% to nearly half of such cases. Along with more involved evaluations comes greater complexity in interpretation of the diagnostics, specifically evaluation of the "incidentaloma." What is the next step when you don't believe the CT result?

Deep thoughts:

1. When can patients with undifferentiated abdominal pain be safely discharged?
2. When should a surgical consultation be obtained?
3. Are there times when the diagnostic test is more reliable than the history and physical examination?
4. When is scheduled ED re-evaluation appropriate?

PART 1—MEDICAL

I. The Patient's Story

Kelli Collins is a married 38 year-old woman. She is an illegal immigrant, but she has been in the country long enough that she does not even have an accent; her English is perfect.

Several days after a steamy Southern July Fourth, she begins to experience abdominal pain. It initially comes and goes, but on Saturday, July 15, she awakens at 4 AM with upper abdominal pain severe enough that it causes her to vomit. Just after noon, Kelli finds herself at the triage desk of University Hospital.

II. The Doctor's Version (the following is the actual documentation of the provider)

Date: Saturday, July 15, 2007
Chief complaint: Abdominal pain and vomiting
Nurse's note (12:40): The pain comes and goes for one week, and she started vomiting this morning. No fever. Pain scale 10/10.

HISTORY OF PRESENT ILLNESS: This [pain] started 1 week ago and is still present. It is described as epigastric and sharp and radiating to the back. At its maximum, severity described as severe. Modifying factors-Not worsened or relieved by anything. The patient has had nausea and vomiting with 6 episodes of non-bloody emesis. No loss of appetite or diarrhea. Pain initially came and went. At 0400 am pain was constant. Pain is sharp. Last BM was today. She has flatus. No fevers, dysuria or hematuria. She states this feels like her gall bladder pain but she already had her gall bladder removed. No chest pain, problems breathing or cough. No black stools, hematemesis, difficulty or pain with urination. No urinary frequency, bloody stools, fever, headache or chest pain. All systems otherwise negative, except as recorded above.

PAST MEDICAL HISTORY:
Allergies: Tylenol
PMH: GERD, NIDDM
PSH: Cholecystectomy
Meds: Metformin and Prevacid
Social history: No alcohol or tobacco use
FH: Negative

EXAM:

VITAL SIGNS								
Time	Temp(F)	Rt.	Pulse	Resp	Syst	Diast	Pos.	O2 sat RA
12:40	98.0	O	90	18	155	103	U	N/A

RESIDENT'S ASSESSMENT WITH ATTENDING SUPERVISION:
APPEARANCE: Alert. Oriented X3. No acute distress.
EYES: Pupils equal, round and reactive to light.
CVS: Normal heart rate and rhythm. Heart sounds normal. Pulses normal.
RESPIRATORY: No respiratory distress. Breath sounds normal.
ABDOMEN: Scar present. Tenderness in the epigastric area. Abdomen soft.
BACK: Normal inspection. No CVA tenderness.
RECTAL: Rectal exam normal. Rectal exam nontender. Stool heme negative.
NEURO: Oriented X 3. No motor deficit. No sensory deficit. Reflexes normal.

ED COURSE:
LABS: CBC is normal except as noted, WBC 15. Chemistries: Normal; Total bilirubin normal; AST normal; ALT normal; Alkaline phosphatase normal. Lipase normal; Urinalysis normal. Urine pregnancy negative.

14:18 – Nursing reassessment: Pain 10/10
14:57 – Morphine 4mg; Phenergan, 12.5mg IVP
16:38 – Nursing reassessment: Pain 5/10. No nausea or vomiting
18:13 – Care transferred from resident #1 to resident #2 at shift change. Progress note from resident #1: Differential concerning for possible retained stone or possible intraabdominal abscess s/p cholecystectomy vs gastritis or abdominal pain NOS.

19:27 – Physician reassessment: Patient stable but experiencing more pain. She is drinking contrast
19:36 – Fentanyl 100mcg IV
21:11 – Nursing reassessment: Pain 2/10

Abdominal CT (preliminary report): "Normal liver, pancreas, adrenals and kidneys. Appendix normal. spleen with heterogeneous perfusion (possible infarct), diverticuli without diverticulitis, filling defect in abdominal aorta." The abdominal CT was independently viewed by me and discussed with the radiologist.

Progress note (resident #2): "Plan to reassess and follow up on CT results. Initial verbal dictation of CT was questionable splenic infarct and aortic defect of unknown acuity. When discussed with the Radiologist over the phone, possible heterogeneity due to contrast filling and timing of contrast dye. Correlate clinically. Patient well appearing on my exam. Patient had no tenderness and was tolerating PO without difficulty. Clinical significance and acuity of preliminary abdominal CT report finding unclear given clinical exam and improving course. Young Age without risk factors for thromboembolic disease.

22:43: Nursing reassessment: Pain 5/10; Fentanyl 100 mcg IV
23:48: Physician reassessment: Patient is stable; CT is negative; Belly soft and non-tender; She is tolerating P.O.

DIAGNOSIS: Abdominal pain of unknown cause

PLAN: Discharge home with 12 hour recheck in ER and follow up with vascular clinic to further evaluate. Patient instructed to return sooner if symptoms worsen.

Don Chowning, MD
Gillian Schmitz, MD

III. The Errors—Risk Management/Patient Safety Issues

➤**Authors' note:** This physician was not fooled by a quirky patient. She was not too busy to adequately evaluate the patient and incorporate diagnostic information. She is a well-trained doctor, at the time a resident at one of the top EM residencies in the country. She looked at the whole picture … one which didn't make sense within the symptomatic presentation of the patient, and she arrived at a plan in the best interest of the patient. This is how medicine is supposed to be practiced—primary consideration of the long-term interests of the patient and not the short-term legal fears of the physician.

Is there a legal risk when the unusual diagnosis *is* actually occurring? What happens when the consultant makes a decision which turns out to be incorrect? How much responsibility for follow-up care rests with the patient?

The astute reader can guess that this diagnosis did not turn out to be gastritis, since it is included in this book of "very bad outcomes." In the course of our normal ED shifts, we often are confronted with unexpected findings. The safest approach is to admit *everyone* and cover our butts, but there is a problem with that approach; we have a MD/DO behind our names and took an oath to advocate for the patient. Please read the risk management points below with this in mind.

Risk management/patient safety issue #1:

Error: Disbelief of CT findings.

Discussion: Abnormal test results must be addressed during the emergency department encounter. In low-risk entities (i.e., minimally elevated SGOT in a patient with abdominal pain, questionable non-displaced, lateral maleolar fracture in a splinted patient, a potassium of 3.2 incidentally noted in a patient with cellulitis), the decision to defer resolution of the abnormality to an outpatient referral/evaluation is appropriate. Is the risk increased in these clinical scenarios? Not likely.

However, in high-risk entities (i.e., negative grey zone troponin in a patient with chest pain, a WBC count of 20,000 in a patient with abdominal pain or even a patient with persistent, unexplained abdominal tenderness despite adequate analgesics), the issue at hand must be resolved prior to discharge, since these items are both time-sensitive and likely to result in disastrous outcomes if serious pathology is actually present. Neither the provider nor the patient can afford a missed appendicitis or missed myocardial infarction. Mesenteric ischemia is one of those high-risk, time-sensitive diagnoses.

✔ **Teaching point:** Abnormal findings must be disproved prior to discharge.

Risk management/patient safety issue #2:

Error: Reliance on improved symptomatology.

Discussion: A skill acquired with experience is being able to differentiate when H&P is helpful and when a test is necessary. Certain entities such as evaluation of abdominal pain or bleeding in pregnancy can not be adequately distinguished with bedside exam alone.[1] Sometimes symptom relief may be helpful (the two year-old running around and playing after Acetaminophen), but other times it is misleading (pain relief with headaches associated with subarachnoid hemorrhage). In fact, in relation to headache, ACEP specifically states that response to therapy should not be used as a diagnostic criteria.[2]

The treatment of abdominal pain should be approached with the same perspective; when symptom relief occurs after appropriate analgesics, cautious optimism is appropriate. However, if the patient required extensive analgesics or has intractable pain, this may indicate a surgical entity is occurring.

In this case, the patient was observed for an extended period of time, approximately 11 hours. Her pain improved with narcotic analgesics, but it did recur. Conservatively, one must consider the possibility that the etiology of her pain may not be benign. In combination with the concerning CT findings, her pattern of pain should be viewed with greater scrutiny than if her pain was the only positive finding in her evaluation.

✔ **Teaching point:** If the patient has intractable or recurrent symptoms, concern for significant pathology should be heightened.

Risk management/patient safety issue #3:

Error: Lack of surgical consultation.

Discussion: This issue reflects back to the first, dismissal of the CT findings. As stated previously, if the diagnosis being considered is time-sensitive, life-threatening or both, the question at hand must be resolved prior to discharge. If this cannot be accomplished, then admission is indicated. In this particular case, the diagnosis in question is surgical and a consultation is reasonable. Although consultation doesn't entirely insulate the emergency physician from liability, it will certainly help.

✔ **Teaching point:** Don't hesitate to ask for help when needed.

Risk management/patient safety issue #4:

Error: Decision to discharge.

Discussion: Coupled with the decision to obtain consultation is the decision to discharge. In this case, the physician employed an excellent risk management tool, 12-hour scheduled ED follow-up. Re-evaluation of RLQ pain with scheduled ED return in 8–12 hours is appropriate. In contrast, such a time frame may not be acceptable for an imminently life-threatening condition, such as abdominal aortic aneurysm (AAA).

✔ **Teaching point:** If such a high-risk, time-sensitive diagnosis cannot be reasonably excluded, admit or consult.

IV. The Bounceback

Sunday July 16, 2007
  14:28: The patient returns as instructed, and is triaged soon at 14:39.
Chief complaint: Abdominal pain

HISTORY OF PRESENT ILLNESS (resident): This started yesterday and is still present but is improving. Pt had 10/10 pain yesterday with N/V-today, pain has improved and pt reports 3/10 pain and is eating well today. No fever/chills. Reviewed workup from yesterday. It is located in the epigastric area and left upper quadrant. No nausea, loss of appetite, vomiting or diarrhea. No constipation, black stools, hematemesis, fever or chills. All systems otherwise negative, except as recorded above.

EXAM: Vital signs: BP: 142/110, HR: 97, RR: 20, Temp: 37.5 oral
Normal except: Abdomen: Mild tenderness in the epigastric area and left upper quadrant. Abdomen soft. No guarding or rebound tenderness.

DIAGNOSTICS: WBC: 13.0, basic metabolic profile (BMP): normal
PROGRESS NOTE: Reviewed CT report from last night and filling defect of questionable acuity. Benign clinical exam. Plan to dc home with strict return precautions and follow-up as outpatient.

Attending Note: I supervised care provided by the resident. We have discussed the case. I have reviewed the note and agree with the plan of treatment. I personally interviewed the patient and examined the patient. She was here yesterday with abd pain, neg ct, returns for recheck. Pain still present but improved, no longer vomiting. Pain is in the epigastrium and luq. She has some tenderness in the luq without peritoneal signs. review of ct showed ? splenic infarct, ? acutity. Has flu PHS this wk or return here sooner if worse.

Treatment: Percocet

Disposition: Discharge and maintain previously scheduled appointments. D/C home with husband as driver

V. Outpatient Appointment: Vascular Surgery Clinic—Friday, July 21, 2006

(6 days after initial ED visit). Note: Pt. seen by attending vascular surgeon board certified in general surgery and vascular surgery.

- HPI: Patient was referred for a three-week history of left upper quadrant pain. The patient was treated in emergency room initially with some pain medicine and eventual workup discovered a thrombus at the origin of the celiac artery and splenic infarction. The patient states over the past 3 weeks, her pain has gotten better. She is able to eat without problems. Her pain has significantly reduced. The patient otherwise has no other significant past medical history.
- CT from 7/15/06 (initial CT – official radiology reading): *"The patient's CT scan shows extensive splenic infarct and thrombus at the origin of the celiac-artery with maintaining peripheral flow in the hepatic regions."*
- It is recommended that she get additional blood work today and an echocardiogram, but she refuses to stay for this work-up.
- Plan: Given that she continues to be asymptomatic and with her benign clinical exam, immediate anticoagulation is not initiated. The patient is to follow up with Vascular Surgery and Hematology for potential etiologies.

➤**Authors' note:** The patient does not make appointments for the rest of the tests.

VI. The Third ED Visit

At 1:30 PM on Thursday, August 17, five weeks after her initial ED visit, Kelly calls her husband at work to "check in;" she is fine. Half an hour later she develops a sudden onset of excruciating abdominal pain. She is in severe distress. She is driven back to the ED and arrives at 15:42.

Unscheduled ED Visit—8/17/06 (5 weeks after initial ED visit)
- History: "It is described as sharp and well localized. Quality not described as burning, dull or migrating and it is described as located in the epigastric area and in the upper abdomen. No radiation. At its maximum, severity described as severe and 10/10. When seen in the E.D. severity described as severe and 10/10. No black stools."
- Physical Examination (shortened):
  o Abdomen: Severe upper abdominal tenderness with rebound tenderness.
  o Rectal examination: Occult blood negative.
- Labs: WBC: 17.5 Hb 8.3, platelets 905

- CT scan: Occluded superior mesenteric artery
- **ED diagnosis:** Acute mesenteric ischemia. Occlusion of superior mesenteric artery.
- Disposition: Admission to surgery

Operative course:
- Taken to surgery for emergent thrombectomy of the SMA.
- The following day required a bowel resection from the ligament of Treitz up to and including a right hemicolectomy.

Hospital course:
- The patient developed short bowel syndrome and required long-term TPN.
- Hematology-oncology consult to evaluate for hypercoagulable state: This entire workup was negative with no source of thrombus identified.
- There is a difficulty arranging home TPN therapy, due to financial reasons

VII. FINAL DIAGNOSES (December 26, 2007)—Four months after admission for SMA occlusion:

1. Mesenteric ischemia
2. Acute thrombosis of superior mesenteric artery
3. Splenic infarct
4. Short gut syndrome, prolonged nausea and vomiting

PART 2—LEGAL

I. The Accusation/Cause of Action

- Misdiagnosis of SMA clot and splenic infarct
- Failure to admit the patient for further treatment and evaluation
- Multiple defendants are named

II. The Depostions

A. *Plaintiff:* The expert witness for the plaintiff was an emergency physician. Analysis:
- He stated the CT findings were consistent with possible splenic infarct.
- He was critical of the discharge disposition.
- A surgical consultation should have been obtained, and he thought the surgeon would have recommended systemic anticoagulation.

B. *Defense:* The defense expert, also an emergency physician, reported that the care provided was appropriate and did not fall below the standard of care.
- The patient's symptoms were consistent with splenic infarct. However, he curiously concluded that even with the finding noted on CT, it was reasonable to consider another etiology for her symptoms due to her young age and lack of risk factors.
- He would not have admitted the patient or anticoagulated her. There was no occlusion present upon presentation and evaluation at the second ED visit or at the vascular surgery clinic appointment.
- The time interval between the second ED visit and the vascular surgery follow-up visit was reasonable.

III. What Would Greg Do (WWGD)?

Greg Henry, past president of The American College of Emergency Physicians (ACEP), Professor of Emergency Medicine at the University of Michigan, and CEO of Medical Practice Risk Assessment, has been an expert witness in over 2,000 malpractice cases.

Greg discusses evaluation of abdominal pain and legal strategy.

"If you ask a patient who is improving if they'd like surgery, the answer is generally no"

This case is trouble from the beginning. Whenever you have a veritable cast of defendants, one can always turn against the other. Casual comments placing blame can be the kiss of death. Abdominal pain in a 38 year-old woman is usually not an immediate life-threatening problem. Problems with circulation in the abdomen and ruptured viscus are usually seen in considerably older patients and are rarely subtle for long.

The warning is often given that one should not be dissuaded by improvement—but how else are we to function? To the average emergency physician, improvement is a good thing; it's hard to improve on a patient who no longer has pain. I was taught early on in my career that I should not interfere with patients who are getting better. One can always find cases to the contrary, but I would positively bet on the horse that's ahead.

The strategy for the defense in this case needs to be improvement, improvement, improvement. If you ask a patient who is improving if they'd like surgery, the answer is generally "no". The entire essence of this case is in the follow-up. Patients should not be sent out into the wilderness, but told that if they have a return of pain or they are not completely well in eight hours, they should return to the Emergency Department, as was well done in this case.

Is this case defensible—well, defensible on whose part? The first doctor, the second doctor or the time it took to get her to surgery? The greatest problem in presenting a defense is that the jury is not into nuances. They don't care who actually caused the problem since it is much easier to paint with a broad brush. They just tend to find the entire crowd guilty of something which they find objectionable.

Faced with multitudes of defendants and the difficulty in understanding who is at fault, settlement may not be inappropriate. Settlement does not constitute an admission of guilt but simply says "we aren't going to talk about this anymore." The settlement is a way of resolving a civil dispute in a civil manner. The emergency physician who's involved in the case should never be involved in the decision to settle.

In the best of circumstances, I have seen juries come back with absolutely unpredictable results. A settlement is not an unreasonable approach to this matter.

IV. The Outcome—Settlement or Trial?

➤**Authors' note:** Well, chalk another one up for Greg Henry. After 2,000 legal cases you get good at this! As with almost all of these cases, he was blinded to the outcome of whether the case settled or went to trial, but he hit the nail on the head.

This case ultimately settled at mediation for a large amount, which would allow for life-long TPA. *None of the amount was attributed to the initial ED physician.* Per prior arrangement with the hospital and risk management department, we are unable to disclose the exact amount (but did you ever price TPN at Kroger?).

> **Basis of settlement:** "Even if [the initial ED physician's] decisions with respect to the patient's management were less than ideal, the patient was seen by other health care providers and, more importantly, by the appropriate surgical consult within a week of her ED visit, which eliminates a causal connection between [the initial ED physician's] care and the patient's outcome."

➤**Authors' note:** Due to the economic assessment of this patient's ongoing medical care needs (e.g., TPN for the remainder of her life), it is very reasonable to expect that the defendants would receive an excess limits judgment at trial. This is a jury decision for the plaintiff that includes damages exceeding the monetary limits of the policy. Thus, the parties (the doctor(s) and/or hospital), and not their insurance companies, would be liable for the damages awarded that are in excess of the policy limits. Most policies are $1,000,000 per occurrence. In many cases, excess limits judgments will be negotiated down to policy limits to ensure a more immediate payment and resolution. Surprisingly, the plaintiff will often initiate these negotiations.

In this case, the defendants are at substantial risk since this patient would invoke sympathy from the jury and would clearly have exhaustive medical expenses for the duration of her life. This type of assessment and reasoning leads defense counsel to entertain mediation. While legal counsel prepares their defense and tries their case, their expenses quickly add up to six figures, providing additional reasons to consider mediation.

The necessary elements for any negligence tort claim are:

- Duty to act
- Breach of that duty
- Causation and damages

For the purposes of this case, we'll focus on standard of care and causation (but all are discussed in detail in the final section of this book, "Help! I am being sued").

The *standard of care* is the minimum duty owed to the plaintiff. In medical negligence, the standard of care is what a reasonable physician with similar training in similar circumstances would do. This concept becomes critical to this case when we examine the defense expert's deposition testimony. He stated that he would not have admitted the patient or provided systemic anticoagulation, but this statement does not address the question at hand, which is whether or not a reasonable physician with similar training and in a similar situation, would have admitted the patient. This would be up to a jury to decide. The plaintiff would likely try to discredit the witness on this point in attempting to weaken the defense's case.

There are two necessary elements of *causation*: direct or actual cause and proximate cause.

1. **Direct causation** means that the alleged negligence must be the *direct cause* of the plaintiff's injury or damages.
2. Beyond direct cause, the alleged negligence must also be the **proximate cause** of the patient's injury or damages. In order to meet the element of proximate cause, there can be no superseding or intervening events that relieve the defendant of liability. In other words, if some other unrelated event is deemed to have caused the injury or damages, thus breaking the chain of causation between the alleged negligent act and the injury or damages, there is no proximate cause.

In this case, there are proximate cause issues that would likely be the primary defense strategy for the emergency physicians on both visits one and two. Whether it is deemed luck or not, the fact remains that the patient did not suffer a bad outcome until others, primarily the vascular surgeons, had a chance to intervene. Thus, the alleged negligence of the vascular surgeons may be considered a superseding or intervening event that breaks the chain of causation between the emergency physicians and this patient's injuries. Although this is a viable defense, in most cases in which multiple medical providers commit similar negligence, they will all be found negligent, notwithstanding the possible lack of proof of proximate cause of a defendant.

Depending on the jurisdiction, the doctrine of comparative negligence may be used to apportion the judgment to the defendants, based upon the degree of liability the jury assigns to each.

V. Guest Interview: Gillian Schmitz, MD

- Emergency Medicine Faculty, Georgetown University/Washington University
- 2010 AWAEM Early Career Faculty Award from the Academy for Women in Academic Emergency Medicine
- Gillian is currently ED attending, but actually saw this patient when still an EM resident

Authors: *What is your memory of the case?*
GS: I assumed care of this patient from another ED resident during sign out [Gillian was resident #2]. He was concerned for possible retained stone after her cholecystectomy. Her labs were essentially unremarkable, she was afebrile, he was underwhelmed by her

exam and anticipated her going home. Her belly was soft and non-tender on my exam, and she was comfortable resting when I evaluated her.

Authors: *What was your thought process at the time? Did you consider admission?*
GS: No, I did not consider admission. I never saw the patient in any distress. Although I noted that she subjectively stated she had pain, my exam of her abdomen was benign and she was resting comfortably from the time I assumed care.

The first mistake I made was a knowledge deficit—not equating the term "filling defect" with acute mesenteric ischemia. The fact that there was flow distally led me to incorrectly believe that the filling defect was a result of the way the contrast was administered and was incidental and not related to her diagnosis. If the preliminary read had indicated that this finding was concerning for acute mesenteric ischemia, I think I would have acted differently. There was, of course, some mention of possible infarct on the preliminary CT read.

My second mistake was not expanding my differential diagnosis. I was focused in on the differential and plan from the team who initially evaluated her and was looking for a retained stone or abscess. When I did not see those things, I minimized the other findings that were staring me in the face. My understanding of mesenteric ischemia at the time was that it was a disease of elderly patients … in atrial fibrillation … with pain out of proportion to exam. Here was a young healthy female with a benign belly and pain relieved with a couple doses of narcotics. She was in the ED for 11 hours and was improving, and she wanted to go home.

Because there was some abnormality on the CT read and a final read would be available in the morning, it seemed reasonable to me to discharge her with 12-hour recheck.

Authors: *What would you do differently with a similar case in the future? How has this ordeal affected your practice?*
GS: I'll admit that after this case, part of me wanted to get a CT scan on every 20 to 30 year-old with abdominal pain on the off chance they had acute mesenteric ischemia. Of course, we all know that this is not good medicine and a terrible waste of resources, not to mention radiation exposure … but this case made me question my own clinical judgment and exam skills. I learned with time that clinical gestalt is accurate most of the time, but that I have to pay attention to abnormal findings, even if they are unexpected or incidental, and adequately address them.

If I had this to "do-over," I would have obtained a surgical and vascular consult on her initial ED visit and had them document on the chart to support the disposition and management decision. I would have also impressed upon the patient the serious findings and implications of her CT scan and the importance of follow-up. If the consulting team had decided, however, to work her up as an outpatient (as they decided when they saw her six days later), I would still consider discharging her from the ED if she was pain free, tolerating PO and had close outpatient follow-up.

Authors: *What were your thoughts when you first heard about the outcome?*

GS: My first reaction was probably denial … no way could I miss such an important diagnosis; there must be some mistake somewhere. This quickly turned into guilt, fear, and apprehension. Did I hurt someone and was this entirely my fault because I discharged her? There was also some component of anger that the patient refused further diagnostic testing and follow-up after seeing both her primary medical doctor and vascular. Shouldn't she take some responsibility for her own health?

I was informed that the patient was an illegal immigrant and an attorney had told her that she would be eligible for damages and to stay in the U.S. if she filed a suit, which was enraging. I was aware that a claim would likely be made and all the physicians who saw her, including residents, would be named. I was terrified about how this would affect my future and did not know if I needed to find my own attorney. Nothing in my residency had taught me how to handle the stress of litigation, what resources were available and what the process would be. [Gillian discusses her "ordeal" at length in the October 2009 issue of *Risk Management Monthly*.] The process of case review and settlement took over two years. I felt I had very little input and was kept in the dark most of the time. I found out after the fact that the case was settled, though I never consented to that. I felt very alone and intimidated throughout the process as I was not allowed to talk to anyone about it. It affected my sleep, my confidence, my family and my well-being.

I have tried to use this experience to help others to learn from my mistakes. I have improved my documentation and medical decision-making and encourage my residents to do the same. I have given some lectures on risk management and warn residents that they are unfortunately not immune to lawsuits. I try not to let lawyers change the way I practice, but I do make a concerted effort to address any abnormalities I find both to the patient and in my documentation.

I serve on our practice committee and review charts at our hospital to help look for better ways to protect our patients and physicians from bad outcomes. I have learned, however, that bad outcomes are an inevitable part of what we do; it does not mean that you are a bad clinician. I have slept much better knowing how many patients I have helped. Although no one can be perfect, there are strategies to minimize risk, and those have helped in my daily practice.

Authors: *Other thoughts?*
GS: As a physician who has practiced in both an academic and community hospital setting, I now often have the responsibility of overseeing residents or physician assistants. Although they often document on the chart, I realize that ultimately I am responsible for reviewing their documentation and evaluating the patient myself. This can be challenging in a busy department when I am overseeing many learners at one time.

I don't know that the outcome of this particular case would have changed if the ED attending had reviewed the preliminary CT result, and I take responsibility if I did not adequately communicate my decision-making. It is inherent to trust people we work with, but it is another opportunity to catch near misses to have a second person review the data. I think it is important for attendings to try and review the labs and imaging results themselves, when possible, to try and reduce any potential errors made by those still learning.

VI. Guest Interview: Peter Rosen, MD

- Father of Emergency Medicine
- Senior Lecturer, Medicine, Harvard University School of Medicine
- Attending, Emergency Medicine Beth Israel/ Deaconess Medical Center
- Founding editor of *Rosen's Emergency Medicine: Concepts and Clinical Practice*

Dr. Rosen's original comments:

Dear Gentlemen,

Reading the case, my problem is that this is such a rarity that there can be no standard of care to deviate from. I have seen in 51 years, only one patient with spontaneous SMA thrombosis, and it wasn't really spontaneous. He was a cyclist who rode many hundred miles per week; and the flexed cyclist position caused the thrombosis. Trying to outguess the argument the plaintiff attorney will use to obtain financial compensation is an exercise in futility. I think the attorney is correct that the case is completely defensible, but there still might be a plaintiff verdict.

Yours truly,

Peter

Peter Rosen, MD

We wouldn't let Dr. Rosen off the hook with such brief comments, so he was called for some follow-up questions:

- Would he have sent this patient home?
- Would he have settled?
- On a personal note, has he ever been sued?

Authors: *You said previously that there can be no standard of care for such a rare presentation. Rubber meets the road: The resident checks out the patient to you, what do you recommend doing next?*
PR: I would have called the radiologist and asked for an explanation for what he thought the CT showed. I would need to know if the findings are firm or merely a consideration. If it is just a shadow, I would send the patient home. Additionally, consideration should be given to specialty consultation.

Authors: Did the treating resident deviate from the "standard of care?"
PR: When you are dealing with a unicorn, you don't know how to tame it. To try to hold someone to a standard of care when one doesn't exist ... it's something that the legal system does, but it makes no logical sense medically. That's what makes this defensible of course and juries understand that. If no one has ever seen one before, there can't be a standard.

Authors: *The vascular service asked her to get further testing, but she didn't follow-up. How much responsibility do patients assume for their own medical care?*
PR: Most patients will do what they are told:

- "I'm glad your abdominal pain is better; we can do another CT scan to see if there are any changes."
- "I am concerned because there might be a blood clot in a major vessel."

When we put the uncertainty in the patient's lap, I think they would come back. Part of what they do is dependent on how clear we demonstrate the importance of our instructions, as well as the arrangements for follow-up care. For example, if we say, "Go see a vascular surgeon," and we don't arrange the appointment, it's unlikely the patient will be able to find one, let alone get in to see one. That's part of our responsibility.

Authors: *Now to the legal part of things; another scenario: the plaintiff's attorney requests you to review the record. Was there negligence?*
PR: I would tell them what I am telling you. This is a unicorn masquerading as a zebra—it's not negligence. Do not pursue the case.

Authors: *You hang up the phone and five minutes later it is the defense attorney.*
PR: If I am on the defense side, I *would* pursue it as it's a defensible case.

Authors: *Were you surprised the defense settled without a trial?*
PR: No. Depending on the amount of the settlement, sometimes it's not worth going to trial. Often it makes good business sense to settle. One of the things we forget as physicians is that the insurance companies represent themselves, not you. They are their own clients.

Authors: *Any pearls on evaluation of abdominal pain?*
PR: I think the most common error is to look for a common cause of the pain and to stop when that search is negative. If there is no explanation after your evaluation, the next most important part is to arrange for follow-up, particularly if you're dealing with a patient population that can have something serious that does not present in an easily-recognizable fashion. For example, if I am dealing with a child with possible intussusception and the testing is normal, it may have resolved, and I need to figure out follow-up.

Authors: *On a more personal note, how do you balance overtesting with legal risk and how has that changed during the course of your career?*
PR: I am a strong believer in logic. The only biologic test that we possess with a high sensitivity and high specificity is a pregnancy test, and some of the reasons it is so accurate is that we don't screen people who cannot be pregnant. Neither patients nor doctors understand this, but feel that more tests give us more information.

In medicine we are asked to do an impossibility—to prove a negative. What we need to do is to assemble a combination of positive and negative evidence to support a diagnosis and move on from there. As I get older in medicine, I see a need for ordering more tests, but do not find the information improving [in a corresponding manner]. Sometimes you need to compromise and order a test due to patient demands or the referring physician.

But you need to be very careful as sometimes it takes you down a totally different pathway to a disease you weren't even considering.

Authors: Have you ever been sued?
PR: Yes, probably a half a dozen times. I have never had a trial and never needed to settle, but I have had a lot of aggravation. Sometimes it takes two years to have the case dismissed, leaving you with an obligation to notify the board. When I moved from Wyoming to Massachusetts, I needed to report a case from California. Just to show the absurdity— it was an 82 year-old woman struck by a car who refused transport, so they called me. I told them to take her to a trauma center [since she was in such bad shape]; she wasn't able to make her own decision. She turned out to have 12 broken ribs and didn't want to pay her bill, so the hospital sued her, and then she turned out and sued me. I was finally dismissed two years later.

I can see why doctors don't want to have judgments against them, but there is no less aggravation if you pay actual dollars or nothing. So my advice is don't worry about the legal system, it is for its own convenience, not for the protection of the medical system. Do what you have to do. Sometimes I would rather settle cases than go through a trial, even if I pay money out.

Authors: *Have those six allegations changed your practice?*
PR: No. In every single case I was able to say there is a debate about the practice of medicine, and I am not going to change a good practice to a bad one. I may occasionally be found guilty, but I know that I did the right thing. I think I've been lucky as I'm sure I have made my fair share of errors. I will give one more piece of advice—when you make your final disposition ask one more question: "Is it safe?" And if it's not safe, then do something else. For example, when I am sending home a patient with abdominal pain, did I tell her to see her doctor if her symptoms recur, did I make an appointment for her, did I tell her to come back if her symptoms don't resolve in eight hours, did I recommend a consultation and did I arrange it? Or did I just say, "She is a whole lot better, so I don't need to worry about it."

Authors: *Thanks so much for talking to me*
PR: Any way I can help I'd be happy to. Nice talking to you.

VII. Guest Commentary—The Legal Analysis: Karl Schedler, JD

- Principal Attorney, Office of the Ohio Attorney General
- Court of Claims Defense Section
- Defense of Malpractice Claims against Ohio State University Medical Center

Mr. Schedler's practice involves medical litigation in a teaching facility. He discusses how liability differs between residents and attendings, thoughts on this case, and if he would have settled.

Resident Liability: Generally, residents are viewed as trainees, and their "standard of care" is measured by their level of responsibility. Residents usually work-up the patient and then present the case to their attending physician, who is ultimately responsible.The ultimate decision is disposition of the patient, and that is almost always the responsibility of the attending. However, if the resident assumes the responsibility of an attending then he or she is expected to act in accordance with their accepted standard of care and assume the liability of an attending.

Hospitals generally have vicarious liability for acts or omissions of an employee, including a resident, that occur in the course of the employee's duties. Resident liability generally arises from failing to provide pertinent information to the attending physician that would alter the management of the patient's care. An example is when a nurse reports a change in the patient's condition to the resident, but he or she decides not to communicate the change to the attending. Sometimes a resident may incur liability by making a decision to send a patient for a diagnostic test when the test is contraindicated (e.g., sending a patient with renal failure for a CT study with contrast), or when the patient's condition mitigates against transport (an unstable patient who decompensates in the CT scanner).

In this specific case, the resident conducted an initial work-up under the supervision of the attending, which is consistent with the standard of care for a resident. Unless the resident was instructed to do something that she realizes is a clear departure from the standard of care, she is unlikely to have liability. There is a progress note written by the resident regarding a discussion with the attending radiologist. Even though the note was written by the resident, presumably the ED attending was aware of the information in the note. The outcome might be different if the communication was strictly between residents.

The hospital could also have exposure through the attending physician because some states impose liability on the hospital for malpractice by the ED attending, even if he or she is not an employee of the hospital. This liability has been founded on the notion of "ostensible" agency, where the public relies on the hospital to select the physician in the ED and courts have held that the hospital is liable even if the attending physicianis not an employee.

Legal analysis: In this case there was a missed diagnosis, and there was a bad result; a classic scenario in emergency medicine. In retrospect, it is possible to see that the patient had a diagnosis with significant morbidity and mortality. If the plaintiff's lawyer could get the ED attending to acknowledge that a SMA infarct is part of her differential diagnosis (and the progress note documenting the discussion between the ED team and radiology seems to reflect it was), then the ED attending is left to defend her decision to discharge the patient without definitively ruling out that diagnosis.

In this case illustration, the ED attending would be hard-pressed to defend herself with the contention that this was such an odd presentation that the real diagnosis never crossed her radar screen, because apparently it did. Moreover, since an arteriogram most likely would have identified the occlusion, and lytic therapy or surgery would likely have resolved the clot, the plaintiff has a solid argument on causation. So, it is understandable that the defendant would consider settlement.

Settlement: The evaluation of settlement involves an attempt to quantify the odds of success at trial and to estimate a likely verdict. In addition when the plaintiff offers to settle within the limits of the policy, and settlement if declined by the defense, the risk of excess judgment must be considered. If the insurance company refuses to accept a settlement within policy limits and the verdict comes back in excess of limits, the insurance company may be compelled to pay the difference. If the physician's policy requires the physician's consent to settle, refusal to settle within limits may expose the *physician* to the excess liability.

Damages: This is a very high damage case with three main elements of damage, including loss of income, cost of medical treatment for life, not a small number, and non-economic damages, including pain, suffering and loss of enjoyment of life.

Some states cap or limit non-economic damages and that could affect the amount of the settlement. In the final analysis, the amount of settlement has to be based on an objective assessment of the likelihood of an unfavorable verdict and the monetary range of a verdict if returned for the plaintiff. To use our case as an example, if the present value of future lost earnings was $1 million and the present value of future medical treatment was $1.5 million, then it is not hard to see a potential verdict in excess of $4 million. This assessment is as much art as it is science, and requires experience in the particular jurisdiction to know what similar cases have settled for in the past. In some jurisdictions, lawyers have collected data on jury verdicts, and there are software programs designed to estimate the value of a potential verdict.

ED physician liability in this case: From the standpoint of the ED physician it seems reasonable that she would not have contributed to settlement. Assuming that the radiologist's communicated assessment of the July 15 study is accurately described in the progress note, the ED physician has a plausible explanation for not doing additional imaging studies or seeking a vascular surgery consult. However, the ED physician's strongest argument is that this patient was seen by the experts, the vascular surgery service, on July 26, almost a month before the infarct came to a crisis. Moreover, given the disposition of this patient following an outpatient office visit, with persistent symptoms and a CT study in hand, it is not likely that a vascular surgery consult would have changed the course of events in the ED. This clearly disrupts the direct chain of causation, and from a "common sense" standpoint makes it hard to blame the ED physician for her discharge decision on July 15.

VIII. Authors' Summary

Though EM residents are some of the smartest folks on the planet, there is no substitute for adequate supervision. Coordinating lab and radiographic results during shift change is no easy manner. Lost in the maelstrom of peristalsis and supratentorial concern is a subset of patients who have an actual diagnosis. The trick is find the diamond in the rough …

References

1. Dart RG, Kaplan B, Varaklis K. Predictive value of history and physical examination in patients with suspected ectopic pregnancy. Ann Emerg Med 1999; 33(3):283-90.
2. Edlow JA, Panagos PD, Godwin SA, et al. Clinical policy: critical issues in the evaluation and management of adult patients presenting to the emergency department with acute headache. Ann Emerg Med 2008; 52(4):407-36.

Additional reading

• Ofer A, Abadi S, Nitecki S, et al. Multidetector CT angiography in the evaluation of acute mesenteric ischemia. Eur Radiol 2009; 19:24-30.
• Ullery, BS, Boyko AT, Banet GA, et al. Colonic ischemia: An under-recognized cause of lower gastrointestinal bleeding. J Emerg Med 2004; 27:1-5.
• Chang RW, Chang JB, Longo WE. Update in management of mesenteric ischemia. World J Gastroenterol 2006; 12(20):3243-7.
• Chang JB, Stein TA. Mesenteric ischemia: acute and chronic. Ann Vasc Surg 2003; 17(3):323-8.
• Kumar S, Sarr MG, Kamath PS. Mesenteric venous thrombosis. N Engl J Med 2001; 345(23):1683-8.

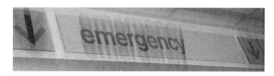

CASE 6

A 32 YEAR-OLD WOMAN WITH HEADACHE: WE OWN THIS DIAGNOSIS

Primary case author Michael Weinstock

PART 1—MEDICAL

    I. The Patient's Story 143

    II. The Doctor's Version (the ED Chart) 143

    III. The Errors—Risk Management/Patient Safety Issues 145

    IV. The Bounceback 147

PART 2—LEGAL

    I. The Accusation/Cause of Action 150

    II. What Would Greg Do (WWGD)? 151

    III. The Trial/Depositions 152

    IV. Additional Comments, Greg Henry 160

    V. Judge Instructions 161

    VI. The Twist 161

    VII. The Verdict 161

    VIII. Legal Insight from Plaintiff's and Defense Attorneys 162

    IX. Legal Analysis—Robert Bitterman, MD, JD 163

    X. Medical Discussion—Jonathan Edlow, MD 168

    XI. Authors' Summary 171

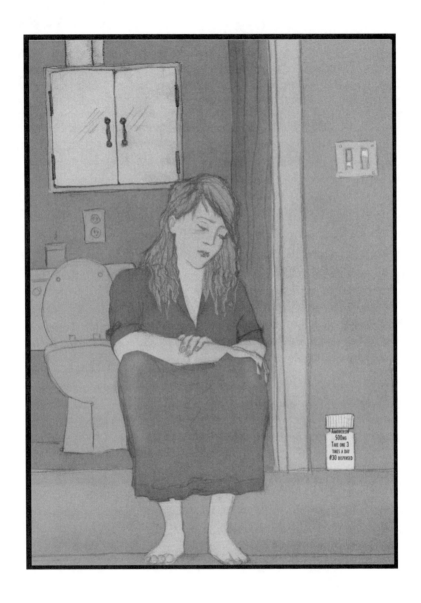

CASE 6

A 32 YEAR-OLD WOMAN WITH HEADACHE: WE OWN THIS DIAGNOSIS

Some days I am so good I can diagnose patients from my workstation; sudden onset flank pain is a stone; positional low back pain is a lumbosacral strain … but sometimes I need to see the patient. Headache is a complaint which causes us to put our guard down, particularly if the patient has a history of chronic pain … or sinusitis. My "big two" in evaluating nontraumatic headaches are subarachnoid hemorrhage and meningitis, but there are a few other causes which need to be included in the differential.

Deep thoughts:

1. *Is the "worst headache of your life" pathognomonic for ANYTHING?*
2. *How do we reconcile positive test results with a conflicting clinical story?*
3. *Have you ever been a victim of "diagnosis momentum?"*
4. *What is the role of advanced line antibiotics in the treatment of sinusitis?*

PART 1—MEDICAL

I. The Patient's Story

Kelli Flood has a good job selling advertising for billboards for Stem Outdoor Advertising, making just under $50,000 per year. She is smart, has a sharp wit and a good work ethic. She and her second husband, Shane, are active parents. They recently married, on October 28, 1998, and took a honeymoon at a *Sandals* resort.

Several days after the birth of, Jacob, on July 30, 1999, Kelli presents to her primary care physician with a headache and is diagnosed with sinusitis; she is placed on amoxicillin. The headaches continue to the point that on August 8th she says her head pain is "indescribable, like my head was going to come off, or split in two."

She presents to an emergency department in rural Ohio.

II. The Doctor's Version (the following is the actual documentation of the provider)

Date: August 8, 1999 at 18:32
Chief complaint: Throbbing head [pain], migraine comes on suddenly

Nurse's note: Headache has happened 3 times in past 7 days, c/o pain in the forehead and back of head. This headache was of sudden onset a ½ hour ago. Had an epidural. Ice to forehead, crying, headache 10/10.

HISTORY OF PRESENT ILLNESS (18:55): This patient is a 32 year-old female, who is 8 days postpartum. She describes this [headache] as the worst one of her life. She has no known history of direct or indirect trauma to the head. Apparently, 5 or 6 days ago, she was identified as having sinusitis and placed on Amoxicillin 500 mg t.i.d. Since that time, the patient has had 2 other headaches, which were not quite as severe as this one. The patient describes frontal as well as bi-temporal discomfort with photophobia and nausea, but no vomiting. There is no phonophobia, numbness or tingling. The patient had been asleep and woke up with the discomfort.

PAST MEDICAL HISTORY:
Allergies: Sulfa (swelling)
Meds: Amoxicillin, Tylenol extra strength, prenatal vitamins
PMH/PSH: Negative
Surgery: c-section 1987, broke arm 16 years ago, laparoscopic surgery 1990
FH: Father - diabetes

EXAM

VITAL SIGNS									
Time	Temp(F)	Rt	Pulse	Resp	Syst	Diast	Pos	O2 sat RA	
18:42	97.0	O	68	18	156	95	S	97%	

CONSTITUTIONAL: She is a well developed and well nourished female, alert and oriented X3. She does appear to be moderately uncomfortable.
SKIN: In general has normal texture and turgor. No lesions are identified.
EYES: EOMI. PERRL. The external lids and conjunctivae are clear. Fundi are normal.
NOSE, MOUTH, AND THROAT: There is minimal nasal mucosal erythema. The pharynx is normal. The uvula is in midline. There is bifrontal region tenderness to palpation and pressure.
NECK: Supple without masses, no lymphadenopathy
LUNGS: CTAB. No respiratory distress.
HEART: RRR without rubs, clicks or murmurs. Carotid pulsations are 2+ and symmetric.
NEUROLOGIC evaluation including sensory, motor, cerebellar, and cranial nerve II-XII examination is intact. No meningeal signs present.

ED COURSE:
19:20 – Brain CT: (reading per ED doctor): No evidence of intracranial bleeding or mass lesion. The bone windows do show evidence for mucoid material within both frontal sinuses with possible ethmoid involvement.
19:50 – After discussing the situation and the possible effect of narcotics on the baby, who is breast fed, mother did agree to an injection of Demerol 75mg IM and Phenergan 25mg IM.
    20:15 – Repeat vitals: Pulse 64, respirations 18, BP 176/50
    20:35 – Meds: Biaxin 500mg PO
    Doctor progress note: The patient had moderate relief of her discomfort after Demerol and Phenergan. The patient has cephalgia, which I believe is related to sinusitis and I will switch

her to Biaxin, Darvocet, and Entex LA. I recommend liquids and rest. Recheck in 3 to 4 days if there is no improvement in the overall symptoms, sooner if there is significant worsening.

DIAGNOSIS:
1. Acute sinusitis.
2. Acute cephalgia.

PLAN: Biaxin 500mg BID #20, entex LA BID #20, Darvocet N-100 Q 6 hours PRN pain #6
Released ambulatory at 20:35

Seth Hockenberry, MD

Note: A later overread by the radiologist finds the brain CT normal.

III. The Errors—Risk Management/Patient Safety Issues

➤**Authors' note:** It is obvious from the note that he cared about his patient. He not only spent a lot of time with her, but also informed her when and why to return. The following are some considerations about the initial evaluation:

Risk management/patient safety issue #1:

Error: Overreliance on test results.

Discussion: The phrase "worst headache of life" means a lot to patients and lawyers, but it is really questionable how much it should mean to emergency physicians. If you are going to document this and do a brain CT, it is important to realize the limitations for diagnosis of subarachnoid hemorrhage (SAH).[1-3] In the first 12 hours, the sensitivity of CT for SAH is over 90%, but at seven days it drops to only 58%. Our patient had already had a week of pain when she presented to the ED. Many Hunt-Hess II and III classification subarachnoid hemorrhages may present similarly to meningitis, often inadvertently discovered following LP for SAH evaluations.

✔ **Teaching point:** If a brain CT is done to evaluate for SAH, an LP should follow.

Risk management/patient safety issue #2:

Error: Anchoring bias and diagnosis momentum.

Discussion: It is difficult to determine exactly which diagnosis was to be excluded with a head CT, but once the physician saw sinus thickening, he anchored on sinusitis. This was likely coupled with *diagnosis momentum,* since the patient was actually taking amoxicillin for a sinusitis diagnosis from the primary care doctor. Curiously, there was no documentation of clinical sinus symptoms such as rhinorrhea, postnasal drip, facial/tooth pain or fever, but the patient did have sinus pain with palpation.

✔ **Teaching point:** When a test shows an unexpected result, historical confirmation should support it as the source of the patient's symptoms or it should be discounted.

Risk management/patient safety issue #3:

Error: Differential diagnosis too narrow.

Discussion: Whereas the two most immediately concerning ED diagnoses in patients with nontraumatic headache remain SAH and meningitis, there are other "can't miss" secondary headaches, including:

1. Brain mass
2. Temporal arteritis
3. Pseudotumor cerebri (idiopathic intracranial hypertension)
4. Carbon monoxide toxicity
5. Acute angle closure glaucoma
6. Carotid artery dissection
7. Cavernous sinous thrombosis
8. Preeclampsia/eclampsia
9. Post-LP headache

Preeclampsia is concerning in our patient since she not only had increased blood pressure when she arrived, but it was actually higher just prior to discharge. Preeclampsia/eclampsia can occur up to 30 days post-partum.[4] The problem is that a headache (pain) can also cause the blood pressure to go up. Additional findings with preeclampsia may include hyper-reflexia/clonus, abdominal pain, proteinuria and lack of a previous history of hypertension.

Another consideration is post-dural puncture headache. These are worse when sitting up and better when lying flat. If this diagnosis was firmly established, the elevated blood pressure could be explained as a response to the often severe pain.

Primary headaches include the following; however, none of these were consistent with our patient's presentation:

1. Migraine
2. Tension
3. Cluster
4. Narcotic withdrawal
5. Stress HAs

In addition to pregnancy and the perinatal period, other high risk factors for headache patients include:

1. Immunosuppression
2. Age over 50
3. Systemic anticoagulation
4. Hypercoagulability (Cancer, Behcet's disease, OCP use, pregnancy, lupus, factor 5 Leiden deficiency, etc.)

✔ **Teaching point:** Maintain a high index of suspicion for high-risk headache patients.

Risk management/patient safety issue #4:

Error: Overreliance on antibiotics for sinusitis.

Discussion: Sinusitis is usually viral, with a "number needed to treat" (NNT) with antibiotics between 8 and 12. When the decision is made to use a second-line antibiotic (macrolide, quinolone) instead of a first-line antibiotic (amoxicillin, TMP/SMZ, doxycycline), the NNT skyrockets to 100.[5] If 100 patients with a diagnosis of sinusitis are treated with advanced line ATB, one patient will get better sooner. Whereas it is OK to "bump up" the antibiotic from amoxicillin to Biaxin with our patient, the fact that she failed an antibiotic in the first place should cause pause in the diagnosis of sinusitis.

✔ **Teaching point:** Sinusitis is overdiagnosed and therapy overrated.

Risk management/patient safety issue #5:

Error: Misreading CT.

Discussion: The ED physician did document a thorough discussion of the CT reading. Unfortunately, his reading was in contradiction to the radiologist's final reading. When there is a question, teleradiology should be employed to confirm the correct interpretation. A mechanism must be in place to identify all ED radiology discrepancies after the patient leaves the ED. Regarding CT scans, the standard of care is for radiology to provide the contemporaneous reading. Providing an interpretation of a CT without the assistance of the radiologist may increase risk for the patient and the emergency physician. Sinus findings on CT are very sensitive, but not specific.

✔ **Teaching point:** Avoid interpreting brain CTs without the input of Radiology.

IV. The Bounceback

August 9th, the day after ED discharge, Kelli, Shane and Jacob are running some errands, but upon return to the house, her headache starts to worsen. She fixes dinner, but doesn't eat anything because "I just can't." She asks, "Shane, [will] you please run me a bath?"

Per Kelli: "I went into the bedroom because that's where Jake was, and I couldn't see him. I yelled for Shane and I said, "Shane, I can't see the baby." He came. I said, 'For that matter, I can't see you.' I rubbed my fingers together clear up by my face and I couldn't see them. So, I sat down on the steps of the bathroom and I just don't remember anything else. That's as far as I go."

Shane noticed that Kelli "seemed to be in somewhat of a daze and was rubbing her hands together." She begins to shake all over, her eyes roll back in her head and she is foaming at the mouth. Shane calls 911.

August 9 (21:05): Quincy County EMS receives a call for a patient having a seizure. At 21:08 they are enroute, arriving on location at 21:10 to find their patient sitting on the steps leading into the bathroom. She does not respond to verbal commands and is disoriented to time and place. Finger stick glucose is 92, monitor shows NSR. On the way to the ED, she begins to respond to questions and asks for her husband. She experiences short episodes of body tremors, lasting less than 10 seconds each. At 21:28 they arrive at the ED.

ED record: August 9, 1999 at 21:32:
- **Chief complaint:** Possible seizures
- **HPI**: The patient had been somewhat fatigued and had fallen asleep at the dining room table. Later this evening the husband was running the patient's bath, and noticed the patient seemed to be in somewhat of a daze, rubbing her fingers together, and then she began shaking all over, with her eyes rolling back, which lasted about a minute. Thereafter, the patient appeared confused, did not respond appropriately, but was screaming about her severe headache.
- **Vital signs**: Temp 97.4, pulse 78, resp 16, BP 172/99, sat 97% (RA)
- **PE**: A well developed, well nourished white female, moaning with pain and shaking her head from side to side and crying. Knows answers to questions at times but sometimes ignores questions. She is having periods when she would shake her head and shake her extremities. Slight pallor. No gross neurological deficits were noted.
  - **Progress note:** Although [a brain CT] was done yesterday, there was question of whether she may have had a herald subarachnoid bleed yesterday [so CT was repeated]. Rule out encephalitis, possibly herpes simplex.
  - **CT brain:** No bleed or shifts. Small ventricles without signs of cerebral edema.
  - **Labs:** WBC 12.8, Hb 14.3, plt 434. Chemistry and coags nl. Calcium and magnesium normal. CXR – no infiltrates. UA normal.
- **ED course**: The patient's BP did go up to 190/115, and the patient's headache seemed to increase with increased shaking of her head and crying. Mental status remains unchanged.
- Lasix 20 mg IVP. Nipride 0.25 micrograms per kilogram per minute. Patient's headache did appear to decrease somewhat, though it was still very severe.
- Demerol 25 mg and Phenergan 25 mg I.V.
- **Discussion:** I stated to the husband that she may have encephalitis, and an LP was indicated. Further, Acyclovir would be started depending upon the results of the LP. I spoke with Dr. Quinn, the neurologist on call and the decision was made not to do the LP since our lab is limited. The patient was admitted to the ICU. Discussed with the husband and the patient, but I am not certain of how much the patient understood of our discussion.

FINAL DIAGNOSIS:
1. Severe cephalgia, with acute mental status change, and possible first time seizures.
2. Consider encephalitis, herpes simplex.
3. Cannot entirely rule out a herald bleed, with undetectable subarachnoid hemorrhage at this time.
4. Rule out other inflammatory Central Nervous System problems.

Robert Carozza, MD

> ➤**Authors' note:** Hmmm ... who has ever called a neurologist and been talked *out* of an LP? There were still several diagnostic possibilities on the table which the second ED physician had not ruled out, including subarachnoid hemorrhage, herpes encephalitis, meningitis and eclampsia. A young, healthy woman with a first-time seizure, and consideration of any of these entities would call for an LP. Of course, we all know she has eclampsia—or does she?

HOSPITAL COURSE:

- MRI showed ischemic changes in the right cerebellar cortex. EEG was unremarkable. LP: WBC 1, RBC 84, protein 77, glucose 46. Bacterial cultures and india ink stain were negative. Urinalysis with trace proteinuria. Sed rates ranged from 16–32.
- Repeat MRIs showed cerebral infarcts in the frontal, parietal and occipital lobes. She was placed on Dilantin and Ativan and high-dose Solumedrol. SBPs ranged from 110–190. She had visual loss and speech delay after the occipital event, but was able to communicate with her husband.
- On 8/19/99, ten days after admission, Kelli is sitting in her hospital bed, playing cards with her husband, when she has another seizure. An emergent CT shows attenuation in right occipital lobe and question of vertebral vasospasm.

TRANSFER TO THE UNIVERSITY HOSPITAL MEDICAL CENTER:

- Initial note: Since arrival has been unresponsive and stuporous with decerebrate posturing.
- MRA showed diffuse arterial "beading" of the small and medium vessels in both the carotid and vertebral vascular distributions.
- At that time the differential diagnosis included postpartum cerebral angiopathy, cerebral vasculitis and eclampsia. She was treated presumptively with high dose IV steroids and magnesium.
- Nicardipine drip was continued to keep her BP 160–170 mm Hg.
- Mental status remained unchanged for the next two weeks.
- On 9/4/99 she developed a temperature of 106°. Indwelling lines were removed, and she was pan-cultured.
- Attempts to reestablish central venous access were unsuccessful, and shortly after those attempts, she developed neck edema and became stridorous, which did not respond to racemic epinephrine.
- Anesthesiology is consulted for difficult airway management, and ENT placed an emergent tracheostomy. The stridor was thought to be secondary to an allergic reaction and the neck manipulation during central line attempts.
- Blood cultures returned positive for Klebsiella → Zosyn and tobramycin.
- Throughout the rest of the hospital course, she had slow improvement in neurological status and at discharge was mildly responsive and occasionally interactive.

FINAL OUTCOME: Kelli is triplegic. Her condition has stabilized but not improved. She lives at home, and is cared for by her husband.

PART 2—LEGAL

Why sue? This patient had a horrible outcome; a young mother now triplegic, requiring life-long medical care and assistance. Before her turn for the worse, she was sitting in the hospital room playing cards with her husband, waiting to go home to be with her family and newborn child. Suddenly, she experienced a seizure from which she would never recover. It is not difficult to see why this family would file suit.

Plaintiff's attorney:

Q. [Kelli,] would you generally describe your family and how it's functioning, in broad terms? What about you and Shane, and Sarah, Lindsey, and Jacob?

A. We're a close family.

Q. As to Jacob, would you describe Jacob for us?

A. He's a wonderful little boy. He's three and a half. He is extremely active. He's just … I can't say enough about him. I'm a very proud mother.

Q. What are some of the things that you like to do with Jacob?

A. I like to play Leap Frog with him. If you have children you'll understand. It's a computer game. I like to help him count and teach him his alphabet. I like to play "This Little Piggy" with him. He climbs up and sits on my lap. I let him brush my hair. He likes to read to me. He can't read, but he likes to tell me stories that he makes up. He pretends. He likes to help me with anything that I ask him to do. If I ask him to get mommy a drink of water, "would you, Jacob", he'll run and get it. If I need a Kleenex, he runs and gets it.

Q. Does Jacob love you?

A. Yes, he does.

Q. How do you know that?

A. Because he tells me so. He throws his arms around my neck and says, "Mommy, I love you."

I. The Accusation/Cause of Action

Barton County, OH Court of Common Pleas 2003: Plaintiff requires the use of a wheel chair and has only the use of her left hand. Prior to this event, plaintiff was the active mother of three children. She sought past medicals of **$561,266**, future medicals of **$10,393,754** and future wage loss of **$1,300,000.**

At trial, plaintiff argued that doctors Hockenberry and Carozza failed to differentially diagnose her with postpartum preeclampsia and/or eclampsia (together PE/E) and failed to presumptively treat her with magnesium sulfate, which led to her ultimate brain injury and related paralysis. Specifically, plaintiff argued that any life-threatening illness which appears on the differential diagnosis should be treated presumptively and/or the patient should be admitted if the diagnosis of a life-threatening illness cannot be ruled out.

There was also a lawsuit against the neurologist, Dr. Quinn, which was dropped several days into the proceedings.

II. What Would Greg Do (WWGD)?

Greg Henry, past president of The American College of Emergency Physicians (ACEP), Professor of Emergency Medicine at the University of Michigan, and CEO of Medical Practice Risk Assessment, has been an expert witness in over 2,000 malpractice cases.

Greg discusses the evaluation of headaches, the role sympathy plays in a jury, and if he would proceed to trial or recommend settlement.

"The road to hell is paved with normal CT scans"

Headache is always difficult in the emergency department. You will see between 150 and 200 headaches before you find something significant. Headaches fall into two groups, something bad or just a pain problem. There is always an intrinsic amount of risk in the evaluation. Everyone does not need a CT scan.

I have seen countless headaches in my career, but the number of the truly unusual cases is few and far between. The fact that the patient is eight days post partum certainly brings certain thoughts to bear, including meningitis, since she had spinal anesthesia performed, and much more common would be post-dural puncture headache.

The patient's vital signs were relatively stable and certainly consistent with pain. It is interesting that actual physical examination has gone out of fashion. Although it is commented that the fundi are normal, I always wonder whether the physician is looking for the same things which I would look for. In a headache patient, you are concerned about two findings:

1. Papilledema
2. Loss of spontaneous venous pulsations (SVPs)

It would almost be extremely unusual to see a patient who had normal venous pulsation and increased intracranial pressure. I don't believe the two can exist in the same patient. I only point this out because whenever the fundi are mentioned it is usually "normal" or "abnormal." It would be much more useful if one specifically commented on SVPs and papilledema.

The normal head CT in this case means essentially nothing; a normal CT scan should never be a surprise to the clinically-talented physician. The road to hell is paved with normal CT scans.

Certainly, rare causes of disease cannot be excluded simply because they are rare. I have never seen temporal arteritis without some tenderness in the temporal arteries, and I've never seen such a case in a 32 year-old. I've never seen a mass effect of a pseudotumor cerebri (idiopathic intracranial hypertension) without physical findings such as papilledema or at least loss of SVPs. Carbon monoxide should be supported by the history. Acute angle glaucoma should have at least some tearing or redness of the eye; I have seen a case where the patient had nausea and vomiting as the chief complaint and upon physical examination, one eye was bloodshot. The diagnosis was made with simple physical examination.

To assume that a 32 year-old who has just delivered a baby had developed a carotid artery dissection goes beyond the pale. I can understand it in a lacrosse player who had been hit in the neck. The concept of post-partum preeclampsia is extremely rare, but with this patient's elevated BP, missing it would be hard to defend. I've only seen one case of venous thrombosis present de novo to the emergency department, and this patient was not difficult to diagnose.

At this point in time, not knowing the outcome of the legal decision, all I can say is the emergency physician has one major factor going against him, sympathy. Don't try this case two weeks before Christmas. There but for the grace of God go all of us. The decision to proceed or not to proceed would depend on two things:

1. The amount of money being sought by the family.
2. The creditability and believability of the doctor. If the doctor appears to be someone who did not truly do the examination and was not truly invested in the outcome of the case, you could have a problem.

Doctors are not required to be right all the time; if that were the case, none of us would be allowed to practice medicine. He needs to show he did the usual and customary evaluation. If I were the defense attorney in this case and felt my client was trustworthy, I would move ahead to trial.

➤**Author's note:** Right again, Greg! Blink your eyes and flash forward a few years— "Ladies and Gentlemen of the jury, all rise!"

III. The Trial (January 2003)

Judge's instructions to jury: Good morning ladies and gentlemen. Today is the 15th of January, 2003. We convene in Flood vs. Hockenberry.

Opening statements will give you a preview of what the respective attorneys believe this case will show. Opening statements are not evidence. These are given by the attorneys to assist you and to set the frame work, the table of contents, or the coming attractions. Ultimately, the decision of what the evidence [shows] is yours.

Now, in any lawsuit, the plaintiffs go first because they have the burden of proof. They get to go first in presenting evidence. The plaintiffs [also] will get to go first in closing arguments.

This is not a criminal case and the burden of proof that you may have heard of about "beyond a reasonable doubt" does not apply. In a civil lawsuit the plaintiffs have the burden of proving their suit by a *preponderance of the evidence,* which is the greater weight of the evidence. That is evidence that you believe because it outweighs in your mind the evidence opposed to it. Are counsel ready to proceed with opening statements?

Cast of characters (names changed, except where noted):

The patient: Kelli Flood
ED physician defendant #1: Seth Hockenberry
ED physician defendant #2: Robert Carozza
Plaintiff's attorneys: Mr. Lutz and Mr. O'Neil (actual attorney)
Plaintiff's expert (ED physician): Dr. Geller
Defense attorney: Lawrence Huffman (actual attorney)
Defense expert witness (neurology): Dr. Baja Sabdur
Defense expert witness: Dr. Stan Kapplan

Opening Statement—Mr. Lutz (plaintiff's attorney)

Good morning ladies and gentlemen. I want to first start out by talking a little bit about some rules that doctors follow, rules they learn them in medical school and apply every day. Doctors have a duty to use ordinary care; what a reasonably cautious doctor would do in the same situation. Those are rules you'll follow, too, when you decide this case. There's going to be a word mentioned by every doctor that testifies in this case. That word is eclampsia. It has been known for many, many years.

A couple of things about eclampsia. Number one, fifty thousand people a year die from eclampsia. Number two, that's in the world; okay? In the United States, ninety thousand to a hundred thousand are diagnosed with a condition called preeclampsia. It is the second leading cause of maternal death in the United States. Every textbook talks about it. Every doctor knows, or should know, what it is.

What is eclampsia? Eclampsia is a disease. These are not disputable things. Any woman that is pregnant or has recently delivered a baby can get it. Some people used to think that it was a toxin, a poison that would go through your body. That's why it was called toxemia. I look at it like a snake bite. If you get a snake bite you've got to do something quick. If the poison goes through, well, what do you do? You go get the serum, right, to stop the poison. Well, there's a serum [for] eclampsia. It's a drug called magnesium sulfate. Doctors say "drug of choice." It's *the* drug. In a study published in the New England Journal of Medicine, there were 1,049 patients that had eclampsia. They gave them magnesium sulfate. Guess how many of the thousand forty-nine continued to have seizures? Zero. It's in every emergency room. It's been known for a hundred of years. It's the drug of choice.

Now, I mentioned preeclampsia; you have preeclampsia before you have eclampsia. The body gives out warning signs. There's not much dispute here. Number one, you've got to be pregnant or postpartum. Number two is high blood pressure. There's often a severe headache, visual disturbances like [sensitivity to light], protein in the urine, nausea and upper quadrant [abdominal] pain.

How does a doctor go about finding these signs? Easy. He takes a history. What happened? Are you pregnant? Recently been pregnant? Have you had headaches? Visual disturbances? Nausea? What's the second way they do it? Lab tests, for example proteinuria. What's the third? An exam. So, history, exam and testing.

Some other things about eclampsia that will be interesting to you. I call them truisms. Number one, it gets worse if untreated. It can move from preeclampsia to eclampsia in a short amount of time. That's why it's a medical emergency. How do you treat it? Mag. Sulfate.

Okay. July 30th, 1999 we've got a couple proud parents. Kelli Flood delivered a baby. It was a pretty happy time. July 31st, Kelly and Jacob leave the hospital. On August 8th, eight days postpartum, it's the first opportunity to help Kelli. Kelli is seen by the first emergency room doctor, Dr. Hockenberry. Kelli was in bad shape on August 8th. It was Sunday night at 6 PM. She was crying. She had the worst headache of her life. She had visual changes, photophobia, nausea. He takes a blood pressure. It's 156/95. Dr. Hockenberry thought that a cold was causing the most severe headache of her life and that the high blood pressure was caused by the pain. So, he gave her a shot of Demerol. The headache got better, but the blood pressure went up. The pain was less, and the blood pressure was more. It went from 156 to 176.

Do you know what he didn't do? Order a urinalysis. This is no big complicated test; you pee into a bottle and check it with a dipstick. He didn't do that. He didn't check her reflexes. He didn't refer her to her OB.

When Kelli returned to the ED, the second ED doctor did two things that the first ER doctor didn't do, he ordered a urinalysis for protein which was abnormal. He also checked her reflexes, which were hyperactive. He didn't call her doctor of the last nine months, her OB. He thought that it was herpes. So, that's the first opportunity and the second opportunity.

On the 14th, they finally got around to calling Doctor Garcia [the obstetrician]. He was there within minutes. He looked at Kelli and diagnosed eclampsia. At this point, it was too little, too late. She left the hospital on the 21st near death. Her family was told to hope for the best and prepare for the worst. She was life-flighted on August 21st to University Hospital. She was 20 days in a coma.

They're going to have doctors come in and in hindsight say it [was not eclampsia]. The discharge summary from St. Margaret's says postpartum eclampsia. Doctor Garcia, the obstetrician [diagnosed] eclampsia. The discharge summary at University Hospital and the Specialty [rehab] Hospital admission [was for] eclampsia. They're going to say in hindsight, it wasn't eclampsia.

They're going to say it was something else; Call-Fleming. Hypertension isn't part of the diagnosis. Proteinuria isn't part of the diagnosis. Seizure is not part of the diagnosis. It comes on all at once.

Kelli was a career woman. She made $45,000 a year. She hasn't worked since and will never work again. This is a picture of her family, her kids (shows picture to jury). She can do a few things. She can read to them if the print is big or if she has a magnifying glass. She can count numbers a little bit. But, she can't throw a ball. She can't drive to soccer. Kelli is frozen in her own body and it was preventable.

> **Authors' note:** If I ever get eclampsia (which is highly unlikely), I want this guy working for me! Though it seems clear the diagnosis was preeclampsia, the defense is about to throw a wrench into the mix; they argue the patient did not even have preeclampsia, but a syndrome called Call-Fleming, a *progressive* disease resulting in large cerebral infarcts. Ever heard of it? Neither have I.

Opening Statement—Mr. Huffman (defense attorney)

Well, good morning ladies and gentlemen of the jury. As we promised you yesterday when we opened this trial, there are, of course, two sides to every story. Mr. Lutz has presented the side of the story represented by the plaintiffs. I'd like to talk to you a bit about the side of the story that has to do with my clients Drs. Hockenberry and Carozza.

First, I'd like to have you meet my clients. Dr. Hockenberry is the gentleman in the center who has just nodded to you. He did a combined internal medicine and pediatrics residency. He's been doing emergency room medicine since then. He's a highly qualified and a highly skilled emergency room physician.

My other client is Dr. Carozza [the second ED physician], who is seated there on the left, in the gray jacket. He practiced family medicine for a number of years and then became board-certified in emergency medicine.

Mr. Lutz stated the occurrence of eclampsia is 50,000 world-wide. The facts are that eclampsia is a disease solely limited to pregnant women. The treatment of choice for preeclampsia is delivery of the baby. Almost every time, when the baby is delivered, preeclampsia is over. That's it. You're finished.

Postpartum preeclampsia is very, very rare, and all the witnesses are going to [confirm this]. Furthermore, it is even rarer for her to have postpartum preeclampsia or eclampsia if she had no symptoms during the pregnancy, and Mrs. Flood had no symptoms whatever of preeclampsia during her pregnancy.

As each day goes by after the delivery, the prospects of her having preeclampsia get even more distant.

The only witness who will say that Dr. Carozza or Dr. Hockenberry did anything wrong is Dr. Geller. He's going to say, yes, they should have recognized this disease in the emergency room. I asked Dr. Geller when we took his deposition, I said, "Dr. Geller, how many cases have you ever seen in your professional life of a woman who had eclampsia after the birth of the child?"

Do you know what he said? "One." That was back in the early nineties. He saw one case. My expert witness, Dr. Wendel Johnson, who is the head of the emergency room service at [his] hospital testified in the depositions, "I have never seen a case of eclampsia postpartum. I haven't seen it." Dr. Kevin LaHue, who is a second emergency room expert witness says, "I think I may have seen one or two cases years ago when I was training in [a big hospital] in New York City." That's how rare this disease is. So, keep in mind when people are talking about eclampsia; are they talking about before birth or after birth?

Plaintiffs contend that there's kind of a magic bullet here of magnesium sulfate. But it can be a very dangerous drug, causing respiratory distress and death. Mr. Lutz mentioned a study in which 1,049 people who were given mag sulfate and none of them proceeded to have seizures. In the same study, there were a similar of number of patients who had the same symptoms and who were not given magnesium sulfate and 12 of them may have proceeded on to a seizure. So, whether mag sulfate is a magic bullet that heals everything will be open to serious question. There are some countries, for instance England and Canada, that never use magnesium sulfate; it's unheard of.

All of this talk about eclampsia makes good theatre, but in fact, doesn't really mean anything if, in fact, Mrs. Flood did not have postpartum eclampsia. It's going to be part of our evidence that she did not have postpartum eclampsia. She had a condition which is known as postpartum cerebral angiopathy; a disease lumped together called Call-Fleming syndrome.

We will bring in a physician named Baha Sabdur who is the Chairman of the Department of Obstetrics and Gynecology at the University of Cincinnati Medical School and when you hear him state his qualifications, you will recognize why he is considered the world's leading expert on eclampsia. He's written 40–50 articles which are "the Bible" of eclampsia.

We will also present to you the testimony of Dr. Louis Kapplan, Chairman of the Department of Neurology at the [very prestigious] Medical School. He is considered to be the leading expert in America on Call-Fleming syndrome.

Dr. Kapplan [will explain] that the reasons she had Call-Fleming syndrome is that the arteries were found to have "beading," similar to an old-fashioned handful of frankfurters. You do not have that in postpartum eclampsia.

Dr. Kapplan indicates that in Call-Fleming syndrome you have large infarcts of the brain, but in postpartum eclampsia you have some brain swelling and maybe some small infarcts. In Call-Fleming syndrome the brain damage is extensive and is in the cortex part of the brain. In postpartum eclampsia, it's mostly in the white part of the brain. Magnesium sulfate may prevent seizures, but it does not prevent the brain damage in Call-Fleming syndrome. There are clear distinctions between the two diseases.

One other distinction in the two disease processes, which will be pointed out by Dr. Sabdur, is that eclampsia is not a progressive disease. This is the crucial issue in this case. You do not get it on October 8th and then get worse and worse and worse and worse and worse and worse and worse, as Mrs. Flood did. That's not the way eclampsia acts. In the Call-Fleming syndrome, you get progressively worse, as she did.

In the end, she didn't have postpartum eclampsia. She was suffering from Call-Fleming syndrome, a rare condition with some of the same symptoms as postpartum eclampsia, for which there is no known treatment. The unfortunate physical situation in which she is now is not the result of any medical malpractice on the part of my clients, Dr. Hockenberry and Dr. Carozza.

➤**Authors' note:** So, it is a bit curious. What seems so obvious on initial read of the ED chart (preeclampsia) has now been drawn into question by the alleged world's leading experts on eclampsia and Call-Fleming. His argument is not so farfetched. Has anyone seen someone become quadriplegic after a simple seizure? How about the "beading" in the carotid and vertebral vessels? Is there even consensus on how to treat postpartum eclampsia? Does a patient need to be admitted and placed on a magnesium drip until they reach the "magic number" of 30 days postpartum?

In the end, a "standard of care defense" is always preferable to arguing "proximate cause" (we missed the diagnosis, but that miss was not the sole cause of her quadriplegia). I.e., "we screwed up but it wouldn't have mattered.

The deposition is a way for each side to see how its witnesses will respond to questions and to discover each other's strategy. The deposition is how the plaintiff's attorneys in this case knew the defense was going to argue Call-Fleming and their subsequent attempt to preempt it in their opening statement.

Let's travel back in time to the deposition of the main plaintiff's witness, Dr. Geller. He seems sure of himself during the plaintiff's "direct," alleging the first three items on the differential were eclampsia, but is then blindsided by the clever defense attorney, who grills him on the progressive nature of the disease process. Dr. Geller seems taken by surprise about the importance of this distinction. In fact, it seems as if he doesn't even understand the question.

The Depositions

Deposition (direct) of plaintiff's expert witness Dr. Geller by plaintiff's attorney Mr. O'Neil (June 21, 2002):

Q. You would agree that Mrs. Flood had a condition difficult to diagnose?
A. No, I wouldn't agree to that actually

Q. I take it that you have criticisms of the emergency physicians?
A. That's correct

Q. In your review, were you able to formulate a diagnosis as to Mrs. Flood's condition?
A. Yes.

Q. And would you please tell me what your diagnosis was in that regard?
A. I believe at both times she had eclampsia. It is a continuum of the disease, and she presented in two different stages.

Q. Did you make a differential diagnosis?

A. Yes. First was eclampsia, second would be eclampsia, third would be eclampsia, fourth would be other causes of an intracranial process. And I'm going to lump them together for you; various forms of stroke, vasculitis or infection, but that would fall far beneath that. Given the symptom complex and its findings, [eclampsia] is far and away the most likely diagnosis.

Cross-examination of plaintiff's expert witness Dr. Geller by defense attorney Mr. Huffman:

Q. Is it your understanding that her brain films became progressively worse?

A. I'm not sure what you mean by brain films.

Q. Is it your understanding that the strokes which appear on the serial brain films became progressively worse as time went on?

A. It is my interpretation from the record that both her clinical course and her radiographic studies showed increasing injury to the brain. How we characterize them, whether it's strokes or other events isn't really fundamentally the issue. She did become worse both subjectively and objectively over time.

Q Are you aware of whether or not a progressively worsening condition is consistent with postpartum eclampsia?

A. I didn't review the records to seek to draw an opinion about that in either direction so I can't offer you an opinion.

➢**Authors' note:** Oops! Defense goes on to ask about the "beading" of blood seen in the vasculature. He is continuing to build the case for Call-Fleming, to the seemingly unaware plaintiff's expert.

Q. Are you aware that "beading" of blood was manifested on the MRAs?

A. I'm not sure what you are asking me exactly.

Q. Are you aware of whether "beading" of blood on MRAs is consistent with postpartum eclampsia?

A. I did not review the records seeking to draw conclusions or opinions about that so I can't offer you anything.

Authors' note: The defense is using the witness' own description of symptoms of preeclampsia against him. Earlier, the witness had discussed abdominal pain as a component of preeclampsia/eclampsia. He is now forced to admit the patient did not have this symptom.

Q. Another sign of postpartum eclampsia is abdominal pain; would you agree with that?

A. That's one sign along with nausea or vomiting.

Q. She had no abdominal pain?

A. She had no abdominal pain but again that is not an invariant finding in patients with eclampsia even at severe forms.

➢**Authors' note:** How about edema?

Q. Alright, when Dr. Hockenberry saw her on the 8th, she did not have any edema. Did she?

A. He did not document any excessive amount of edema. I don't know whether or not there was the absence of edema in its totality. That would be a very rare event in someone who had just delivered a baby recently.

Q. When she was admitted to St. Margaret's on the 9th, Doctor Quinn (the neurologist) specifically noted at that time that there was no edema. Didn't he?

A. I believe that's correct.

Q. Okay. So, if it was specifically noted on the 9th on her admission history and physical that there was no edema, you don't contend that there was probably or might have been edema on the 8th, do you?

A: Yes. I believe that there might have been. I can't possibly … all I know is that it wasn't directly assessed. It's not possible for me to offer an opinion about something that's not clearly sought after and documented.

Q. You can form an opinion based upon the circumstantial fact that we know there was no edema on the 9th. Why would there be edema on the 8th?

A. All I know is that one physician believed there was not edema to meet his individual criteria for abnormal. That doesn't mean that it was absent in its totality on either day, and I wouldn't be able to offer you an opinion about it. There's not enough information to even offer conjecture about it.

➤ **Authors' note:** We have heard from the attorneys and some of the experts. How does the physician defend himself?

Cross examination of physician defendant Dr. Hockenberry by plaintiff's attorney Mr. O'Neil:

Q. Now, with headaches, especially severe headaches, there are some conditions that can become very serious and others that are just transient.

A. That's correct.

Q. And as part of the triage of emergency room medicine the doctor is to find out if any of the short list of items on the very bad list are present, isn't that correct?

A. That's certainly part of the job, sir.

Q. Okay. And what items are on the short bad list for severe headache?

A. The bad list includes such things as meningitis, encephalitis, brain abscess. It would include various forms of intracranial bleeding whether it be from aneurysm or intravenous malformation—trauma, but that's usually pretty obvious when the patient presents.

Q. Okay. What about with a woman who is just recently postpartum, is there a list of serious conditions with a severe headache that you have kind of a check-off sheet in your mind?

A. With a headache, you always have to think about any of those things that are listed. Could the headache be associated with something like eclampsia or pre-eclampsia? What I remember is that pre-eclampsia and eclampsia are generally diagnoses of pregnancy and the treatment is delivery. I also recall there have been some reported cases 24 or 48 hours after delivery.

Q. And based on that memory, did you not then consider the issue of pregnancy-induced hypertension, pre-eclampsia and eclampsia?

A. It was something that I considered, but based on historic elements and the physical examination, I felt it was much lower on the list of items in the differential diagnosis.

➢**Authors' note:** This is tricky terrain. The physician doesn't want to appear stupid or give the impression that he wasn't thorough, so he says he considered pre-eclampsia. The problem is that, in a legal setting, consideration of a diagnosis can imply that that diagnosis, especially if potentially life-threatening, should be further explored. See comments below by Bob Bitterman, MD, JD, on the "believability" and advisability of this line of testimony.

I was taught in medical school that if you consider a diagnosis (the classic example was pulmonary embolism) you needed to test for it. I categorically disagree with this line of reasoning. Putting this case aside, I contend that every patient with chest pain needs to have the emergency evaluation start with a consideration of the differential diagnosis of the five life-threatening causes of chest pain, which can be rapidly whittled down based on the history and physical exam. Does the 45 year-old with onset of chest pain while lifting a refrigerator have angina from the exertion or a muscular strain from the lifting? Both need to be considered, but all patients with chest pain do not need to be admitted—we are *doctors* after all, not robots.

IV. Additional Comments from Greg Henry

➢**Authors' note:** Greg is now aware the case has proceeded to trial. He discusses defense and plaintiff strategy and use of expert witnesses.

The plaintiff has to bring in the patient and emphasize the problems that the family faces with a "day in the life of" video. This establishes "damages," a necessary component of any lawsuit and the strongest component of the plaintiff's case. Sympathy is sympathy.

The defense has an equally simple job. It's to show that the physician cared for and evaluated the patient in a way which a reasonable physician of like or similar training would do under like or similar circumstances. That is the standard of care. If you are looking for perfection, find another Universe.

The expert witnesses were used effectively. It is always easy for a plaintiff's attorney to say to the jury that if the physician had only admitted the patient, everything would be good at this time. On that basis, we have to admit 100% of our patients. Judgment is still what separates qualified from unqualified physicians, and the judgments made in this case were good. It is my prediction that because of the huge amounts of money that would have been asked for in this case, the insurance company would have been willing to try the case simply because a reasonable financial settlement could not be obtained.

I would have advised the physician if he wished to settle within his policy limits, to have stated such in a letter to the insurance company. This is referred to as a "bad faith" letter and it would be required should an excess verdict be obtained which would threaten the personal assets of the physicians. If the defendant is willing to settle and tender policy limits, but the insurance company proceeds with the case, losing it for a judgment larger than the policy limits, it has done so in "bad faith," against the client's wishes and that will likely obligate the insurer for the excess limits judgment.

➤**Authors' note:** Greg's advice is good. The trial proceeded over more than two weeks with multiple experienced experts as Greg's recommendation of a plaintiff plan for sympathy (a short segment was reproduced at the beginning of the "Legal" section of this case); what did the jurors think?

V. Judge's Instructions to Jury (January 29, 2003)

The Court has given you the instructions on the law applicable to this case. In a civil case, at least six members of the jury [out of a total of eight] must agree upon a verdict. When you have reached a verdict you will select and complete the verdict forms according to your decision. In fulfilling your duty as jurors, your efforts must be to arrive at a fair and just verdict. Each of you must decide this case for yourself, but, you should do so only after a discussion of the case with your fellow jurors.

VI. The Twist

As the jurors leave the courtroom to deliberate, there is a flurry of activity on both sides. A defense offer of $500,000 to settle had already been declined, but an emergency call from the insurance company reaches the defense attorney, cell phone in hand; their new offer is increased to $750,000. This is conveyed to the plaintiff's attorney who, after deliberating with the client in a hotel room across the street, declines the offer. Panic ensues as the insurance company is told of the rejection and the ante is upped to $1,000,000. Additional telephone calls are placed, but the offer is again rejected by the plaintiff.

Per the defense attorney, Mr. Huffman: "I felt from a scientific standpoint we had a winner, but I kept looking at a lady in a wheelchair. I was not confident [the jury] would walk away from her. They were asking for almost $15 million, which I did not think they would get, but I would not have been surprised with $4–5 million. Our defendant was very good."

VII. The Verdict

THE COURT: It's January 29th, 2003. The record should reflect that the parties are all present, with counsel. The jury has indicated that they have reached verdicts. Mr. Spino, I understand you were selected as the foreperson.
JURY FOREMAN: Yes, your Honor.

THE COURT: Congratulations. Have you reached verdicts?
JURY FOREMAN: Yes, we have, sir.

"We, the jury, being duly impaneled, sworn and affirmed, find for the defendants with respect to the claim against the defendant:

Number One—Seth Hockenberry [ED doctor first visit]: "Do you find that defendant Dr. Seth A. Hockenberry was negligent?" It's circled "no." The same seven jurors signed that verdict form.

Number two—Robert Carozza [ED doctor second visit]: The second verdict is signed by seven jurors. "Do you find that defendant Dr. Robert Carozza was negligent?' The answer circled is 'no.' "

THE COURT: Ladies and gentlemen of the jury, this obviously was a long case and a very difficult case. Throughout the trial, as I would look over and watch you folks, I know you you didn't take your job lightly. I appreciate your willingness to sacrifice the time that you put into this. The parties had a dispute they couldn't resolve. Our system says that we call upon eight citizens to help resolve the issues. You did everything you were called upon to do—you should be proud of your service.

You are now free of any obligations. You can discuss this case now with anyone you want. That's entirely up to you. You are free from any of the other restrictions that I have been saying throughout about discussing the case or talking it over with anyone. Anything else from any counsel before I excuse the jury from the case? Plaintiffs?
MR. O'NEIL: Nothing, your Honor.
MR. HUFFMAN: No, sir.

➤**Authors' note:** The jury split 7–1, voting for the physicians-defendants. After the trial, the lead defense attorney was standing in the hall and saw the plaintiff being wheeled out of the courthouse. The wheelchair was being pushed by two people, one was the lone juror who voted for the plaintiff. When they exited the courthouse, she helped load the defendant into the van.

VIII. Legal Insight per Attorneys in this Case

Thoughts from defense attorney:

- The jury didn't buy whether two ED doctors ought to have been able to diagnose postpartum eclampsia when an OB who has testified at 450 trials had only seen it once.

Thoughts from plaintiff's attorney:

- I think about this case at least once a week.
- The ED docs won the case as they [the jury] thought "if neurologist couldn't diagnose it, how could we expect an ED doc to [make the diagnosis]."
- Once the case was settled with the neurologist, the case against the ED docs was lost.

➤**Authors' note:** The "Empty chair" defense is an excellent tool when available. Although it is inadmissible, it is glaringly obvious to the jury when a critical defendant is missing, such as the neurologist in this case. The jury is free to draw their own conclusion, which is often that liability was alleged and a settlement reached, thus pointing the finger of liability at the empty defendant's chair (that was vacated by the neurologist).

IX. Guest Author—The Legal Analysis: Robert Bitterman, MD, JD, FACEP

- President, Bitterman Health Law Consulting Group, Inc.
- Chairman, ACEP Medical Legal Committee
- Member and Immediate Past Chairman, Board of Governors, EPIC RRG
- Contributing Editor, Emergency Department Legal Letter

My perspective stems from 30 years practice in busy inner city emergency departments, as well as being the attorney, director of risk management, and faculty member of a large academic emergency medicine teaching program. Additionally, I am an owner, board member, chair of claims committees and chairman/CEO of malpractice insurance companies which insure only emergency physicians.

I'll comment on five aspects of this case:

A. How does knowledge bias influence retrospective review of cases?
B. What were the four main diagnostic failures in this case?
C. Should EPs interpret CT scans?
D. Is the EP's liability resolved when the patient is admitted?
E. Which factors determine the outcome of medical malpractice lawsuits?

A. How does knowledge bias influence retrospective review of cases?
Everything is easier in retrospect, especially when you are biased by knowing the ultimate outcome of the case. Unscrupulous plaintiffs' attorneys are particularly adapt at intentionally inducing *knowledge bias* in their experts; they hurriedly tell you the negligence, adverse consequences and poor medical outcome before you can inform them you really only want to know what the emergency physician knew at the initial encounter. If the care at an initial ED visit is what's in question, as it is in this case, I think it's much more valuable and fair to all parties to provide an expert opinion without knowing the eventual outcome. The government is frequently guilty of inducing the same bias when obtaining peer review for physician quality improvement hearings.

That said, I hope, but can't guarantee, that my comments on the two emergency department visits described herein would be the same even if I hadn't been provided the second visit data, the ultimate medical facts, expert opinions, trial evidence and author comments.

B. What were the four main diagnostic failures in this case?
I don't know if either emergency physician should have made the correct diagnosis, but a few things are certain. First, the diagnosis of sinusitis should not have been made; it was clear error. Second, the physicians should have done an LP. Third, the patient's obstetrician should have been involved. And fourth, better medical decision-making would have led either physician down a different pathway, and may have led to an earlier diagnosis.

1. Sinusitis?
Three distinct episodes of head pain described as sudden, spontaneous and "worst of her life," woke her from her sleep, and "indescribable, like my head was going to come off, or split in two" just *isn't* sinusitis. No way. To even entertain that diagnosis may be an

error, and non-improvement after treatment should cause the provider to question the diagnosis. The sinuses on the CT scan were completely normal; the described findings are routinely seen and provide no evidence of sinus infection, let alone a sinus infection sufficiently rip-roaring to cause severe headaches.

2. No lumbar puncture (LP)
The first physician clearly entertained the diagnosis of subarachnoid hemorrhage (SAH), and even wrote in his progress note that "at this time, I can find no evidence of intracranial bleeding." Well, it's hard to find evidence if you don't look properly. The scientific literature is crystal clear: any time a CT is done to look for SAH it is mandatory that a LP be done if the CT is non-diagnostic. I've seen at least half a dozen cases of negative CTs but positive LPs; these are the most important cases to catch early—those with subtle sentinel leaks.

The second physician considered the diagnosis even more and still didn't do the LP. He notes in the chart that there was a question of a herald SAH bleed yesterday, so he repeated the CT, and then as a final diagnosis writes, "Cannot entirely rule out a herald bleed, with undetectable subarachnoid hemorrhage at this time." This alone mandated a LP.

Furthermore, on the second visit the patient is postseizure, with no clear diagnosis, and the physician entertained encephalitis as a possibility, going so far as to even put on the chart, "I stated to the husband that she may have encephalitis, and an LP was indicated." Ouch.

To skip the LP because he was dissuaded by a consultant or "since our lab is limited" is also clear error and faulty reasoning, particularly in a confusing case where more data may be helpful. The CSF may reveal SAH blood, cells or protein and can be sent for cultures and saved/frozen for later testing with a lab less "limited."

3. Failure to involve the patient's obstetrician
In an otherwise healthy woman with no significant past history, new onset severe headaches, hypertension and no clear etiology, the obvious question is what's different in her life that is temporally related that could be causing her symptoms? Pregnancy, delivery, epidural anesthesia and recent hospitalization jump out as obvious considerations! The obstetrician's knowledge of those events may be invaluable.

If the first physician truly considered postpartum preeclampsia as stated in his deposition (I'll comment more on this assertion below), he had even more reason to talk with the patient's obstetrician. The second physician, though, was faced with a still more confusing picture in a much sicker patient; there's no excuse for not utilizing the obstetrician's expertise. There is every reason to believe the obstetrician would have suspected a vascular event and advised the emergency physician to obtain an MRI, which likely would have revealed the culpable pathology.

4. Failure to consider less common disorders
Emergency physicians should continually ask themselves the question, "What if I'm wrong—what serious diagnoses can be causing the patient's symptoms?" This is especially true

when considering whether to accept the diagnosis of "sinusitis" in a patient with symptoms that could be from a lethal disease, such as SAH, preeclampsia or other intracranial vascular pathology.

The emergency physician doesn't need to know all the odd or rare diseases, but should know enough to consider that this patient is in the sphere of the unusual and needs to be evaluated for an uncommon disease or an uncommon presentation of a more commonly-seen problem (such as SAH).

To make a diagnosis, you must first think of it. Pain from ischemia with hypertension as a reflex autoregulatory response to maintain tissue blood flow should be considered, particularly postpartum. Whether it's an odd vascular event or some rare cause of ischemia, such as "Call-Fleming syndrome" isn't the point. What matters is that the emergency physician recognizes that the clinical picture isn't in the ordinary category and that it needs further investigation to determine the etiology, including specialty consultation.

C. Should EPs interpret CT scans?

Should emergency physicians read head CT scans themselves? Absolutely not! First, it is not standard practice for EPs to read CT scans. So if you do read your own head CTs, no matter how good you think you are, you had better be formally credentialed by the hospital, and you had better be right—every single time. In this case, the physician's misinterpretation of the CT led to an incorrect diagnosis.

Second, certain deadly conditions, such as subarachnoid hemorrhage (SAH), can be quite subtle, particularly early on; precisely when you need to catch it. It can also be subtle later in its course, when blood becomes difficult to detect. Patients rightly expect someone with the training, expertise, experience and appropriate hospital privileges to read studies that can make the difference between life and death.

Where was the ED Medical Director, the hospital's risk manager or the insurance carriers which insured the hospital or the physician group? How could they allow the emergency physician to interpret head CT scans and discharge the patient without first obtaining a reading by a qualified radiologist? The plaintiff's attorney should have sued the hospital, the ED administrator, and the ED Medical Director right along with the emergency physicians; these individuals were equally to blame for the CT error, and it would have made the care provided look "sloppy" (just another word for "negligent").

Skilled radiologists make enough errors, and their interpretations or communication of their interpretations creates a great deal of liability for emergency physicians. It might surprise emergency physicians to learn that about 20–25% of hospitals don't even keep a copy of the preliminary reading in the patient's permanent medical record. Instead, they discard the preliminary interpretation and replace it with the final interpretation, which is contrary to recommendations of the American College of Radiology.[22]

This practice is medically and legally untenable. It doesn't honestly or accurately reflect the true course of events related to the patient's care, and it unnecessarily creates additional risk for the emergency physicians and the hospital. We frequently make very consequential medical decisions based on these preliminary interpretations.

With today's digital technology, all special studies (CT, MRI, etc) should be read by a radiologist in real time while the patient is still in the ED—not the next morning—and any acute significant findings communicated immediately by the radiologist directly to the physician. The preliminary interpretations must be *in writing*, must be *signed* by the radiologist interpreting the images and must be *maintained in the patient's permanent medical record*, exactly like the final reading of that same study is kept in the patient's records.

D. Is the EP's liability resolved when the patient is admitted?

Admitting the patient, even to an ICU as in this case, does not necessarily relieve the emergency physician of malpractice liability. There are a whole host of reasons that emergency physicians are successfully sued related to admissions, such as:

- Failure to admit to the appropriate level of care
- Failure to timely order the clinically indicated diagnostic studies
- Delay in consulting the appropriate specialist
- Delay in starting treatment in the ED
- Failure to communicate the seriousness of the patient's condition to the admitting physician

In this instance, failure to do the LP, failure to consult with the patient's obstetrician and perhaps even failure to order an MRI prior to sending the patient to the ICU, all fall squarely into this category. Failure to administer parenteral antibiotics in the ED to admitted patients with serious infections is perhaps one of the more common theories of litigation against emergency physicians related to admitted patients.

Whenever you know what a patient needs, "just do it"—don't assume it will get done in a timely fashion, or get done at all, by the admitting physician.

E. Which factors determine the outcome of medical malpractice lawsuits?

Physicians routinely underestimate the influence of non-medical issues on the outcome of malpractice suits. Good medicine is not good enough to prevent lawsuits, or to win lawsuits. Only 20% of lawsuits filed contain negligence; the vast majority of cases are focused on the care provided. Were you nice to the patient and family, did you answer all their questions, did the hospital systems break down?

The degree of damages incurred by the patient has a much greater correlation with the amount of settlement payment or jury award than the presence of negligence. The universal mantra of medical malpractice reinsurers is "how bad are the damages," prodding claims managers to set aside reserves.

In most cases, however, the prime factor in the outcome is the credibility and believability of the defendant. In this case, the emergency physician was not very credible. The comment made at deposition (which, by the way, is where defendants-physicians win or lose most malpractice cases) that "I thought of [preeclampsia]" is not logically consistent with his actions. Any physician who actually considered preeclampsia would have checked for peripheral edema and hyperreflexia, obtained a urinalysis for proteinuria, documented their presence or absence and likely discussed the issue with the patient's obstetrician. It sounds too self-serving to say that and likely wouldn't sit well with the jury.

Why didn't the case settle during jury deliberations when the defendants made a million-dollar offer?
Many factors impact settlement decisions, including the amount of money sought and the unpredictability of juries. But a major factor is sympathy for the plaintiff, especially when coupled with terrible damages. The woman in this case was smart, had kids and a husband, and a good job, but now is triplegic, requiring life-long care. As the defense attorney noted, "I kept looking at a lady in a wheelchair." The lone juror who favored the plaintiff and helped push her wheelchair out of the courthouse evidences the sympathy that the plaintiff attorney hoped to engender, which would lead to a multimillion-dollar award. The attorney had reasonably good expert witnesses, some medical issues to chew on and physician credibility issues to bolster his case. He chose to seek the $15M megascore, and ended up leaving a million bucks on the table.

The defense attorney was clearly concerned with the sympathy factor, but the settlement offers were forced by the insurance carrier or the defendants-physicians themselves. The physicians may have been concerned that they would be personally liable for any amount over their policy limits, typically $1M each, and demanded that the insurance company attempt to settle the case within policy limits. The plaintiff's rejection and failure to offer an amount within policy limits forced the verdict, and also saved the insurance company a potential "bad faith" claim from the doctors if it didn't accept a counteroffer within policy limits. (For additional discussion of a "bad faith" claim, see final chapter: "Help! I am being sued.")

Why did the physicians "win" at trial?
First, whatever this patient had was extremely rare, regardless of whether it was postpartum preeclampsia/eclampsia or a progressive postpartum cerebral angiopathy. Second, as the two attorneys involved opined, the jury didn't expect two small-town emergency physicians to be able to diagnose something so rare that the plaintiff's obstetrician expert had only seen once a zillion years ago, or that the neurology "specialist" wasn't able to diagnose either. Lastly, the jury may have believed the causation defense, that even if the physicians and hospital were negligent, their actions didn't materially affect the patient's preordained clinical outcome.

This case, in essence, presents poor physician care, lousy medical decision-making and incompetent, or at least inattentive, ED administrative leadership but a lucky legal result. It didn't have to end up that way.

X. Guest Author: Jonathan Edlow, MD, FACEP

Associate Professor of Medicine, Department of Emergency Medicine
Harvard Medical School

Vice Chairman, Department of Emergency Medicine
Beth Israel Deaconess Medical Center

Dr. Edlow is Chair of the June 2008 American College of Emergency Physicians (ACEP) Headache Clinical Policy Task Force

In addition to clinical duties, Dr. Edlow has authored two books for the general public: *Bull's Eye: Unraveling the medical mystery of lyme disease*, which was featured on Terri Gross' NPR show *Fresh Air*, and his newest book, *The deadly dinner party and other medical detective stories.*

I will start out by disclosing that I act as an expert witness on medical malpractice cases, both for plaintiff and defense. From the outset, there are two features about this case that draw my attention. The obvious one is the differential diagnosis of headache in postpartum (and pregnant) patients, which includes all the usual diagnoses, plus some less common but important ones. The second is a bit more mundane—how often does sinusitis really cause headaches?

Let's examine the second issue first. Sometimes, the most dangerous thing a patient can bring to the ED is a diagnosis, especially if it's a wrong one. The misconception about sinusitis being a common cause of headache is pervasive amongst both patients and doctors.

Despite the fact that patients often use the term "sinus headache," most headache specialists think that sinusitis is a very uncommon cause of acute headache.[6-9] The antibiotic that the first doctor started is not working, so the second doctor falls into the trap of "upgrading" the therapy for an incorrect diagnosis. In fact, many patients with self-diagnosed "sinus headaches" improve with triptans and most have migraines.[7,10] And photophobia, if it occurs at all with sinusitis, is neither prominent nor common. Acute sinusitis with undrained pus can cause headache, but chronic sinusitis never does.

Interestingly, the emergency physician uses the word "migraine" in the chief complaint. Maybe the patient used it, maybe not. But either way, be cautious about the words that patients use. It's one thing to dutifully document "sinus headache" or "migraine" if that's what the patient said, but it's quite another to assume it is true. Migraine headache has certain definitions: *At least five episodes of a specific type of headache that interferes with daily activities.* The doctor records that is has happened three times in the past eight days, but to assume that this new, "worst of life headache," beginning postpartum and associated with new high blood pressure, is a migraine or sinusitis is an unequivocal error.

The emergency physician then records a very complete physical examination; kudos for examining the fundi! The physical examination shows "minimal nasal mucosal erythema" and the "tenderness to palpation" over the frontal sinuses. What is "mild" nasal mucosal erythema? Is it the same as calling "mild TM redness" in a crying febrile six-month old so that there is a "source?" In a systematic review, sinus tenderness was not found to be predictive of acute sinusitis and mucosal color has never even been studied.[11] I cannot help but wonder whether these "findings" are recorded to buttress the diagnosis of sinusitis. Whether they were or not, they do not substantiate that diagnosis.

The emergency physician chooses to read the CT scan himself, not standard EM practice. If you are going to do so, you ought to be sure of your skills and understand what findings mean; the presence of "mucosal thickening" or "mucous retention cysts" should never lead to a diagnosis of acute sinusitis. An air-fluid level is one thing, but chronic mucosal changes are quite another. In this case, the radiologist reads normal sinuses, which drives a final stake through the heart of the incorrect diagnosis of "sinusitis."

So now we have a postpartum woman without sinusitis and with a new unusual headache associated with photophobia and new high blood pressure. Of course, the blood pressure could be due to pain or anxiety; however on re-exam, the pain is better, yet the systolic blood pressure is higher, eliminating that theory. In fact, in this case the elevated blood pressure suggests a brain abnormality that is triggering autoregulation, an increase in blood pressure to maintain flow to an ischemic (or injured) region.

So this brings us full circle.

A young postpartum woman, without a significant headache history, presents with episodes of severe headache for whom there is no clear-cut diagnosis. It is obvious from reading the chart that this physician was thorough, caring and a good documenter. But he was sunk from the outset by accepting the previous erroneous diagnosis of sinusitis and was the victim of diagnostic anchoring, a pitfall into which we have all fallen.

For this particular patient, in addition to the usual list of serious causes of headache, several specific diagnoses need to be considered. One ought to pose the question, "How likely are these other possibilities, given the epidemiologic context and the absence of another plausible diagnosis?" If one can rule out some of these diagnoses by history and physical examination, great, but if not, further testing is warranted.

Postpartum headaches have a large differential diagnosis.[12] On the first visit, I hope that I would have at least considered preeclampsia, PRES (posterior reversible encephalopathy syndrome), cerebral venous sinus thrombosis, SAH, pituitary apoplexy (was there any hypotension during delivery?), RCVS (reversible cerebral vasoconstriction syndrome— which can be triggered postpartum) and an arterial dissection. I can hear the reader saying, "really?" But I have seen all of these diagnoses at one time or another, and one must have a different checklist for pregnant or postpartum patients.

In addition, the epidural, if it punctured the dura, could have led to a subdural (which should have been seen on the CT), meningitis (for which there are lots of clinical reasons to exclude) and a postdural puncture headache (was the headache positional?). Clearly, further exam (reflexes), imaging (MR) and testing (UA and probably LP) were necessary to make many of these diagnoses.

On the bounceback, two additional symptoms develop, visual loss and seizures, and it is now clear that something bad is happening. The disposition (an ICU) is obvious, but what about the issue of in what hospital should that ICU admission be? We still do not have a diagnosis. Some of what the patient needed, an MR, a neurologist and probably an intensivist and obstetrician, was available at the first hospital. I would have done the MRI, with MRA and MRV first, since this would help quite a bit with a number of the potential diagnoses listed above.

As for the LP, although I admit that I was not thinking about encephalitis when I read the case, the reason for not doing an LP—that the lab at this hospital was limited (which I assume means could not do viral tests given the context in which it is mentioned)—does not make sense to me. Why not do the tap to see if there are cells or elevated protein or high or low ICP? Refrigerate some CSF for later testing. Or if the CSF was normal, then it takes some of these diagnoses off the table. Unless there was a focal lesion on the scan contraindicating an LP, then why not get more information in this diagnostically ambiguous case?

An MRI was eventually done and the first one showed some cerebellar ischemia, but why not do one up-front? If this required transfer of the patient, then she should have been transferred. She is a complicated patient who will benefit from the input of various specialists. She was in the first hospital for 10 days before getting transferred out, only after she was having decerebrate posturing.

Simply admitting a patient to an ICU does not necessarily get you off the hook. One wonders if this hospital had the resources to adequately care for this patient. PRES and RCVS are esoteric diagnoses. There is probably overlap and definitely uncertainty with respect to the relationship between eclampsia (pre- or postpartum), hypertensive encephalopathy, PRES and RCVS. The average emergency physician does not need to know all the details (though if interested, see the references 13–21) but does need to know when to ask for help. I would argue that this case is one of those instances. This is a very complicated case, at least by the second visit (if not the first)—why not consult other specialists?

On the first ED visit, one can understand why the expert witness considers eclampsia so likely, even if he did so over-dogmatically. The documentation, which was not skimpy, suggests that the treating doctor never considered eclampsia; otherwise he would have checked the reflexes, examined for edema and done a urinalysis. It is interesting to listen to the opening arguments and how a good lawyer will "spin" facts in either direction. Making these distinctions (between prepartum and postpartum eclampsia) is important.

Bottom line for me: Be very skeptical about the notion of sinusitis causing headaches; don't accept sinusitis as a cause of a new headache without air-fluid levels in the sinuses. If an antibiotic is not working, consider the possibility that you have the wrong diagnosis in the first place, not that you need a "stronger" antibiotic. In the postpartum setting, the differential diagnosis of headache widens to include many MRI-dependent diagnoses. Don't let a consultant talk you out of an LP if *you* think it will help. It's one thing to have never heard of PRES or RCVS, but it's another to not recognize one's institutional limitations. Some patients need tertiary care.

XI. Authors' Summary

Is there harm in getting unwarranted tests? Does this "therapeutic radiation" increase patient satisfaction? (I had a great doctor—he was really concerned—ordered tons of tests!)

Our patient's CT may have harmed her in another way; forget the radiation, the brain CT wasn't falsely *negative*, it was falsely *reassuring*.

Let's try and follow the thought process of the initial EP who ordered the scan. He has a patient with a severe headache and CT seems a logical choice—it's a headache, let's image the head—*but what was he looking for?*

1. Brain cancer—This would be a bizarre coincidence in a post partum woman with less than a week of headaches and no neurological symptoms. Has it happened in the history of the world? Yes. Was it happening here? No.
2. Subarachnoid hemorrhage—With around a week of symptoms, sensitivity of CT is just over 50%; if this life threatening diagnosis was a legitimate concern, an LP should have followed.
3. Meningitis—Well … would need some awfully good resolution.
4. Carbon monoxide toxicity, acute angle closure glaucoma, pseudotumor cerebri, temporal arteritis, carotid artery dissection, dural sinus thrombosis—if these serious entities are seriously considered – a brain CT is not the test.

Was this radiation therapeutic or misleading? Did it help the patient—did it help the doctor? You be the judge …

This case strikes to the heart of the EM encounter; how do we find bad disease in the routine complaint? As our contributing authors point out, there were more than several elements of this ED visit which were not routine, including the severity of the headache, the increased blood pressure and the "special-population" patient, a woman eight days postpartum. Headaches are usually nothing. But as EM physicians, we will see 150–200,000 patients over the course of our careers … playing the odds is not good enough.

References

1. Edlow JA, Caplan LR. Avoiding pitfalls in the diagnosis of subarachnoid hemorrhage. N Engl J Med 2000; 342:29-36.
2. Vallejo van Gijn J, Rinkel GJ. Subarachnoid haemorrhage: diagnosis, causes and management. Brain 2001;24:249-78.

3. Edlow JA, Malek AM, Ogilvy CS. Aneurysmal Subarachnoid hemorrhage: update for emergency physicians. J Emerg Med 2008; 34(3):237-51.
4. Chames MC. Late postpartum eclampsia: a preventable disease?Am J Obstet Gynecol 2002; 186[6]:1174-7.
5. Anon JB, Jacobs MR, Poole MD, Singer ME. First-line vs second-line antibiotics for treatment of sinusitis. JAMA 2002; 287: 1395-6.
6. Silberstein SD. Headaches due to nasal and paranasal sinus disease. Neurol Clin 2004; 22(1):1-19.
7. Eross E, Dodick D, Eross M. The Sinus, Allergy and Migraine Study (SAMS). Headache 2007; 47(2):213-24.
8. Jones NS. The prevalence of facial pain and purulent sinusitis. Curr Opin Otolaryngol Head Neck Surg 2009; 17(1):38-42.
9. Jones NS. Sinus headaches: avoiding over- and mis-diagnosis. Expert Rev Neurother 2009 ;9(4):439-44.
10. Kari E, DelGaudio JM. Treatment of sinus headache as migraine: the diagnostic utility of triptans. Laryngoscope 2008;118(12):2235-9.
11. Williams JW, Jr., Simel DL. Does this patient have sinusitis? Diagnosing acute sinusitis by history and physical examination. JAMA 1993; 270(10):1242-6.
12. Stella CL, Jodicke CD, How HY, et al. Postpartum headache: is your work-up complete? Am J Obstet Gynecol 2007;196(4):318 e1-7.
13. Singhal AB, Bernstein RA. Postpartum angiopathy and other cerebral vasoconstriction syndromes. Neurocrit Care 2005; 3(1):91-7.
14. Calabrese LH, Dodick DW, Schwedt TJ, et al. Narrative review: reversible cerebral vasoconstriction syndromes. Ann Intern Med 2007; 146(1):34-44.
15. Chandrashekaran S, Parikh S, Kapoor P, et al. Postpartum reversible cerebral vasoconstriction syndrome. Am J Med Sci 2007; 334(3):222-4.
16. Gocmen R, Ozgen B, Oguz KK. Widening the spectrum of PRES: series from a tertiary care center. Eur J Radiol 2007; 62(3):454-9.
17. Katzin LW, Levine M, Singhal AB. Dural puncture headache, postpartum angiopathy, pre-eclampsia and cortical vein thrombosis after an uncomplicated pregnancy. Cephalalgia 2007; 27(5):461-4.
18. Lee VH, Wijdicks EF, Manno EM, et al. Clinical spectrum of reversible posterior leukoencephalopathy syndrome. Arch Neurol 2008; 65(2):205-10.
19. Fletcher JJ, Kramer AH, Bleck TP, et al. Overlapping features of eclampsia and postpartum angiopathy. Neurocrit Care 2009; 11(2):199-209.
20. Fugate JE, Claassen DO, Cloft HJ, et al. Posterior reversible encephalopathy syndrome: associated clinical and radiologic findings. Mayo Clin Proc 2010; 85(5):427-32.
21. Roth C, Ferbert A. Posterior reversible encephalopathy syndrome: long-term follow-up. J Neurol Neurosurg Psychiatry 2010; 81(7):773-7.
22. Monico EP, Forman HP, Goodman TR, et al. A survey of policies and procedures on the communication and documentation of radiological interpretations. Amer Soc Healthcare Risk Mgmt 2011; 30(2):23-7; and Practice Guidelines and Technical Standards. Reston VA: American College of Radiology; 2005.

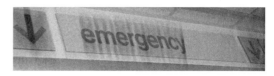

CASE 7

A 52 YEAR-OLD WOMAN WITH A COLD: *WHY VITAL SIGNS ARE VITAL*

Primary case author Kevin Klauer

PART 1—MEDICAL

    I. The Patient's Story 175

    II. The Doctor's Version (the ED Chart) 175

    III. The Errors—Risk Management/Patient Safety Issues #1–3 177

    IV. The Bounceback 178

    V. Additional Risk Management/Patient Safety Issue #4 178

PART 2—LEGAL

    I. The Accusation/Cause of Action 180

    II. Expert Witnesses Review of Case 180

        A. Plaintiff's Expert Witness 180

        B. Defense Expert Witness 180

        C. Treating ED Physician 180

        D. ED Nurse 180

    III. What Would Greg Do (WWGD)? 181

    IV. The Legal Proceedings: Depositions/Settlement vs. Trial—Outcome 182

    V. Legal Analysis—Daniel Malkoff, JD 183

    VI. Medical Discussion—David Andrew Talan, MD 185

    VII. Authors' Summary 189

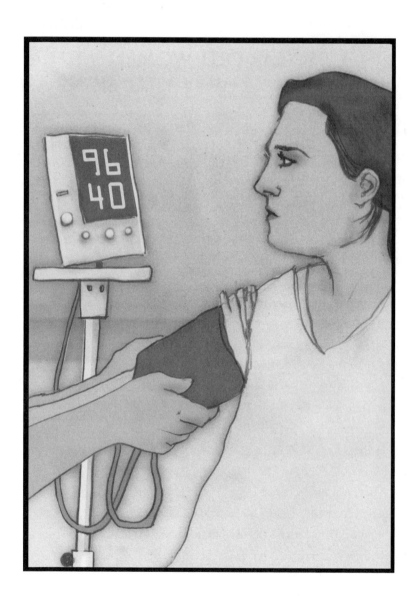

A 52 YEAR-OLD WOMAN WITH A COLD:
WHY VITAL SIGNS ARE VITAL

You know? The reality is that most of what we see in the emergency department is routine. Amongst those ankle sprains, prescription refills, rhus dermatitis, diarrheal episodes and upper respiratory infections are a few cases requiring us to check back in. The issue is recognizing when to hear the call to action. Considering serious pathology, while swimming in a sea of benign presentations, is critical.

Deep thoughts:

1. What are availability errors, and how do we avoid them?
2. Who is responsible when the nurse charts information after the physician has completed an exam?
3. Is a chest radiograph necessary in every patient with a cough?
4. How do we apply the diagnostic criteria for systemic inflammatory response syndrome (SIRS) in clinical practice without over treating patients?

PART 1—MEDICAL

I. The Patient's Story

Cindy Williams is married with three children, the youngest in the ninth grade. She and her husband both work full-time and share child-care responsibilities. Cindy has had bad colds in the past, but this time her symptoms are not improving. Initially she is not concerned, so upon presentation to the ED does not even ask her husband to come. Just after 4 AM, she presents to Faith Hospital.

II. The Doctor's Version (the following is the actual documentation of the provider)

Date: January 20, 2006

Chief complaint: Fever and cough for three days

Nurse's note (04:05): The patient aches all over, specifically her muscles and joints. She complains of a cough without sputum production. She denies sore throat, nausea and vomiting.

HISTORY (04:30): 52 year old female with flu-like symptoms for several days. Myalgias, cough w/o blood or sputum, feels weak and has poor appetite. Non-smoker, no history of asthma. No one else sick at home, couldn't sleep at all in spite of taking Advil.

PAST MEDICAL HISTORY:
  Allergies: NKDA
  Meds: Advil
  PMH/PSH: Negative
  FH: Negative

EXAM

```
VITAL SIGNS
Time  Temp(F)  Rt.  Pulse  Resp  Syst  Diast  Pos.  O2 sat RA
04:05 102.5    O    106    18    115   46     U     96%
```

CONSTITUTIONAL: Febrile, complaining of pain
THROAT: Normal pharynx with no tonsillar hypertrophy.
NECK: Supple; non-tender; no cervical lymphadenopathy.
CARD: Regular rate and rhythm, no murmurs, rubs or gallops
RESP: Breath sounds clear and equal bilaterally; no wheezes, rhonchi or rales.
ABD: BS+, soft, Non-distended
SKIN: Normal for age and race. Warm and dry. No apparent lesions
NEURO: Alert, interactive

ED COURSE:
05:00 – Toradol 60mg IM, 1gm Tylenol
05:45 – Physician Reevaluation: "Feeling better"
06:00 – Repeat vitals (RN) BP-96/40, HR-92, RR-18, T-101.6, Pox-96%, patient ambulatory, improved

DIAGNOSIS: Viral syndrome

PLAN (05:45) – The patient received pre-printed discharge instructions for "viral syndrome." In hand writing, the physician adds: Return if feeling worse, Tylenol or Advil for pain, see your doctor for recheck 2-3 days if not improved.

Scott Kelly, MD

III. The Errors—Risk Management/Patient Safety Issues

➤**Authors' note:** How could *this* case ever end in a lawsuit? It's just another URI, right? The patient had a normal examination and a clinical picture that could easily be explained as a benign viral illness.

Risk management/patient safety issue #1:

Error: Unaddressed abnormal vital signs.

Discussion: Vital signs are used for screening; this is the one universal test that all emergency department patients get. And just like other ordered tests, we are responsible for the results. In some circumstances an abnormal vital sign will prompt a test or further HOPI, while other times it will not alter the evaluation. The only wrong option is to summarily dismiss an abnormal finding, without noting that it has been identified and how its presence factors into the medical decision-making process.

✔ **Teaching point:** Acknowledge abnormal findings and discuss in a progress note.

Risk management/patient safety issue #2:

Error: Not recognizing the potential for cognitive error.

Discussion: Cognitive errors are common in medicine. The key to avoiding them is recognizing that they exist and knowing when they are likely to occur. The *availability heuristic* refers to a cognitive error generated by recent experience with a diagnosis. When physicians see the same pattern over and over again, we are likely to leap to this available diagnosis. Further compounding this pattern is that during cold and flu season, the "availability heuristic" is positively reinforced by the fact that most respiratory symptoms are from benign viral syndromes.

Pat Croskerry has termed CDRs, *cognitive dispositions to respond*. The availability heuristic is one such CDR predisposing "flesh and blood" (blink response) response without formal diagnostic evaluation. Some strategies to reduce CDRs are:

- **Insight:** Awareness that this type of process may result in error—the mere knowledge of this type of error reduces its impact on providers.
- **Considering alternatives** (an adequate differential diagnosis): Even the development of a brief differential will force consideration of alternative diagnoses, avoiding latching onto the "available" diagnosis."
- **Heightened metacognition:** Actively stepping away from the situation and examining the thought process. This technique forces the provider to consciously take control of the approach to problem-solving.

✔ **Teaching point:** Recognize that cognitive error is often at the root of medical error.

Risk management/patient safety issue #3:

Error: Not checking the discharge vital signs.

Discussion: Often patients have two sets of vital signs, one at intake and another at discharge. It is ludicrous to think that such an important piece of information is left for the physician to discover.

This case is an excellent example of failing to communicate critical results. This patient was discharged with a blood pressure of 96/40, decreased from 115/46. Although the wide pulse pressure could be easily overlooked, this may be a sign of vasodilation secondary to sepsis or merely a return to the baseline BP. In conjunction with a repeat blood pressure that is declining, sepsis should be strongly considered and a third BP documented to "break the tie." Another approach would be to reassess patients to see if they are symptomatic; in this situation an inquiry about dizziness.

✔ **Teaching point:** Maintain a high index of suspicion for high-risk headache patients.

IV. The Bounceback—Three Days Later

- Upon returning home, Cindy's condition remains unchanged; she continues to cough and experience intermittent fevers. On the third day after her ED discharge, her situation takes a turn for the worse with the development of shortness of breath, particularity at night, with accompanying dizziness. Awakening, she tells her husband that she needs to see the doctor. They call and get a "sick visit" appointment with their primary care provider, and this time he drives her there.

January 23, 2006
- AM: She is seen by the primary care doctor as an emergent "add-on" visit. She is breathing fast and doesn't look well. Husband is asked to drive her to the ED.
  - o Mental status – Alert and oriented
  - o Lungs – Bilat. rhonchi and rales
  - o CV – Tachy and regular
  - o Abd – Soft, nt
  - o Skin – Pale
- 10:30 AM – Cindy presents to a second ED in respiratory distress with complaints of pleuritic chest pain.
- **Physical Exam:** T – 100 (o), P-110, RR-28, BP-115/65, Pulse ox-86% (RA)
- **Testing:** Chest radiograph reveals multilobar pneumonia
- **ED Course:** Intravenous fluids, oxygen and broad-spectrum antibiotics.
- **Diagnosis:** 1. Pneumonia 2. Hypoxemia

HOSPITAL COURSE:
- Admitted to the ICU
- Develops ARDS, DIC
- Mental status declines and CT reveals a large intracerebral hemorrhage
- She is made DNR
- Dies three days after admission

V. The Errors—Risk Management/Patient Safety Issues

Risk management/patient safety issue #4:

Error: Not addressing the concepts of SIRS and sepsis.

Discussion: With the advent of early goal-directed therapy for sepsis, a new light has been shed on the assessment of patients who may be septic. The harsh reality is that the assessment and treatment of sepsis has evolved quicker than most providers have been able to adapt. What used to be a fever and tachycardia is now someone who could be septic. Tests aren't necessarily the answer. However, intellectual consideration of this diagnosis and documentation of your thought process is. Not only will this prompt consideration of the diagnosis, but will also prompt the improved delivery of care. The documentation should confirm that the diagnosis was adequately considered and explain why it was either dismissed or why additional diagnostic and/or therapeutic decisions were made.

✔ **Teaching point:** Consider sepsis in infected patients with hypotension.

VI. Initial Discussion of Sepsis and SIRS

To diagnose sepsis, you must first diagnose systemic inflammatory response syndrome (SIRS). SIRS, in combination with a source of infection, equals a septic patient. Although there is some debate regarding whether early goal-directed therapy is useful, early broad-spectrum antibiotics with aggressive volume resuscitation are not controversial.

The criteria for SIRS were established in 1992 by the American College of Chest Physicians and the Society of Critical Care Medicine:

1. Temperature $< 36°C$ or $> 38°C$
2. Heart rate > 90 beats per minute
3. Tachypnea ≥ 20 breaths per minute; or $pCO_2 < 32$ mmHg
4. White blood cell count < 4000 cells/mm^3 or $> 12,000$ cells/mm^3; or $> 10\%$ immature neutrophils (bands)

Any two of the above will meet the diagnostic criteria for SIRS. In this case, both the temperature and heart rate requirements were met. Since no laboratory data was ordered, we won't know if the WBC parameter would also have been fulfilled.

There are certainly issues of over inclusion with this broad definition of SIRS (see guest author commentary by Dave Talan below). We do treat and discharge many patients that actually meet the definition of SIRS. However, this does not obviate or mitigate our newly-found responsibility to address the issue in our medical decision-making and documentation.

Though a 17 year-old patient with an ankle strain, tachypneic and tachycardic from the pain, meets SIRS criteria, if there is an eventual diagnosis of sepsis, it would serve us well to document the chart around the potential missed case. For example, document why you elected not to pursue positive diagnostic findings for SIRS. The evaluation and documentation should reflect that there are other plausible reasons for the findings, such as dehydration, tachycardia from fever, or that the presentation does fit a clinical picture of sepsis. Documenting that your patient responded to the symptomatic treatment provided and that the positive SIRS criteria have resolved further strengthen your case.

PART 2—LEGAL

I. The Accusation/Cause of Action

- The allegation was wrongful death from inadequate evaluation and missed diagnosis.
    o Pneumonia and sepsis were both present at the time of the first ED visit as evidenced by the low blood pressure at discharge.
    o The patient should have had a chest radiograph and laboratory evaluation performed.
    o The low BP at time of discharge required re-evaluation by the physician.

II. Expert Witness Review of Case

A. **Plaintiff's expert witness:** In deposition, the plaintiff's expert described the low blood pressure as a "Smoking Gun." He also stated that this was likely never reported to the physician. Not performing a re-assessment fell below the standard of care. The patient probably had pneumonia and SIRS at the time. The physician should have obtained blood work and a chest radiograph, which are both readily available and inexpensive. Treatment at the time of the initial ED visit would have been life-saving.

B. **Defense expert witness:** The defense expert gave a favorable review. Although he acknowledged that there had been a change in, at least terminology, regarding sepsis and SIRS, this patient presented as a run-of-the-mill viral syndrome that should not have warranted further concern. The patient was doing well for several additional days after ED discharge before following up with her primary care physician. He inferred that she was stable at time of discharge.

The expert further discussed the low blood pressure and felt that it was not a "smoking gun for sepsis." The patient's normal blood pressure was in the 100s when she visited the primary care physician (per their records) and that this BP, with a reduced heart rate and improved symptomatology, represented nothing more than a "relaxed" patient. It appeared that the physician was never advised of the blood pressure. However, had he been, nothing different would have been done.

C. **Witness statements—ED defendant physician:** The ED physician stated that he didn't recall the patient. However, based on his documentation, she appeared well at the time of discharge and responded very well to the treatment provided. He does not recall being told about the blood pressure or any discharge vital signs. However, based on her condition, he was fairly certain that he would have discharged her despite the blood pressure if she "looked good."

D. **Witness statements—Nurse:** The RN reported that she did not specifically recall this patient. However, she confirmed that she would not routinely report such a blood pressure to the physician if the patient was clinically doing well. She doubted that she advised the physician, since she normally documents in the record: "physician informed [of repeat vitals]." There was no such documentation in this medical record.

III. What Would Greg Do (WWGD)?

Greg Henry, past president of The American College of Emergency Physicians (ACEP), Professor of Emergency Medicine at the University of Michigan, and CEO of Medical Practice Risk Assessment, has been an expert witness in over 2,000 malpractice cases.

Greg opines on vital signs, legal strategy and if he would settle.

If you're not going to defend this case, which one are you going to defend?"

A 52 year-old with a "cold." Stop! Enough! This is the quintessential ED case. There is a time when anyone, including your mother, can diagnose disease; there is also a time when no one can make a diagnosis because the disease hasn't yet appeared.

Clearly, this patient presented with a URI, everything says that. The emergency physician took reasonable history, did a reasonable physical examination and referred the patient for follow-up care. If you think that *this* case needs some sort of gigantic work-up—then all cases do. Even if you had the Star Trek machine (where you push the patients through the "diagnose-o-meter" and the disease prints out at the other end) you still wouldn't have found the diagnosis on the first visit—because it was not yet present!

This set of vital signs can be seen on any number of patients. "All patients need two sets of vital signs?" Horseshit! Are you actually doing a second set of vital signs on every finger lac? There is not even clear science on the first set of many patients, unless you are going to use it as a screening mechanism to improve public health. Be careful what you wish for—judgment is still required. I do agree that the blood pressure variation in this case is worth noting since 115/46 is a wide pulse pressure, but it is not uncommon in certain small and ectomorphic individuals. To assign this directly to a hypovolemic shock when the pulse rate is normal would be a stretch.

The defense strategy needs to point out that the patient did see her own physician in a reasonable time frame as instructed and was not septic at that time. They should also highlight that we cannot crucify every physician based on one vital sign reading.

Using my insurance company lens, I would recommend to the defense that they should be very slow to settle. If you're not going to defend this case, which one are you going to defend? The only way I could be convinced to settle is if it was an amount less than it would cost to take the matter to trial. I have a very hard time believing that a jury with some common sense would not recognize the fact that early on this disease entity can be very difficult to diagnose. Everyone on the jury has had a fever, cough, and chills—and most of them didn't even go to the doctor.

As a side note, the question is always brought up as to whether a settlement is truly damaging to the physician. Settlement is an economic as well as a social decision.

Some physicians need to have their cases settled because they will be no good in court. I have seen physicians who on the stand would admit to the Sacco and Vanzetti killings, break down and cry, and plead for mercy for their incompetent souls.

The decision to settle is complex. The insurance company bases its rates on what a group has cost them. The group itself, as an entity, wants to have the lowest expenses possible to be competitive in their bid to obtain insurance quotes. Doctors who think that taking cases all the way through trial is essential for their professional reputation are wrong.

IV. Settlement or Trial?

Was Greg right? This case never saw the light of a courtroom.

It was settled for an undisclosed amount, estimated to be between $35,000 and $50,000. From one perspective, it is comforting to know that the physician did not have to withstand the grueling process of a trial; but it is also a tragedy. If this were a card game, the hand was folded prematurely. Despite its minimal weaknesses, it is a defensible ED case. The plaintiff's focus on the "smoking gun" blood pressure is her ace in the hole, but the ED physician is able to counter that a report on the second BP was never received, an undisputed fact.

The hospital's liability is different. A nurse working as an employee of the hospital creates substantial vicarious liability under the *ostensible agency* theory. Nurses are hospital employees, not independent contractors. Their practice is controlled by the hospital, and their subsequent liability is then assumed by the hospital.

Knowing that most tried cases find for the defense (85% of jury verdicts in one recent study[6]), a strong argument can be made to try this one. A complicating factor in this case is that the physician and hospital shared medical malpractice insurance carriers and were represented by the same defense counsel. Herein lies the problem; despite the fact that this case would very likely be decided for the defense, the physician's case is much stronger than that of the hospital. When the hospital and insurer consider the aggregate liability and the possibility of expenses and indemnity exceeding $50,000, the estimated settlement is easy. But from the physician's perspective, having to pay indemnity and have a mandatory entry into the National Practitioner's Databank, it is simply not fair when his liability was so limited.

Some policies require the physician's consent for settlement. If an insurer can settle a case for $50,000 and the physician is not willing to provide consent, the physician will have to sign a receipt of a disclosure and acceptance of any judgment or settlement that extends beyond the settlement amount ($50,000). What if, on the small chance, this case is decided in favor of the plaintiff with a judgment against the defendant-physician for $150,000? You guessed it. The physician will be responsible for paying the $100,000. When one's personal assets are at risk, the decision to settle becomes easy.

V. Guest Author—The Legal Analysis: Daniel Malkoff, JD

- Senior Assistant General Counsel, Attorney General of Ohio
- Ohio State University Medical Center

Mr. Malkoff manages and coordinates litigation for The Ohio State University Medical Center. In his previous position as Senior Deputy Attorney General, he was responsible for overseeing legal actions filed in the Ohio Court of Claims against state agencies and state colleges and universities.

He summarizes important facts which will be considered in a settlement decision, how assessments of settlement are entertained, and how these battles are waged in a university setting.

"Smoking Guns" and *facts* in this case

A "smoking gun" is typically meant to refer to a piece of evidence that is conclusive. This characterizing is often done to make a piece of evidence appear more important than it really is. While it is debatable whether there are any smoking guns in this case, there are several important facts that may be *perceived* in this manner:

- The plaintiff's declining blood pressure may have been suggestive of sepsis. Was this pressure (both wide and low) normal for this patient? The patient's low blood pressure at discharge is at the heart of the controversy between the two experts and is not a good fact for the defense.
- The defense will need to contend that the physician was not aware of the abnormal vitals at discharge.
- A curious statement is the deposition claim by the ED physician that he was "fairly certain" he would have discharged her despite the blood pressure findings. The physician is trying to say that if he knew of the lower BP he still would have discharged her, but falls far short of saying "I would have discharged her even if I saw the repeat vitals." This equivocation moves the BP closer to a "smoking gun" category.
- A chest radiograph and CBC may not have been indicated, but they are cheap tests and a jury could be swayed to this fact. The defense will need to answer the question of why they were not ordered.
- The plaintiff will argue that there were several pieces of information pointing to sepsis and SIRS, which should have led the physician to order this additional testing:
    - Low and declining BP
    - Tachycardia
    - Fever

Are these smoking guns? Hard to say. But either way, they cannot be overlooked in the settlement analysis.

Should this case be settled?

The decision to settle a case is far from an exact science; reasonable minds may differ concerning the interpretation of the facts. But an informed prediction of success or failure can be accomplished through a careful and thorough review of:

- The medical record
- Depositions of health care providers
- Depositions of experts

In medical malpractice claims, determination of standard of care is largely a battle between experts retained by the parties. In addition to the substance of the expert's opinion, there is a less quantifiable factor: effectiveness in communicating an opinion to a jury. The expert may be a brilliant physician, but be perceived by a jury as smug, arrogant and unlikable. The deposition of the expert will assist counsel in assessing the demeanor, credibility and overall effectiveness of the expert.

The juries' perception of the defendant-physician is often the wild card in the trial setting. Even with hours of witness preparation, it is sometimes difficult to know how the physician will hold up in the face of relentless cross-examination and the stress of trial. For example, in our bounceback situation, counsel will need to take into consideration how well the ED physician and nurse will testify in court.

Will the physician come across as a caring, careful and experienced practitioner who made a reasonable clinical decision to discharge the patient? Or will he be perceived as a physician who paid minimal attention to this patient on a particularly busy night in the ED? His defense counsel will try to ensure that he is a charming, likable and credible witness in the face of the expected melodramatic spin that we might hear from plaintiff's counsel at trial: "He didn't even look at the vitals before discharging this incredibly ill mother of three who obviously had signs of sepsis."

Another unknown is the testimony of the patient's husband, with the potential to evoke great sympathy in a jury and inch them closer to opening up the proverbial checkbook. On the other hand, he may be viewed as an uncaring husband who didn't even bother to accompany his wife to the ED.

Other factors impacting a settlement decision include:

- Trial outcomes for similar cases within the jurisdiction
- Experience and ability of plaintiff's counsel
- Tendencies of the judge (if the case is a bench trial)
- The amount of setoffs (if available under the law of the jurisdiction)
- The amount of caps for non-economic damages in the jurisdiction

From the facts presented in this bounceback, my impression is that this may be a tough case for the plaintiff, but not a slam-dunk for the defense. I would consider settlement much like the defense did in this case. The patient presented to the ED with what appeared to be a run of the mill "cold," with fever, aches and pain. She had a cough but no chest pain, and she felt better after the administration of Toradol and Tylenol. Because of her improved clinical picture, she was discharged with the perfectly reasonable instruction to come back if "feeling worse" and to see a primary care physician for a recheck in 2–3 days if not improved. The fact that she was stable at discharge is borne out since she did not return for several days.

From the defense standpoint, it was reasonable for the physician to conclude that she had a benign viral syndrome. From the plaintiff's standpoint, demonstrating "causation" will be a challenge. In order to prevail, the plaintiff will need to prove by a preponderance of the evidence that quicker treatment would have saved her life. Nevertheless, with the benefit of 20/20 hindsight, the plaintiff has a story to tell and that story may compelling and persuasive to the jury.

Settlement/University Teaching Setting
In this case the physician and the nurse shared the same counsel and insurance carrier, which may be helpful to the defense because it will prevent public finger pointing, otherwise known as "the blame game." This is a game that plaintiff lawyers love; they can sit back and watch co-defendants point a finger at each other until the jury is convinced that one or both are negligent. The defendants become "crabs in a barrel," each trying to escape but ending up pulling the other back in.

In a university setting where the hospital, staff and physician-faculty members are insured by the same company, it is far easier to create a unified defense. Depending on the jurisdiction in which the suit is filed, university-employed healthcare providers may be entitled to immunity from personal liability for medical malpractice events; in other words, the university would be the sole defendant because it is responsible for the conduct of its employees. In this scenario, finger-pointing can be hashed out behind the scenes with counsel, and not in front of a jury. Such a unified approach to litigation maximizes the chance of success. It also makes it easier to analyze a case for settlement since defense counsel has more control over the testimony of parties.

VI. Medical Discussion—Evaluation of Respiratory Complaints/Diagnosis of Sepsis
Guest author: David Andrew Talan, MD, FACEP, FIDSA

- Professor of Medicine, UCLA School of Medicine
- Chair, Department of Emergency Medicine, Olive View—UCLA Medical Center
- Faculty, Division of Infectious Diseaes, Olive View—UCLA Medical Center

Dr. Talan serves on the editorial boards of the *Annals of Emergency Medicine, Emergency Medicine News* and *Pediatric Emergency Care* and is a reviewer for *Clinical Infectious Diseases, JAMA* and *The Medical Letter*. Dr. Talan has written and researched extensively on infectious diseases. He is triple boarded in emergency medicine, infectious diseases and internal medicine.

I review cases both for plaintiffs and defense. I have opined and testified for both sides, although my opinions often do not support the case of the referring attorney. My academic niche is the intersection of emergency care and infectious diseases. I am primarily an emergency physician, but occasionally practice as an infectious diseases consultant; as such, I am frequently asked to review medical-legal infectious disease cases that involve emergency department care.

As in this case, infectious disease medical malpractice cases often present with a similar prodrome; a previously healthy patient who has symptoms compatible with a non-specific viral illness. Sepsis, which I will address in more detail later, typically arises from a focus, except in the case of bacteremia related to certain conditions like endocarditis and neutropenia. In this case, the patient had earlier symptoms of fever and cough, and pneumonia was the primary infection found later. Therefore, a main issue in this case is whether there was evidence to suspect pneumonia at the first ED visit.

I have co-authored the pneumonia chapter in *Rosen's* textbook for many years, and this chapter is frequently quoted as a court exhibit.[1] In it, the symptoms and signs suggestive of pneumonia are discussed. In support of the defense's position, none of the findings that correlate with confirmation of pneumonia on chest radiograph were present in this case; specifically, increased respiratory rate, abnormal auscultatory findings and low oxygen saturation. Nor did the patient complain of chest pain, another finding suggestive of pneumonia. Therefore, a chest X-ray was neither indicated nor likely to demonstrate an infiltrate had it been taken at the time of this visit. Antibiotics are not only ineffective for bronchitis in otherwise-healthy individuals, but major public-health campaigns have been waged to encourage avoiding unnecessary antimicrobials with their associated cost and adverse effects.

The patient's symptoms certainly were consistent with influenza. We are not provided any details concerning the ultimate infectious etiology of her demise, but one possibility is a preceding influenza complicated by bacterial infection. This would be consistent with this patient's apparent minor illness for several days prior to her rapid deterioration. Delayed treatment of influenza was probably not as much of an issue at the time of this case. However, medical malpractice cases have recently increased related to the heightened public awareness of deaths associated with the H1N1 pandemic of 2009. In May of that year, the Centers for Disease Control and Prevention (CDC) recommended that anti-viral treatment (oseltmivir or zanamivir) be extended to include not only people with severe respiratory illness requiring hospitalization, but also those at high risk of complications from seasonal influenza, regardless of duration of symptoms.

This included children younger than five years-old (later modified to less than two years-old), pregnant women, people with chronic medical conditions and people 65 years and older. For healthy patients, anti-virals were recommended as a consideration if symptom onset was within 48 hours, which would not apply to the woman in this case who had symptoms for several days. However, had the patient been found to have influenza but had not been treated during her hospitalization, negligence could have been contended.

Another issue in this case is whether or not the patient had signs of sepsis at the time of the initial emergency department visit. Although it was not intended to, the creation of the term, Systemic Inflammatory Response Syndrome or SIRS, seems to have spurred a cottage industry of sepsis-related negligence claims against emergency physicians attempting to judiciously manage the sea of patients with seemingly benign viral illnesses.

In 1992 the American College of Chest Physicians (ACCP) and Society for Critical Care Medicine (SCCM) published a formal definition of sepsis to provide a practical framework to standardize the term in anticipation of future clinical trials.[2] This definition of sepsis required, in addition to presumed infection, evidence of SIRS, i.e., at least two of these four criteria:

1. Temperature $< 36°C$ or $> 38°C$
2. Heart rate > 90 beats per minute
3. Tachypnea ≥ 20 breaths per minute; or $pCO_2 < 32$ mmHg
4. White blood cell count < 4000 cells/mm^3 or $> 12,000$ cells/mm^3; or $> 10\%$ immature neutrophils (bands)

Any doctor can readily see that these criteria are so generous as to include most patients with benign infections and are completely unhelpful in discriminating a sick patient. I have been so infuriated by the misappropriation of this term that I wrote an editorial addressing SIRS in the Annals of Emergency Medicine.[3] The editorial accompanied an article that concluded that among emergency department patients suspected of infection, SIRS criteria did not confer a worse prognosis. I asked that, since hypotension, organ dysfunction, and elevated lactate levels have been correlated with prognosis and have been enrollment criteria of pivotal treatment trials (such as for the Early Goal-Directed Therapy study), we should return to the clinical and colloquial use of the term "sepsis" and abandon SIRS.

Indeed, the revised definition of sepsis by the same critical care societies now is more consistent with severe sepsis (i.e., organ dysfunctions) and septic shock.[4] As senior author of expert guidelines for sepsis management in the emergency department, I have emphasized that even these sepsis criteria only describe the presumed existence of an infection and at least a minimal systemic response, and therefore would not necessarily imply the existence of hemodynamic compromise or a bacterial cause, as is often suggested by the still-common usage of this term.[5]

In this case, we could expect to see plaintiff's attorneys with complicit experts circle an initial pulse of 106 and temperature of 102.5° and blow these up with a chart of SIRS criteria the size of the courtroom. Having said this, a little additional explanation of one's medical decision-making, documentation of a re-evaluation and follow-up instructions go a long way to avoid needing the help of an expert like me. To the providers' credit, both the doctor and nurse documented that the patient felt better just prior to discharge.

It was contended that the patient's blood pressures were concerning because of the wide pulse pressure and the decrease between initial and discharge vitals signs. The patient's systolic pressures were not below 90mmHg, the level typically used to designate concern for shock, and her accompanying pulse was not so high as to suggest impending circulatory collapse. The low diastolic pressure is somewhat concerning, but so non-specific as to be of little importance in a previous-healthy woman with other normal vital signs who looks well and has no findings to suggest a localized bacterial infection.

Of note, the most recent critical care societies' sepsis definition mentioned above only lists systolic blood pressure thresholds, but it also lists a mean arterial pressure (MAP) of < 70, and it was approximately 60 in our patient. However, these blood pressures are not atypical for many individuals, as supported by the patient's past blood pressures, and the "decrease" in blood pressure between emergency department admission and discharge was consistent with normal blood pressure variability. The fact that the patient felt better and was ambulatory upon discharge, despite not getting any fluid supplementation, supported the conclusion that she was not under-perfused.

Finally, it would be highly unlikely that this patient had untreated septic shock at the time of her initial visit since she reportedly was unchanged for another two days. For similar reasons, had blood work been obtained, it was unlikely to have demonstrated evidence of organ dysfunction, and white blood cell counts are notoriously non-specific and insensitive for diagnosis of bacterial infection.

In medical malpractice cases there typically is a yin and yang between negligence and causation. The plaintiff's attorney will attempt to argue that the patient was so sick that any reasonable doctor would have suspected the missed diagnosis, but not so sick that had appropriate therapy been initiated, the patient would not have been saved. The defense attorney will attempt to argue the converse; the patient was not sufficiently sick such that reasonable physicians would miss the diagnosis, but sick enough that had therapy been initiated, the patient still would have died. Sometimes, the facts support both negligence and causation.

The reason that infectious disease cases are among the most common malpractice suits is that they are potentially curable, provided that the diagnosis is suspected early enough. No studies exist in which patients with suspected life-threatening infections are randomized to immediate or delayed therapy and then followed for their outcome. Therefore, causation is largely expert opinion based on known outcomes of disease in general, the health and condition of the host and extent of the infection at the time of the possible earlier diagnosis, the virulence and susceptibility of the infecting organism(s) and the time between the possible earlier and actual treatment.

In this case, a strong argument can be made for causation since the patient was previously healthy, she appeared relatively well at the first emergency department visit, and the time between the proposed earlier and actual treatment with antibiotics was approximately three days. The defense would attempt to find an expert who might contend that her low mean arterial pressure, while not sufficient to have caused suspicions of impending septic shock, indicated that her disease process was far enough along that even earlier treatment would have been futile.

VII. Authors' Summary

To emergency physicians, this case is infuriating. But the take home "big close" point still rings true; how the patient looks on the way out the door will be the "bridge" of the plaintiff's attorney's argument.

References

1. Moran GJ, Talan DA. Pneumonia. In: Marx J, Hockberger R, Walls R, et al, eds. Rosen's Emergency Medicine: Concepts and Clinical Practice. 6th ed. St. Louis: Mosby, 2005.
2. American College of Chest Physicians, Society of Critical Care Medicine. American College of Chest Physicians/Society of Critical Care Medicine consensus conference: definitions for sepsis and organ failure and guidelines for the use of innovative therapies in sepsis. Crit Care Med 1992; 20:864-74.
3. Talan DA. Dear SIRS: it's time to return to sepsis as we have known it. Ann Emerg Med 2006; 48:591-2.
4. Levy MM, Fink MP, Marshall JC, et al. 2001 SCCM/ESICM/ACCP/ ATS/SIS international sepsis definitions conference. Intensive Care Med 2003;29:530-8.
5. Nguyen HB, Rivers EP, Abrahamian FM, et al. Consensus guidelines for the treatment of severe sepsis and septic shock in the emergency department. Ann Emerg Med 2006; 48:28-54.
6. Brown TW, McCarthy ML, Kelen GD, et al. An epidemiologic study of closed emergency department malpractice claims in a national database of physician malpractice insurers. Acad Emerg Med 2010; 17(5):553-60.

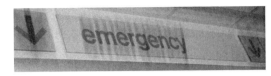

CASE 8

A 15 YEAR-OLD GIRL WITH RLQ ABDOMINAL PAIN: IT *IS* AN APPY ... *RIGHT?*

Primary case author Michael Weinstock

PART 1—MEDICAL

    I. The Patient's Story 193

    II. The Doctor's Version (the ED Chart) 193

    III. The Errors—Risk Management/Patient Safety Issues 195

    IV. Guest commentary—Patient handoffs: Ryan Longstreth, MD 198

    V. The Bounceback, as told by

        A. The Patient's Mother 199

        B. The Primary Care Physician 199

        C. The ED Physician (at the Second ED Visit) 199

        D. The Specialist 200

PART 2—LEGAL

    I. The Accusation/Cause of Action—Why Sue? 201

        A. Patient's Father 201

        B. Patient's mother 202

    II. The Legal Proceedings: Settlement v. Trial 202

    III. What Would Greg Do (WWGD)? 203

    IV. Legal Analysis—Karen Clouse, Esq. (Interview) 205

    V. Additional Greg Henry Comments—Defense Strategy 205

    VI. The Legal Proceedings: Depositions/Trial 206

    VII. Legal Analysis—Karen Clouse, Esq. (Interview): Continued 211

  VIII. The Verdict 213

    IX. The Motion for New Trial 213

    X. Medical Discussion—David Andrew Talan, MD 215

    XI. Authors' Summary 217

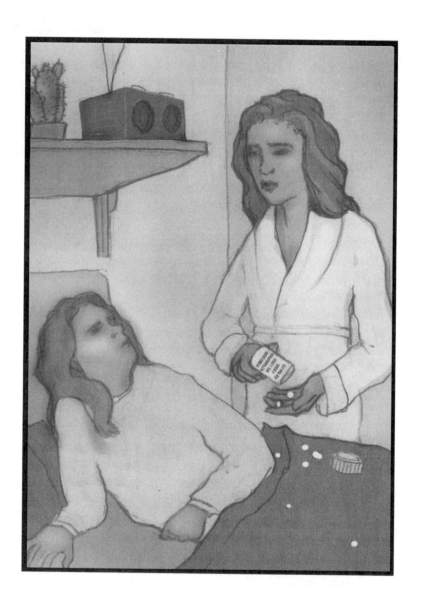

A 15 YEAR-OLD GIRL WITH RLQ ABDOMINAL PAIN: IT *IS* AN APPY ... *RIGHT?*

One of the red flags for a missed diagnosis occurs when the primary complaint could be serious, and there is no alternative diagnosis. For example, in a patient with fever and headache and absolutely no other symptoms, how can we say it is *not* meningitis without doing a lumbar puncture? This patient had symptoms suggestive of appendicitis with a positive WBC count "kicker." Enter the alternative diagnosis ...

Deep thoughts:

1. *Does a 15 year-old girl with pelvic pain who is not sexually active need a speculum exam?*
2. *What is the real medical and legal risk with end-of-shift turnover of patients? Does the data suggest a method to decrease it?*
3. *Is there a legal risk in getting a WBC count when the results are ignored in light of more specific tests, such as a CT scan?*
4. *Why do patients decide to sue?*

PART 1—MEDICAL

I. The Patient's Story

Ashly is a healthy, bright, and active 15 year-old girl; daughter and sibling, tons of friends. She enjoys movies, going to the mall, and is thinking of going out for cheerleading. But sometime in January or early February, like many 15 year-old girls, she was a participant in a seemingly innocuous event, a rite of passage. This action will have profound implications, not only for her, but for others in her community for years to come.

Our story begins on Monday, February 17, 2003, with nonspecific symptoms of fatigue, dizziness and abdominal pain. On Wednesday, February 19, Ashly goes to the school nurse and is sent home, but later in the evening the symptoms become unbearable. Her mother decides to take her to the hospital.

Close to midnight on Wednesday, February 19, Ashly and her mother present to the Emergency Department.

II. The Doctor's Version (the following is the actual documentation of the provider)

Date: Wednesday, February 19, 2003 at 22:59

Chief complaint: Abdominal pain

EXAM

```
VITAL SIGNS
Time  Temp(F)  Rt.   Pulse Resp  Syst  Diast Pos.  Pain Scale
00:12  99.8    T      124   18    100    64    S      10
```

TRIAGE (22:59): "pt mother states abd pain, dizzy, fever, passed out at school"

HISTORY OF PRESENT ILLNESS (01:12): The pt is a 15yo who is in good general health. No history of abd surgeries. No h/o ovarian cysts or endometriosis. LMP just finished. She states that she has had fatigue and dizziness in the past few days. Today the pt noted gradual onset of rlq aching which has worsened over the day. The pain is worse with movement and walking. + nausea without emesis. No diarrhea. No urinary sx. No vaginal bleeding or discharge. + fevers/chills. No earache, sore throat, sinus, cough, cold. No rash.
ROS: AOSN [all other systems negative]

PAST MEDICAL HISTORY:
Allergies: NKDA
Meds: None
PMH/PSH: Negative
SH: Non smoker, no alcohol

EXAM (03:42)
CONSTITUTIONAL: tired appearing; well nourished; A&O X 3, in no apparent resp distress.
THROAT: Normal pharynx with no tonsillar hypertrophy.
NECK: Supple; non-tender; no cervical lymphadenopathy.
CARD: Regular rate and rhythm, no murmurs, rubs or gallops.
RESP: Breath sounds clear and equal bilaterally; no wheezes, rhonchi, or rales.
ABD: BS+, soft, Non-distended; + tenderness in the rlq, which is reproducible , no rebound, rigidity or guarding. No CVAT.
SKIN: Normal for age and race; warm and dry; no apparent lesions.

ED COURSE:
01:09 – Orders for CBC and triple contrast CT scan to r/o appy. Demerol 25mg, phenergan 12.5mg.
01:52 – Labs return: WBC count 17.2, Hb 11.6, plt 230. Urine pregnancy test and dip - negative
02:09 (RN) – Pt. with about 600cc of emesis of food product. Dr. advised. Additional phenergan 12.5mg ordered. **Repeat VS: pulse 100, resp 24, BP 100/50**
03:01 (RN) – Pt. continues to c/o abdominal 6/10. Dr. advised.
03:42 – Patient care transferred from *DOC 1* to *DOC 2*. EMR records: "This chart has been electronically signed DOC 1. The receiving Physician accepted the transfer." At 3:58 DOC 1 orders another 50mg Demerol and 12.5 mg phenergan
04:00 – (sometime just after 4AM): CT "wet-read" results per radiologist: The appendix is normal in size without surrounding inflammatory change. Within the right adnexal area, there

are several greater than 1 cm ovarian cysts visualized. The largest is about 3 cm in dimension with hazy attenuation suggesting a recent hemorrhage.

04:59 – Repeat VS: pulse 88, resp 16, BP 98/48, pain scale 2/10

05:40 – Progress note *DOC 2*: "Patient resting comfortably. Family aware of results of CT scan for ovarian cysts on right. Will d/c with pain meds and f/u with GYN"

DIAGNOSIS *DOC 2* (05:40): Cyst – ovarian.

AFTER CARE INSTRUCTIONS: Follow-up with your physician in 2–3 days. Rx Vicodin #20, Phenergan PO and suppository. Instructions for ovarian cyst

Pamela Ramsey, MD
Kristen O'Donnell, MD

III. The Errors—Risk Management/Patient Safety Issues

➤**Authors' note:** The evaluation and management of this case was actually well done. A young woman with short duration RLQ pain and a CT scan showing a normal appendix is reassuring. Additionally, there was an alternative diagnosis: hemorrhagic ovarian cyst. The patient felt better, and she was discharged with a reliable caregiver, her mom. Her vital signs had returned to normal, and there was every reason to believe the management of her cyst could be completed as an outpatient. But a few red flags were waving … not waving high … not waving strong … but still waving …

Risk management/patient safety issue #1:

Error: Not repeating the abdominal exam before discharge.

Discussion: Abdominal pain is a high-risk complaint; we find a definitive diagnosis less than half the time. We are flying in the dark, using instruments (including our hands) to assess what is occurring in the abdominal cavity. Though many tests can "rule in" diagnoses, there are few tests short of surgery, which can definitively exclude life-threatening causes.[1] Ashly's CT scan showed ovarian cysts, but typically these cause symptoms mid-ovulation, not at the completion of menstruation. The radiologist noted findings "suggestive of" hemorrhagic ovarian cyst, but a definitive diagnosis remained just that, *suggestive*. Repeating the abdominal exam prior to discharge would have gone a long way toward confirming that a serious illness wasn't occurring, especially in a young patient who had received multiple doses of pain medications.

✔ **Teaching point:** Perform and document repeat focused examinations on all abdominal-pain patients.

Risk management/patient safety issue #2:

Error: Ignoring an abnormal test result.

Discussion: Current (and past) research is clear on the disutility of WBC counts, even suggesting that the mere act of obtaining a WBC count can lead doctors away from the correct diagnosis.[2,3] But if you do order a WBC count, an abnormal test result needs to be acted upon or explained in a progress note. Documenting a "real-time" progress note that the elevated WBC count was likely from stress demargination could have gone a long way toward explaining that a non-infectious explanation was suggested.

✔ **Teaching point:** It is easier to defend not ordering an inappropriate test, than not acting on an abnormal result.

Risk management/patient safety issue #3:

Error: Not addressing documented complaints, i.e., syncope.

Discussion: This is a recurrent theme in malpractice cases as well as a recurrent theme in this book. Why would a patient tell the nurse about a symptom but fail to mention it to the doctor? It is not all the patient's fault; the patient feels that after medical information is conveyed to a medical-care team member, it is accessible to everyone on the care team, particularly in the age of electronic medical records (EMRs). The fallacy is that the doctor often doesn't spend the time sorting through the tremendous amount of extraneous material in a chart to find the pertinent information, but is still responsible.

A good habit is to at least read the nursing triage note; it is hard to feign ignorance of this integral part of the chart. The nurse documented a syncopal episode, but this is not mentioned in the doctor's history, and a neurologic evaluation was not performed. Syncope is easily evaluated with a thorough H&P in a patient who is now alert and oriented, without current subjective or objective neurologic symptoms, and usually the only indicated testing is an ECG to evaluate for cardiac causes such as:

1. Brugada syndrome
2. Prolonged QT
3. Tachy- or brady-arrhythmia
4. Wolffe-Parkinson-White (WPW)/Lown-Ganong-Levine (LGL) syndrome
5. Hypertrophic cardiomyopathy (HCM)

Recognition of documented chief complaints does not necessarily require testing since many can be explored with H&P alone, and if a discrepancy exists, this can be documented in a progress note (e.g., it was documented that this headache patient had a fever, but I confirmed that their recorded temperature at home was 99.0° ... stated to be "a fever for me.")

✔ **Teaching point:** Address all chief complaints documented by the nurse/triage.

Risk management/patient safety issue #4:

Error: The patient's sexual history is just that, the *patient's* sexual history.

Discussion: For most patients, asking about sexual activity is a waste of time; can you imagine not doing a pregnancy test or a pelvic exam in an adult female patient with abdominal pain? A young virginal patient who denies history of sexual activity presents a different issue. Is it appropriate to have a young girl's first pelvic exam done in a curtained room at 3 AM with an obscenity-shouting drunk hand-cuffed to the bed next door? This decision needs to be made with the patient and her parent(s). If they refuse they need to understand the risk of misdiagnosis and the discussion documented. These doctors felt they had a cause when the CT returned a radiologic diagnosis of hemorrhagic ovarian cyst, but in light of recent sexual activity this would change the differential. Consideration should have been given to other causes:

1. Ovarian torsion (sudden onset of pain severe enough to cause syncope)
2. Pelvic inflammatory disease (PID) or tubo-ovarian abscess (TOA). Unilateral PID is unusual but not unknown and TOA can be diagnosed with an ultrasound (US).
3. Ectopic pregnancy is extremely unlikely with a negative pregnancy test. Consider heterotopic in patients undergoing fertility therapy, a history of PID or tubal ligation; none present with our patient.
4. Appendicitis missed on CT. Though the appendix was seen and noted to be normal, there remains a small percentage chance of false negativity for CT.

✔ **Teaching point:** If a pelvic exam is not done, document your recommendation and the risks of misdiagnosis. Document sexual history, particularly in young patients.

Risk management/patient safety issue #5:

Error: Failure to inform the patient and her family that the diagnosis is not definitive.

Discussion: Patients like to be told a specific diagnosis, prescribed a specific therapy, and then get better; who wouldn't? Unfortunately, this is rarely possible in the ED setting. Over 90% of our chest pain patients turn out to have a non-cardiac etiology; even the ECG diagnosis of STEMI is not 100%. Abdominal pain is a hazy, swirling habitat of peristalsis and visceral pain in close proximity to "big red" and a couple of very important "beans." The pain is subjective and often linked to psychological stress, but frequently a sanctuary for a life-threatening process—clearly an area in which to "proceed with caution." When a patient with abdominal pain is discharged, these simple instructions may be helpful:

- "We think your pain was from [some bleeding into an ovarian cyst], but we're not a 100% certain."
- Return after 12 hours if you have any pain whatsoever.
- Return immediately with fever, worse pain, blood in the stool or any other concerning symptoms.

✔ **Teaching point:** Informing the patient of "diagnostic uncertainty" will encourage returning if symptoms worsen or do not resolve.

Risk management/patient safety issue #6:

Error: Not taking "ownership" of a hand-off patient.

Discussion: In February, 2010, Cheung, et al., explored failures in a well-known high-risk area of emergency medicine, the patient handoff. This is discussed at length below. When a patient is accepted in a handoff, a focused exam and brief progress note will ensure that the initial physician's assessment was correct and that the patient's condition has not changed.

✔ **Teaching point:** Beware of handoff patients.

IV. Guest Commentary—Patient Handoffs: Ryan Longstreth, MD

- Co-author *Bouncebacks! Emergency Department Cases: ED Returns*
- Attending ED physician, Immediate Health Associates, Mt. Carmel St. Ann's Hospital, Columbus, Ohio

Patient handoffs in the ED are a fact of life, occurring between EM physicians and to the inpatient team. Unfortunately, these "sign-outs" may lead to potential medicolegal liability.

A landmark 2000 publication by the Institute of Medicine, *To Err Is Human: Building a Safer Health System,* concluded that Emergency Departments are susceptible to "high error rates with serious consequences." Errors in communication led to 70% of ED errors, while treatment delays were a direct result of poor communication 84% of the time. Nearly two-thirds of these treatment delays involved handoffs.[5,6]

Based on this 2000 IOM study, the Joint Commission (JC) established a list of patient safety goals, stating "The primary objective of a "handoff" is to provide accurate information about a [patient's] care, treatment and services, current condition and any recent or anticipated changes. The information communicated during a handoff must be accurate in order to meet [patient] safety goals." The JC's intent was to standardize the handoff process, making it clear and concise, allowing the opportunity for both providers to ask and answer questions.[7]

A February, 2010 article in the Annals of Emergency Medicine, *Improving Handoffs in the Emergency Department,* also dissected the handoff process. The authors looked to provide "up-to-date evidence and collective thinking about the process and safety of handoffs." The authors noted that improper sign-outs were implicated in 24% of malpractice claims. The article addressed both legal issues and risk management concepts with the following recommendations:

- Reducing the number of unnecessary handoffs
- Limiting interruptions and distractions during the handoff
- Providing a succinct overview
- Communicating outstanding tasks, anticipating changes and conveying a clear plan
- Having information readily available for direct review
- Encouraging questions
- Having a clear moment of "transition of care" from provider number one to number two

The authors do acknowledge the fact that there are few studies addressing the handoff process and little data suggesting the key points of a good sign-out.[8,9] Thus, the JC's intent of standardization of the handoff process is difficult at the present time.

Could these conepts have improved the care Ashly received in the ED? During visit #1 at 03:42, there is a note stating care was transferred from **DOC1** to **DOC2**. Unfortunately, it is unclear how well this transition was made since there was no note from the second provider as to when care was assumed and no repeat exam documented. A more delineated transition of care could have occurred with a phone consult to the PCP or GYN to review the work-up and ensure timely follow-up.

V. The Bounceback

➢**Authors' note:** The following excerpts allow us to trace the events in "real time." The story of Ashly's "bounceback" is told per interviews or deposition testimony by those involved in her care.

Ashly's mother, Linda Green: (from deposition testimony)—Early Thursday morning Feb. 20 to Friday morning Feb. 21:
- "[When we got home] I tried to feed her soup. She didn't keep it down. She was sleeping all day. She was cold. She was freezing, wrapped up in a blanket like you wouldn't believe. I knew she was in pain. She said, "Oh, my stomach hurts." She tried to get up and use the bathroom and she was just "uhhhh.""
- "I slept with her through the night. She would wake up in pain and I would try to comfort her. I didn't want to give her the narcotics no sooner than 4–5 hour intervals. When she got up to get dressed I had to hold her up. She was not feeling well enough to do things on her own. I was holding her in the bathroom.
- "I called my [family practice] doctor Friday morning [February 21]. I was giving her Vicodin, you know, I thought maybe it was because the cyst ruptured, I really don't know. I told them, 'She's really sick, she's bad off. You can either get me in there this morning or I'm taking her to ER.' They came back on the phone and said to have her there by 11:00.""

Jim Alexander, Family Medicine Resident: at 11:00 AM Friday, February 21, 2003:
- "I was asked to see Ashly and had never seen her before. When she arrived, she was in a wheelchair, quite ill appearing. Her skin color was an off shade of grey, and her head was bobbing. She could barely hold it up. She had diffuse abdominal pain, which was not clearly rebound. I was not able to get her up to the exam table. She was writhing and moaning in pain.
- "She was clearly beyond outpatient management. I contacted the Emergency Department and let them know that she would be coming over. We are fortunate that the ER is right across the parking lot. She was wheeled over and left in the hands of the ER doc."

Greg Decker, Attending Emergency Medicine Physician at ED #2: at 12:30 PM Friday, February 21:
- "I remember the details … I remember everything about this case; I can't get it out of my head. I was in there right when she arrived. I think I beat the nurse in the room. She was tender in the right lower quadrant, and I thought: should be a missed appendicitis. I figured we would get another scan and it would show a missed appendicitis. Didn't expect anything a whole lot worse. I'm sure we'll figure out what this is. The radiologist called me and she said, 'This is kind of strange. There is inflammation, but appendix looks OK. I don't know exactly what it is.' "

- "I figured I would do a pelvic exam. She had said she was not sexually active, and she was tender in the right adnexal. But there was no discharge or cervical motion tenderness (CMT) so we get an ultrasound (US) … it's got to be her ovary."
- "We did the US and really didn't come up with answer there either."
- "Her white count was low. I don't remember, maybe 2.5."
- "Looking at her now, she had been there for hours and was steadily worsening. I was watching this process happening in front of me, and I still don't have a good answer with all the medical technology I can throw at her. Something has to be done. So, I figured someone is going to have to open her up. I called surgery and OB."
- "The surgeons got there first and they said 'We don't think it's an appendix,' and I knew they were going to say that because the [CT] scan showed it was normal. They wanted to watch her overnight. The OB/GYN residents said, 'We don't think it's a pelvic problem, we think it's her appendix.' "
- "Tom Harmon was the OB attending, and Tom stepped up to the plate. He said, 'I'll take her to surgery and if it turns out to be abdominal, surgery is going to be standing by. We'll see what's what.' "

Tom Harmon, OB/GYN attending: at 7:00 PM, Friday, February 21:
- "I was just getting ready to go off call when I got the call from Greg [Decker]. I told him I would come and look at her. Ashly was lying on the gurney and looked very sick, and there was no doubt she had diffuse peritonitis and needed to go to the OR for a diagnostic lap."
- "I had a moment of time with the patient and bent down and whispered in her ear and asked her if it was true she wasn't sexually active and she said that she was [active]."

To the OR:
Friday, February 21 at 20:15 – [Blood pressure remains in the 80's–90's systolic]
- Per Dr. Harmon: "In the OR I started with a diagnostic lap, and pus just poured out through the trochars, and I realized there was no way I was going to do it laproscopically, so I converted to an open lap. The most amazing amount of purulent material extruded through the surgical incision and in her pelvis. The right ovary was spewing pus and there were exudates over tubes bilaterally and the left ovary."
- "The decision was made to copiously irrigate. As she had just been put on ATB, my hope was that we would be able to salvage her pelvis."

➤**Author's note:** Postop, Dr. Harmon informs the family that she may need to go back for further surgeries but as the ATB had just been started, they would first give them a chance to work.

Postop:
- **Friday, February 21 at 21:30** – PACU—Continued on broad-spectrum ATB including cefotan, doxycycline, flagyl and gentamicin. She continued to do poorly and remained hypotensive.
- Pressors are started.

Early the next morning:
- **Saturday, February 22 at 02:45** – Ashly is admitted to the ICU. Per her nurse, the family cannot be interviewed as "they were too emotional."

- **07:15** – The family practice service is walking up the stairs to see the patient when a code is called overhead. They arrive in the ICU to find Ashly in full arrest with the father yelling, "No, no … this is wrong!"
- Ashly is initially resuscitated and regains a pulse.
- A few minutes later she arrests again and is unable to be resuscitated.
- **07:45** - Tom Harmon (OB surgeon) arrives and speaks with the family

FINAL DIAGNOSIS: Ruptured ovarian abscess with sepsis and cardiopulmonary arrest

PART 2—LEGAL

I. The Accusation/Cause of Action

Why sue? The answer seems obvious; two loving and engaged parents have lost their daughter. But every day brings adverse outcomes and deaths and not all the doctors are sued. In a sentinel study published in Lancet, Vincent, et al. found that the decision to take legal action was determined not only by original injury, but also by insensitive handling and poor communication after the original incident.[4] Four main themes highlight the reasons for litigation:

1. Standards of care: both patients and relatives wanted to prevent similar incidents in the future
2. Explanation: to know how the injury happened and why
3. Compensation: actual losses, pain and suffering or to provide care in the future for an injured person
4. Accountability: a belief that the staff or organization should have to account for their actions

Several factors likely accounted for the decision of Ashly's parents to sue. The initial doctors were not able to give an explanation after the bounceback visit, since the patient went to a different hospital for the second visit. Additionally, the family may have misinterpreted a discussion by the surgeon Tom Harmon at the second visit concerning the elevated WBC count at the first visit (see father's testimony below). Finally, an internet search by Ashly's mother found information which, taken out of the context, suggested that antibiotics would have saved her daughter's life.

Following is deposition testimony of Ashly's father and mother (note: family names are changed).

Steve Smith (Ashly's father):

Q: Did anyone ever explain to you, any health care provider at [ED #2] the cause of Ashly's death?

A: The only thing I recalled him [Tom Harmon] saying was, he said something about the infection, said if we would have caught it earlier, and I told him we had been at [ED#1] 2–3 days ago, and he seemed surprised, He called and had them fax him the information. I recalled him, I believe, responding that her WBC count was elevated, and the way I took it is he was upset that they didn't notice that she had infection, the way I took it.

Q: Did he say that any of the physicians at ED#1 did something wrong?
A. No. I don't recall

Q: Has any health care provider told you that physicians at ED#1 did something wrong?
A: No, not that I'm aware of.

Q: And you feel that something more should have been done when Ashly was at ED#1
A: I do.

Q: And what do you feel should have been done?
A: [She] should have been kept overnight and watched and, if she had an infection, given antibiotics.

Q: Anything else?
A: No

Lucinda Smith (Ashly's mother)

Q: Has any health care provider told you that the ER physicians at ED #1 did something wrong?
A: No.

Q. What prompted you to file this lawsuit?

Plaintiff's attorney: Object. You're not to relate anything you learned from any of your counsel, me or anyone else in this office. But if you want to go ahead and answer, then that's OK.

A: Me and her father had discussed, you know, we talked a lot. "Do you think this should have happened," just conversations with other people. Boy, I had an ovarian cyst that ruptured and I was kept overnight and things like that and I kind of got to wonder if something else should have happened and that's just a concern I had.

Q: What kind of things do you believe should have happened?
A: I believe they should have kept her overnight.

Q: Anything else?
A: Knowing her white blood count level, I'm not a doctor or anything like that, but there's information "on-line," things like that that indicate to me that there was infection. I wish they would have just treated her with antibiotics. Of course, that's my belief.

Q: Do you recall what Web site?
A: I read it. I can always go back to it. It's right there.

II. Settlement or Trial

On October 12, 2004, approximately 1½ years after the initial visit, plaintiff's attorney Todd Stanley laid out his arguments and presented a demand to settle:

"Quite simply, given Ashly's presentation at ED#1 and with PID/TOA in the differential diagnosis, a pelvic exam should have been performed, which would have revealed adnexal pain and cervical motion tenderness which would have resulted in antibiotic administration and admission. Had this been done, it would have avoided this young lady from going into septic shock and she would have in all probability survived. While defendants claim they were led astray by a negative response regarding sexual activity (curiously the only piece of information in the case not charted) common sense would dictate not relying on such an inherently unreliable bit of information to rule out a potentially life threatening condition. I have conferred with both parents and have been authorized to communicate a [settlement] demand in the amount of $1.25 million.

So, now the allegations are clear:

1. The elevated WBC count should have prompted the initial doctor(s) to realize there was an infection and to start antibiotics.
2. Omitting a pelvic exam hampered the ability of the initial doctor(s) to make an accurate diagnosis.
3. She should have been admitted.

Would you settle?

Though honor and pride are at stake, many doctors will be surprised to find that their insurance company makes the decision to settle, not them. A contract signed just out of residency is forgotten 10 or 20 years into treating stab victims and sprained ankles.

➤**Authors' note:** The defendants were surprised to learn that Tom Harmon, the gynecologist who cared for the patient ate ED#2, was sitting across the table as a plaintiff's expert.

He fell into this role as one of his partners was a friend of the lead plaintiff's attorney and was asked to testify. To be clear, Tom is not a hired gun. I have personally known him for years, and he is honest, caring and extremely intelligent. He had never testified previously and has not since.

He described his feeling sitting across the table from the defendants, "I felt horrible. I realized these were two concerned doctors and I just felt horrible." He alleged that there was a delay in care and that a pelvic exam should have been done at the initial visit. Additionally, the patient did not have a firm diagnosis and should have been admitted.

III. What Would Greg Do (WWGD)?

Greg Henry, past president of The American College of Emergency Physicians (ACEP), Professor of Emergency Medicine at the University of Michigan, and CEO of Medical Practice Risk Assessment, has been an expert witness in over 2,000 malpractice cases.

Would he settle?

"Many people in this country have pelvic inflammatory disease. Almost nobody dies of it, unless you give it to my wife.

It should be understood, before I start my discussion, how incredibly tragic this case is. I cannot think of anyone I dislike so much I'd wish upon them the death of their 15 year-old daughter. There are no winners in this case. It is ugly from moment one. It sends shivers down my spine.

I *am* surprised that the barrel of this gun was pointed so directly at the emergency physician, there were many people involved. I am also shocked that the OB physician would give testimony against the emergency physician. This absolutely undermines the defense. The outrageous testimony of the OB physician would force me to think long and hard before taking this case to trial.

It is fair to view this case in an insurance company mode. Emergency physicians and physicians in general all want to try the science of the case. Courts don't care about science. Lawyers know nothing about science, and even if they did know something, couldn't give a wit. What they want to know is "what is it worth?" In a case like this, you have a grieving family who has lost the affection of a teenage child. The good news is this is not a 25 year-old with three children at home. There is no one dependent upon this young woman for support. This is not a 10 million dollar case. But we need to ask painful questions which go along with every malpractice encounter: How is a jury going to view this case? Is the doctor sympathetic? These are complex issues.

The insurance company will look at how often they would win or lose if this case went to a jury. They then take into account the actual money loss such as income and amount needed to support the family if they are dependent upon that income. All of these get stirred together with signs of the zodiac and whether the ground hog saw his shadow, and a number is derived.

This is the kind of case that I believe you would win six out of ten times. The great bugaboo in this case is the testimony of the OB physician, who in my opinion is the one who is at fault. He should have performed a TAH BSO when he saw the extent of infection. This needs to be taken into account.

Anyone who believes that this trial would not be an emotional experience doesn't understand the jury pool. No one is selected for the jury because of their excellence in integral calculus. The attorneys are looking to make Ashley "live again" in the courtroom. The fact that she has died secondary to a venereal disease can not be the principal issue.

In the hard light of day, knowing I had a physician who would be devastated going through trial, and knowing that I had a physician involved in the case pointing the gun at us, settlement would not be unreasonable. Is this worth $1.25 million? Maybe yes, maybe no. I would certainly get out of this case for $250K–$500K without thinking twice.

There are limits to insurance policies, and monies which go above those policies can come back to haunt the emergency physician. I have been personally involved in a case where the hospital had been dismissed and the verdict went above the insurance limits of the physician and he was forced into bankruptcy.

IV. Guest Interview—The Legal Analysis: Karen Clouse, JD

- Partner with Arnold, Todaro & Welch, Columbus, Ohio
- Defense attorney for this case

Authors: *What factors played into the decision of settlement vs. trial?*
KC: As in any case, there were a number of factors. We had two physicians-defendants who made very good witnesses in their own defense and could do a good job of explaining the decision-making process and treatment. We had good expert witnesses to defend their management. This was an unusual presentation which the subsequent treating ER physician and OB-GYN did not easily diagnose. Since they didn't recognize this as a tubo-ovarian abscess later in its evolution, part of the defense was that the standard of care didn't require our defendant doctors to suspect that "zebra" diagnosis when Ashly presented to the first ER. The entire defense team—attorneys, insurance company and physicians-defendants—were committed to defending the doctors' care rather than settling, and put in the time and resources necessary to do so.

➤**Authors' note:** The plaintiff's settlement offer was refused and the case proceeded to trial. Greg Henry continues his commentary with recommendations for defense strategy.

V. What Would Greg Do (WWGD)? (Continued discussion—defense strategy)

There are three aspects on which the defense needs to focus:

- The first is on the emergency physician herself. She needs to be coached so that at the time of trial her testimony is clear, concise and openly sympathetic to the family. She needs to emphasize the fact that she tried to put together the case and protect the patient in the most reasonable way. There is no way the emergency physician would have been clairvoyant; to know the future is not the way we practice emergency medicine. We have to make a decision based on reasonable probability. The emergency departments of this country discharge home approximately 85% of the patients seen.
- Second, the ultimate harm to this patient was related to surgical decisions on the part of the OB physician.
- Lastly, the complexity of managing disease, particularly when it falls outside the realm usual and customary activity, needs to be emphasized. Many people in this country have pelvic inflammatory disease. Almost nobody dies of it, unless you give it to my wife. The rare nature of the condition would likely have resulted in the same tragic outcome with any well-trained ED physician.

The jury needs to understand that one life has already been sacrificed; it is not up to them to ruin others. This patient was not given the "bum's rush". All good intentions were focused on obtaining the correct diagnosis. The jury has to draw a conclusion as to whether they believe the physicians cared about the outcome. Juries don't know much about science. What they do know something about is, did it "taste good." Did it appear that the doctors were actively involved in solving the problem?

I would like to close this section by highlighting what happens when one treating physician turns on another. This is absolutely unacceptable. First of all, another specialty cannot speak to the standard of care of *our* specialty. Second, as soon as the defendants start arguing and assigning blame, it's all over, but the shouting. This case is a plaintiff's dream; the young and beautiful dying before her time, physicians pointing fingers and a lost life in the midst of a wonderful family. Such cases are always difficult to defend and make for dangerous sympathy verdicts.

VI. The Depositions/Trial (April 2007)

The players: As Ms. Clouse, the defense attorney, previously discussed, the defendants decided to go to trial. It lasted two weeks and involved the testimony of many family members as well as expert witnesses. You may be surprised to learn that Tom Harmon (the gynecologist who cared for the patient in the second hospital) was one of them … for the plaintiff.

Cast of characters (names changed, except where noted):

Patient: Ashley Smith
ED physicians defendants: Pamela Ramsey and Kristen O'Donnell
Plaintiff's attorney: Todd Stanley
Plaintiff's expert witness: Tom Harmon, MD (OB/GYN)
Plaintiff's expert witness: Barbara Noonan, MD (EM)
Defense attorneys: Karen Clouse and Gail Arnold (actual attorneys)

➤**Authors' note:** Let's jump right in with Dr. Harmon's testimony/allegations. Remember how relieved Dr. Decker (at ED #2) was to have a surgeon willing to assume definitive care of the patient? Is an OB/GYN able to speak to a standard of emergency department care? That question will be answered by the jury.

The following is an interesting exchange by the attorney Mr. Stanley, who is revealing his plan to question the witness; the following is a colorful rhetorical comment by the defense.

Mr. Stanley (plaintiff's attorney): I intend to ask Dr. Harmon whether had Ashley been admitted and administered appropriate antibiotic therapy if she would have survived
Mr. Arnold (defense attorney): Do you believe if Kennedy hadn't been in a convertible he would be alive?

Cross-examination of plaintiff's expert witness Tom Harmon (OB) by defense attorney Gail Arnold:

Q. (by defense attorney): … you have certain opinions critical of Dr. Ramsey and Dr. O'Donnell, is that accurate information?
A. Critical of them?

Q. Critical of their care.
A. That's fair to say

Q. What opinion do you have?

A. There were some things that I would have done that were not done in the emergency room.

Q. What?

A. Pelvic exam of the patient primarily.

Q. Anything else?

A. Observation of the patient for a longer period of time.

Q. How long?

A. Twelve to 24 hours.

Q. Anything else that should have been done?

A. Allowed to say in hindsight, empiric antibiotics would have been given provided that her pelvic exam would have confirmed pain and adnexal [tenderness].

Q. So you're saying there may be some conditional action taken depending on what findings were produced by the pelvic exam?

A. That's correct. The outcome might have been different if that had happened.

Q. What do you mean by that?

A. This young lady died from overwhelming sepsis, and I might—I believe I expressed the opinion that if antibiotics were started early, that might not have happened. I do believe this was a very complex case.

Q. When you say it was a very complex case, you mean the manner in which the patient presented was difficult to ascertain exactly what was going on?

A. Absolutely.

➤**Authors' note:** Dr. Harmon is really not saying anything different than what we all know—the patient had an infection and antibiotics could have been helpful. He admits this is a tough case; however, this is a patient we see all the time. His experience with ED patients is selective, since he only sees patients *when we* decide to consult him, and these are not the average group of patients we see.

So how is his testimony refuted? The defense uses two main approaches. First, to show that the obstetrician is not trained in emergency medicine, so is not able to pass judgment on a different specialty.

Continued cross-examination of plaintiff's expert witness Tom Harmon (OB), by defense attorney Gail Arnold:

Q. You are not an emergency medicine physician?

A. No, I'm not.

Q. You're not board certified in emergency medicine?

A. No, I'm not.

Q. Since completing your residency, have you ever practiced as an emergency room physician?

A. Definitely not.

Q. Have you even practiced in the context of an emergency physician other than doing a rotation when you were being trained?

A. Only as a consultant to the emergency department.

Q. As far as triaging patients in the emergency department, you have no clinical experience?

A. No, I do not.

Q. Are you familiar with the standards of care then that are expected of an emergency medicine physician in triaging teenage female patients?

A. Not directly.

➤**Author's note:** This is a clever line of questioning, since there is no other way he can answer. The questions are repeated in a slightly different fashion so the point is not lost by the jury.

The second approach is to cajole Dr. Harmon into admitting that the diagnosis was so difficult to make that even upon entering the OR, a definitive diagnosis was not in hand:

Q. … you said sometimes it's difficult, and I was trying to ferret that out to determine whether or not her clinical situation really was that complex so as to not really know preoperatively which specialty would take her to explore. You're nodding your head. Does that mean you agree with what I've said?

A. There were questions even at the time we took her to surgery as to the exact cause of her condition.

Q. … you were surprised [with what] you found?

A. The extent of what I found, correct.

Q. Can you explain why you were that surprised? … her clinical presentation did not at all suggest the degree of severity of her actual condition?

A. That is correct.

➤**Authors' note:** Another witness for the plaintiff was Barbara Noonan, a board-certified emergency medicine physician. Though she had been hired as an expert in the past, this was her first deposition and her first trial. The initial responses support the care of the ED physicians, subsequent ones do not. Some of her allegations are bizarre, others hit home. How effective was she?

Cross-examination of plaintiff's expert witness Barbara Noonan (EM) by defense attorney Gail Arnold:

Q: Have you served as a medical expert witness in any other case prior to this one?

A: I have.

Q: On how many occasions?

A: Approximately six.

Q: You've been through this process which we're embarking upon today where there's a deposition taken to elicit your opinions?

A: I have never given a deposition in this circumstance.

Q: This is the first time you actually appeared to testify about a case?
A: Correct. I have been retained and asked for my opinions.

Sexual history:

Q: [Was it relevant whether she was sexually active]?
A: The history of sexual activity is well known to be unreliable, especially a young patient giving a history in front of her parents. It's probably not going to provide you with reliable information.

Q: Are you telling me that you don't trust what your patients tell you?
A: In this particular instance, we don't trust what our patients tell us. Patients are not always forthcoming and honest with that information.

Q: Is it below the standard of care for this patient's sexual history to not be documented in the record?
A: No, it is not below the standard of care.

Transition of care:

Q: Do you have criticisms of how the transition was handled?
A: The transition was handled as is typical.

Q: And was appropriate?
A: And it seemed appropriate.

Additional testing:

Q: [Was] additional testing indicated?
A: In my opinion, an ultrasound would have been the logical next procedure.

Q: Hypothetically, if the US had been done, do you believe that would rule out the need for a pelvic exam?
A: I think if a pelvic exam would have been done, it would at least be a reasonable certainty that PID would be diagnosed and she then would have received antibiotics.

Q: How would a pelvic exam be helpful in ruling out appendicitis?
A: It would be helpful to rule in other diagnosis, such as PID.

Q: By what findings?
A: Adnexal tenderness and cervical motion tenderness.

➤**Authors' note:** Attorneys don't know about medicine? How about the this next zinger of a question?

Q: How would that diagnose PID as opposed to ovarian cyst, ovarian abscess, or ovarian hemorrhage?

A: Clearly there is some overlap amongst the conditions. However, the commonly held dogma is that a patient with PID would have bilateral symptoms and tenderness on exam. In a thin patient, you should be able to feel the size of her ovaries. You should be able to feel her fallopian tubes if she's thin enough.

Q: And tell me how a tubal ovarian abscess feels differently from a hemorrhagic ovarian cyst on pelvic exam?

A: It would be hard to distinguish the two. However, in a patient with PID, they're going to have bilateral, adnexal tenderness, which I wouldn't expect in the case of a unilateral, one sided ovarian cyst.

➢**Authors' note:** Ever palpate a fallopian tube? Well, let's give the witness a break … this is her first deposition. The questioning continues:

Disposition:

Q. Should she have been discharged?

A: The patient should not have left the facility.

Q: And the reason specifically why the patient should not have left the facility is what?

A: I feel that the etiology of her pain and elevated WBC count was not fairly evaluated, and she should have been admitted for additional testing and consultation, which is the standard of care for a female with a WBC count of 17,000.

➢**Authors' note:** The following is the defense again hammering home the disutility of the pelvic exam, and the plaintiff's witness standing his ground that the exam was "absolutely required." Maybe it would have been easier to just comment on the pelvic exam at the initial encounter …

Continued cross-examination of plaintiff's expert witness Barbara Noonan (EM) by defense attorney Gail Arnold:

Q. [Had it been done], what would the pelvic examination have showed?

A. Cervical motion tenderness.

Q. Would you expect to find cervical motion tenderness in the presence of a hemorrhagic ovarian cyst?

A. That's certainly possible, yes.

Q. So the physical findings don't really differentiate between cyst and [abscess], do they?

A. No.

Q. All right. But you still think, in your own words, a pelvic examination was "absolutely required?"

A. I believe it was.

Q. "Absolutely" is a harsh word, isn't it?

A. I think that [word is] accurate.

Q. I've heard that in medicine you never say never, and never say always.

A. I've heard that—I'm not talking about a general comment, I'm talking about a specific patient.

Q. So you don't think there's any reasonable discretion to allow for not doing a pelvic exam on this patient?

A. Not the way she presented. It is a reasonably uninvasive procedure that we do in any young lady with lower abdominal pain. Are there exceptions? Yeah. But this one I don't see as an exception.

➤**Authors' note:** Let's drive this train into the station. Though the expert claims that all 15 year-old virginal patients need a pelvic exam, that a fallopian tube could be palpated, or that an ultrasound could have been done at 3 AM seems far-fetched, it is hard to dispense with the fact that a repeat abdominal exam was not done and the patient was not informed of the lack of definitive diagnosis, likely prompting her mother to continue giving Vicodin every 6 hours through the night instead of bringing her back to the ED.

How about the legal strategy of trying both doctors together? After all, they did have different degrees of legal exposure. The interview with the actual defense attorney, Ms. Clouse, continues.

VII. Guest Interview—The Legal Analysis: Karen Clouse, JD (second half of interview)

Authors: The two doctors were tried together. It would seem that the first doctor was placed in unnecessary legal jeopardy. Why did the defense make this decision?

KC: Especially when the care of two defendants is closely connected, as in this case, plaintiffs' attorneys are often unwilling to settle with one defendant, fearing that the remaining defendant will then employ an "empty chair" defense and point the finger back at the defendant who has settled. We believed the better strategy was for both doctors to be fully engaged at trial, defending not only their care, but that of their partner. At trial, the jury was asked to separately determine whether each defendant had met the standard of care in the treatment each provided to Ashly, and to render a verdict in favor of each defendant ER doctor.

Authors': What was the defense strategy?

KC: Our strategy was to repeatedly and consistently portray all phases of this ED encounter as thorough, caring and complete. Dr. Ramsey (ED doctor #1) took an appropriate history, did an appropriate exam and ordered the necessary and appropriate tests. Dr. O'Donnell (ED doctor #2) assimilated all of the clinical, laboratory and radiographic information in coming to a diagnosis and discharging the patient. The care met appropriate standards, and the diagnosis could not have been made at the time of the initial ED encounter, as reflected by the fact that it was not made when Ashly re-presented to ED #2 the next day. While we wanted to win on standard of care, causation was an important part of the defense.

Authors: *How did you refute the allegations that an increased WBC count meant an infection was occurring?*

KC: We argued that the white count can be elevated for reasons other than infection, including stress and inflammation. There was not a left shift which tended to mitigate against presence of an infection and suggested the elevation was due to inflammation, i.e., from the hemorrhagic ovarian cyst. Plaintiffs tried to take that one value out of context to argue that the defendants should have diagnosed infection, while we argued the entire clinical picture, including normal discharge vital signs and an afebrile patient was not suggestive of infection.

Authors: What additional/different documentation would have helped you at trial?
KC: Ashly's sexual history became a big issue in the case, with plaintiff's counsel arguing that the ED doctors mistakenly believed her history and failed to do an adequate exam. In reality, they didn't take her history at face value, as evidenced by the fact that Dr. Ramsey (ED doctor #1) did a pregnancy test, despite the history that she wasn't sexually active. It would have been helpful to have some documentation as to why a pelvic exam was not being done. Additionally, with the CT findings, it would have been helpful to have a progress note documenting that an alternate diagnosis had been discovered.

Authors: How can there be a "standard of care" for a one-in-a-million diagnosis?
KC: That's why medicine is an art as well as a science. If there was just a cookbook or checklist of items to meet the "standard of care," medicine wouldn't be practiced by doctors, it could be practiced by technicians. The standard of care is how to treat the presenting clinical signs and symptoms. A heart attack may not always look like a heart attack, and cases may be defensible if that "garden variety" diagnosis presents in such an uncommon way that the ED doctor cannot reasonably be expected to make the diagnosis. In the same way, the ED doctor needs to use the standard of care of a reasonably-prudent doctor in doing the necessary and appropriate exam and ordering the appropriate tests to try to come to the diagnosis or make the appropriate referral, but in the "one-in-a-million" diagnosis, that may not be possible.

Authors: Are there any colorful memories from trial or working with the defendants you would like to share?
KC: The white count was something that became more of an issue as the case evolved at trial. The plaintiffs were permitted to call a pathologist who had not been previously identified or deposed as a rebuttal expert. He testified that the white count elevation was indicative of infection and not merely inflammation. We then tried to call a "sur-rebuttal" expert to refute the plaintiffs' pathology expert, but the court refused to allow us to do so. One of the keys to success in defending a case at trial is having engaged defendants. Both of ours played an active role both before and during trial discussing issues, brainstorming the approach to presenting medical concepts to the jury and attacking the plaintiff's theories.

➢**Authors' note:** I have had several long discussions with the first ED doctor. She felt that her defense was augmented by sitting in on the depositions. This not only kept the experts "honest" but also helped to point out subtleties of the evaluation and management to the defense attorneys.

VIII. The Verdict

Were the arguments effective in convincing "eight people who couldn't get out of jury duty?" A legal verdict is more than a simple up or down vote. The jury needs to find the physician not only breached the standard of care but that this breach was a direct and proximate cause of the patient's poor outcome/death.

Though a "standards" defense is always preferable to a "causation" defense, the latter was an effective argument in this case. Even if the diagnosis had been made initially, it is hard to say if it would have changed the outcome. Additionally, even at the second ED, neither the pelvic exam nor ultrasound (two of the main allegations of the plaintiff) was diagnostic (in fact she had 3 pelvic exams in ED #2, with none showing discharge or cervical motion tenderness). An effective defense argument is that even if these had been done in ED #1, a diagnosis would have remained elusive.

Instructions to the jury (April 2007)

Do you find by a preponderance of the evidence that Dr. Pamela Ramsey (ED physician #1) was negligent in failing to properly evaluate, diagnose and treat Ashly's condition as it was presented to her at ED #1 on February 20, 2003?

- *8/8 jurors agreed "no"*

Do you find by a preponderance of the evidence that Dr. Kristen O'Donnell(ED physician #2) was negligent in failing to properly evaluate, diagnose and treat Ashly's condition as it was presented to her at ED #1 on February 20, 2003?

- *8/8 jurors agreed "no"*

Verdict: Unanimous verdict for both defendants in less than one hour.

IX. Motion for a New Trial

After a huge sigh of relief, the physicians are surprised to receive a letter on June 5, 2007. Plaintiff's counsel has filed a motion with the court for a new trial.

June 5, 2007

Plaintiff's Motion for New Trial

To the Court, Your Honorable Judge Myron Bender:

As you may recall, the trial of the medical negligence and wrongful death action consumed a full two weeks, involved sophisticated concepts of medicine and science, and involved the testimony of five expert witnesses on behalf of the plaintiffs and six for the defense. Faced with ten days of trial and the testimony of 11 expert witnesses, the jury in this case got a carry out lunch and returned a verdict in one hour!

How eight people could deliberate and consider ten days of testimony and reach a decision in one hour is unfathomable. The simple answer is that they did not even seriously consider the evidence, and rushed their verdict in their haste to get out of the house on a Friday. It is respectfully submitted that this conduct constitutes "irregularity in the proceedings of the jury" and "misconduct of the jury" under Civil Rule 59A-1 & 2. Allegations for appeal:

1. Irregularity in the proceedings of the court, jury, magistrate, or prevailing party by which an aggrieved party was prevented from having a fair trial
2. Misconduct of the jury or the prevailing party
3. The judgment is not sustained by the weight of the evidence

Respectfully,

Todd Stanley

Todd Stanley, Esq.

Defense response:

Response: Defendants Memorandum Contra Plaintiff's Motion for New Trial

While understandably disappointed with the jury's verdict against them, Plaintiff fails to present this Court with any legitimate grounds for granting a new trial. Plaintiff were given a full and fair opportunity to present their evidence.

1. Plaintiffs suggest that a new trial must be granted because of an irregularity in the proceedings as the jury deliberated for only one hour to reach its verdict. First, there is no mathematical formula mandating the jury deliberate a certain number of minutes per witness or days spent in trial. Second, although there were many witnesses, a number of common themes were addressed repeatedly. Third, the trial did span two weeks, but actual trial days were ten, of which the first was spent in jury selection and last in closing arguments. Additionally, six days started late or ended early. Given that the jury decided the defendants were not negligent, the jury did not need to consider testimony related to subsequent care at ED #2 or evidence on any proximate causation issues. Finally, the jury received the case for deliberations at 10:45 in the morning and had the entire afternoon to deliberate— they were not under time constraints. None indicated any conflicts or difficulties with deliberating as long as necessary to find a verdict. They consulted amongst themselves and were able to reach their verdict without long deliberation.

2. ➤**Authors' note:** There were other arguments … but you get the point …

Sincerely,

Gail Arnold

Gail Arnold, Esq.

Trial Court's ruling: On July 20, 2007, the judge dismisses the Motion for New Trial.

So who won? The defendants won the trial, but at the expense of four years of worry, endless hours of depositions and review of documents and likely subclinical PTSD. Who won? You be the judge.

IX. Discussion—Evaluation of Pelvic Pain/Diagnosis of Tubo-Ovarian Abscess (TOA): Guest author: David Andrew Talan, MD, FACEP, FIDSA

- Professor of Medicine, UCLA School of Medicine
- Chair, Department of Emergency Medicine, Olive View-UCLA Medical Center
- Faculty, Division of Infectious Diseases, Olive View-UCLA Medical Center

Dr. Talan serves on the editorial boards of the *Annals of Emergency Medicine, Emergency Medicine News,* and *Pediatric Emergency Care* and is a reviewer for *Clinical Infectious Diseases, JAMA* and *The Medical Letter.* Dr. Talan has written and researched extensively on infectious diseases. He is triple boarded in emergency medicine, infectious diseases and internal medicine.

I review cases both for plaintiffs and defense. I have opined and testified for both sides, although my opinions often do not support the case of the referring attorney. My academic niche is the intersection of emergency care and infectious diseases. I am primarily an emergency physician, but occasionally practice as an infectious diseases consultant, and as such, I am frequently asked to review medical-legal infectious disease cases that involve emergency department care.

This case comes down to whether or not the emergency physicians on Ashly's first visit should have suspected pelvic inflammatory disease (PID) and/or tubo-ovarian abscess (TOA).

The clinical diagnosis of PID is imprecise and many episodes go unrecognized, with consequences of tubal infertility and chronic pelvic pain. Therefore, it is recommended that providers rely on more sensitive but less specific diagnostic findings and err on the side of over-treatment.

This strategy is emphasized in the Centers for Disease Control and Prevention's (CDC) Sexually Transmitted Diseases Guidelines, last published in 2006. The previous guidelines from 2002 are similar to those of 2006 and would apply to the time of this case.[10] These guidelines state:

- "Empiric treatment of PID should be initiated in sexually active young women and other women at risk for STDs if the following minimum criteria are present and no other cause(s) for the illness can be identified: uterine/adnexal tenderness or cervical motion tenderness."

If PID is diagnosed in a stable patient, outpatient care is acceptable. However, if a TOA is diagnosed, then inpatient treatment with parenteral antibiotics is recommended for at least 24 hours. Of course, these recommendations should be applied based on the degree of certainty of the diagnosis and risk of complications if untreated.

In this case, the diagnosis of PID/TOA should have been an initial consideration in an adolescent girl with a history of fever/chills and lower abdominal pain. One criticism was that the charting did not indicate if she was sexually active. When she went to ED #2 she did deny being sexually active, so it is likely that she would have answered similarly at the first visit. The recorded history that Ashley denied vaginal discharge supported the doctor's assertion that she asked about intercourse. The fact that a pregnancy test was done at the first visit also indicated that they were not naive about the possibility that she might not be fully forthcoming about this activity. While one should be circumspect about the veracity of a teenager's response to questions about sex, particularly if a parent is present, a negative response would still logically diminish the likelihood that the patient was having intercourse.

Another criticism is that a pelvic examination was not performed. The likelihood that a pelvic examination would add diagnostic information not otherwise able obtainable by H&P, lab tests and CT scan needs to be weighed against the risk of psychological trauma from conducting this examination in the ED. Ashly denied vaginal discharge, and when a pelvic examination was done during the second ED visit, neither discharge nor cervical motion tenderness were found. One could certainly argue that positive findings would not have been found at the initial ED visit. Of course, documenting why it was not done would have better supported the defense's case.

It was contended that the elevated while blood cell count of 17,200/mm³ should have led to suspicion of PID/ TOA. Interestingly, the white blood cell count is not among the more specific findings listed for the diagnosis of PID in the CDC's guidelines:

- Elevated C-reactive protein and erythrocyte sedimentation rate
- Temperature > 101°F
- Mucopurulent discharge
- White blood cells on wet prep
- Laboratory documentation of *Chlamydia trachomatis* or *Neisseria gonorrheae*

Ashly's temperature was normal during her first emergency department visit. However, since she gave a history of fever and chills and had a significantly-elevated white blood cell count, infection should have been strongly considered.

The radiologist's interpretation of the triple-contrast CT scan is critical. He notes that the appendix is normal without inflammatory change, and there are right ovarian cysts, the largest 3 cm, with some hazy attenuation suggestive of recent hemorrhage. Note that no inflammatory changes are noted around the ovarian cyst. This was important supplemental information that could reasonably lead a physician away from the diagnosis of PID/TOA since:

1. It provided another reasonable explanation for Ashly's presentation.
2. The absence of inflammatory changes mitigated the suspicion of infection suggested by other findings.

Had the radiologist's impression of the first CT scan been "probable hemorrhagic cyst with surrounding inflammatory changes, cannot rule out tubo-ovarian abscess," then I think the emergency physicians would have had an obligation to consider TOA and consult a gynecologist.

Of note, the CT scan done two days later did show inflammatory changes but no "cyst," and in retrospect indicated rupture of the TOA. The defense argued that Ashly's diagnosis was difficult since it was also not immediately clear on the second visit. However, this was in part related to the fact that the abscess had ruptured and the radiologist was not able to compare it to the first CT.

Death from PID/TOA is rare, particularly in young healthy women. Ashly's abscess was 3 cm, relatively small, and in most instances would be successfully treated with antibiotics alone and no drainage. Most mortality associated with PID, rare as it may be, is related with rupture of a tubo-ovarian abscess, which in some even previously-healthy individuals can elicit an exuberant and catastrophic inflammatory response.[11]

No studies exist in which patients with suspected life-threatening infections are randomized to immediate or delayed therapy and then followed for their outcome. Therefore, causation is largely expert opinion based on known outcomes of disease in general, the health of the host, condition and extent of the infection at the time of the possible earlier diagnosis, the virulence and susceptibility of the infecting organism(s), and the time between the possible earlier and actual treatment.

The argument in support of causation in this case is compelling. Had Ashly been hospitalized and started on parenteral antibiotics at the first emergency department visit, it was contended that she would have survived since:

1. Mortality in treated TOA in a young, healthy individual is rare
2. Had she not initially responded or worsened, she could have had drainage prior to rupture
3. Had she ruptured, she would have been in the hospital and could have received earlier operative and hemodynamic support

The argument against causation is that parenteral antibiotics for 36 hours would not necessarily have prevented abscess rupture and its inflammatory consequences.

XI. Authors' Summary

What can we learn from *this* tragic case?

1. It is easier to defend not ordering an inappropriate test than not acting on an abnormal result. We said this in a previous case and it is true here also.

   • Getting a WBC count was destructive to the doctors at ED #1 from a legal standpoint since they had to defend against several allegations that an infection was missed.

When she presented to ED#2, the WBC count was 2.5, prompting the surgeons to recommend admission for observation of gastroenteritis, delaying her care. If you are ordering a WBC count because you think the surgeon will want it (a very charitable thing to do), ask the surgeon first if he/she will testify for you when you send home a "gastroenteritis" patient with an elevated WBC count who ends up having appendicitis *or* a 15 year-old girl with an elevated WBC count who you think has a hemorrhagic ovarian cyst.

2. When accepting a handoff patient, plan on spending 3 minutes per patient; two minutes examining the relevant body part and confirming the history and one minute recording your findings on the chart.
   - The handoff patient is truly a high-risk patient, and relative to the hassle of reevaluation, it is time well-spent. The three-minute technique will allow the receiving doctor to *take ownership* of the handoff patient, to confirm that the first doctor's H&P was accurate, and most importantly, to ensure that clinical progression is discovered.

3. Perform a repeat abdominal exam
   - Before ED discharge, on all patients presenting with abdominal pain, reassess at bedside with a documented repeat abdominal exam. This will serve to pick up progression of disease and to allow for additional discussion time to complete the "big close."

4. Inform the patient and family/friends about diagnostic uncertainty.
   - If Ashly's mother understood the radiologist's reading was *suggestive* of hemorrhagic ovarian cyst and not *diagnostic,* she may have returned earlier to be re-evaluated … and this chapter would never have been written.

➢**Authors' note:** Thanks to both of the initial ED doctors for making this information available and discussing the intricacies of the case, as well as to the multiple subsequent physicians who cared enough to remember the patient and take the time to explain their thoughts.

References

1. Rosen MP, Siewert B, Sands DZ, et al. Value of abdominal CT in the emergency department for patients with abdominal pain. [Journal Article] European Radiology 2003; 13(2):418-24.
2. Snyder BK, Hayden SR. Accuracy of leukocyte count in the diagnosis of acute appendicitis. Ann Emerg Med 1999; 33:565-74.
3. Silver BE, Patterson JW, Kulick M, et al. Effect of CBC results on ED management of women with lower abdominal pain. Am J Emerg Med 1995: 13(3):304-6.
4. Vincent Young M, Phillips A. et al. Why do people sue doctors? A study of patients and relative taking legal action. Lancet 1994; 343:1609-13.
5. Committee on the Quality of Health Care in America, Institute of Medicine. To Err Is Human: Building a Safer Health System. Washington, DC: National Academies Press; 2000:36.
6. WHO Collaborating Centre for Patient Safety Solutions. Communication during patient hand-overs. Patient Safety Solutions. 2007; 1: solution 3.

7. Joint Commission. 2006 critical access hospital and hospital national patient safety goals #2E. Available at: http://www.jointcommission.org/PatientSafety/NationalPatientSafetyGoals/06_npsg_cah.htm

8. Cheung DS. Improving handoffs in the emergency department. Ann Emerg Med 2010; 55:171-80.

9. Apker J, Mallak LA, Applegate EB 3rd, et al. Exploring Emergency Physician–Hospitalist Handoff Interactions: Development of the handoff communication assessment. Ann Emerg Med 2010; 55:161-70.

10. CDC. Sexually transmitted diseases guidelines—2002. MMWR Morb Mortal Wkly Rep. 2002: 51[RR06]:1-80.

11. Mickal A, Sellmann AH, Beebe JL. Ruptured tuboovarian abscess. Am J Obstet Gynecol 1968; 100[3]:432-6.

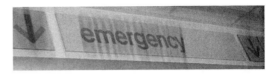

CASE 9

A 46 YEAR-OLD MALE WITH NECK PAIN: POUNDING A SQUARE PEG INTO A ROUND HOLE

Primary case author Kevin Klauer

PART 1—MEDICAL

    I. The Patient's Story 223

    II. The Doctor's Version (the ED Chart) 224

    III. The Errors—Risk Management/Patient Safety Issues 225

    IV. Against Medical Advice Documentation 230

    V. The Bounceback 230

PART 2—LEGAL

    I. The Accusation/Cause of Action 231

    II. The Legal Proceedings: Witness Statements and Depositions 231

        A. Initial ED Physician 231

        B. Patient's Spouse 231

        C. Defense Expert Witness 231

    III. What Would Greg Do (WWGD)? 232

    IV. The Legal Proceedings: Depositions/Settlement v. Trial 233

    V. Additional Greg Henry Comments 233

    VI. Legal Analysis—Jennifer L'Hommedieu Stankus, MD, JD (Interview) 234

    VII. Medical Discussion—Stephen Colucciello, MD 236

    VIII. Authors' Summary 239

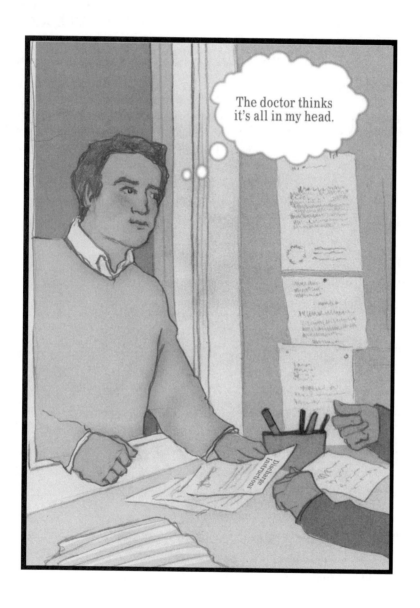

A 46 YEAR-OLD MALE WITH NECK PAIN: POUNDING A SQUARE PEG INTO A ROUND HOLE

The eye does not see what the mind does not know.

We are a proud bunch. Bizarre findings are often converted to a more plausible diagnosis, such as anxiety. The approach, "If I don't understand your pathology, chances are that it isn't real," leaves us with the "spackle" (the putty used for filling holes in dry wall) to fill the gaps in our knowledge. Of these spackling diagnoses, one of the most frequent is "anxiety."

Deep thoughts:

1. *Is the resolution of neurological symptoms reassuring?*
2. *Does diaphoresis suggest a more serious illness?*
3. *When we hear hoof beats, when is it time to go zebra hunting?*
4. *What constitutes adequate documentation of informed refusal?*

PART 1—MEDICAL

I. The Patient's Story

Steven Heller is a 46 year-old man who lives in a rural community. His daily commute is long; 90 minutes each way to the mill, where he works performing skilled heavy labor. He is happily married to Lauren with two children, an 11 year-old son and a 14 year-old daughter, Zach and Carolyn.

While driving home from work one warm, end-of-summer evening, Steve develops neck pain, a feeling his hands are not coordinated and a shaky feeling. Feeling unsafe to drive further, he pulls over to the side of the road and dials 911. While waiting for the medics to arrive, he also calls his wife.

At home with their kids, Lauren receives Steve's call. He is scared—this is not like him. She quickly gets the children in the car and drives them to her mom's house. On her way to the hospital she receives another call from Steve; dialing from the back of the squad. He says simply, "I think I'm dying."

At 9:02 PM, the paramedics arrive at the emergency department:

II. The Doctor's Version (the following is the actual documentation of the provider)

Date: September 6, 2007

Chief complaint: Severe left neck pain, blurry vision, loss of coordination both upper extremities

Nurse note (21:10): While driving home from work, the patient experienced an onset of severe neck pain, shakiness and uncoordinated hands. He pulled over and called 911. Now, without symptoms.

HISTORY OF PRESENT ILLNESS (21:32): 46 year-old male was brought in by ambulance after a frightening episode while driving home from work. He has never had a similar episode. He was fine earlier in the day. He was driving home when he felt hot, felt a sharp pain in left side of his neck, got shaky and felt frightened and uncoordinated. He then pulled to the side of the road, called 911 and was transported to the hospital. His symptoms improved during the ambulance ride. Now he feels normal. He reports no pain or weakness. No fever. However, he did report diaphoresis while in the car.

PAST MEDICAL HISTORY:
Allergies: NKDA
Meds: None
PMH/PSH: Negative
FH: Both parents had cancer
Soc hx: ½ pack per day tobacco use and occasional alcohol use

EXAM (21:34)

VITAL SIGNS									
Time	Temp(C)	Rt.	Pulse	Resp	Syst	Diast	Pos.O2	sat RA	Pain
21:10	37.1	O	76	18	160	90	U	98%	10

CONSTITUTIONAL: Alert and oriented, speaking and answering questions normally. No distress
THROAT: Normal pharynx, no swelling or exudate
NECK: Supple; non-tender; no cervical lymphadenopathy, Full ROM and no JVD
CARDIO: Regular rate and rhythm, no murmurs, rubs or gallops
RESP: Breath sounds clear and equal bilaterally; no wheezes, rhonchi, or rales
ABD: BS+, soft, Non-distended
SKIN: Normal for age and race; warm and dry; no apparent lesions
NEURO: Symmetrical motor and normal sensation, CN 2-12 WNL, gait normal

ED COURSE:
21:45 – The patient's wife arrives in the ED
22:00 to 24:00 – Testing:
- **EKG** – NSR @ 90 bpm, no acute st-t changes, no ectopy, early repolarization

- **CXR** – No acute disease, no pneumothorax
- **CT head** – No intracranial bleed, disease or abnormality (read by tele-radiologist)
- Laboratory results including CBC, BMP, and troponin are all normal

00:00 – Progress note: Patient ambulatory without signs and symptoms of CVA or cardiac disease. Patient prefers to go home and follow up with his doctor.

DIAGNOSIS (00:15)
1. Neck pain of undetermined etiology – suspect musculoskeletal
2. Stress related anxiety reaction
3. Situational stress at work

PLAN: Follow up with Dr. Abby Macerolla in 2–3 days if any recurrence of symptoms. Rx for Ativan 1 mg at bedtime (avoid if driving or at work). Return to ER if any symptom worsens.

Jim Carozza, MD

III. The Errors—Risk Management/Patient Safety Issues

➤**Authors' note:** Though the ultimate diagnosis is not always found at the first encounter, we feel compelled to provide the patient with a final product, a diagnosis. All good things, including ED visits, must come to an end, but that does not mean the *evaluation* is completed. The art is recognizing when a diagnosis is premature.

Risk management/patient safety issue #1:

Error: Inadequate history.

Discussion: Read the HPI again; it is sort of a funny history, a restatement of the triage chief complaint, then a bunch of stuff that is so obvious it is surprising it is included. Unless of course it was dictated at the end of the shift and not much was remembered. "The patient was well until he had symptoms" (really?). "The symptoms brought him to the ED" (really?) "and now the symptoms are better." OK. Additionally, the ROS are a bit brief: "he reports no pain or weakness." What's our differential here?

✔ **Teaching point:** Now at Case 9, we can't even apologize for being a broken record, so we will be succinct: "History is king."

Risk management/patient safety issue #2:

Error: Inadequate neurological examination.

Discussion: A surprising finding is that many cases which proceed to litigation have only a cursory H&P of the chief complaint, the core reason for the alleged negligence. A good rule of thumb is to document the chart, focusing on the chief complaint, as if we *expect* a misdiagnosis to occur—the billing/coding requirements should be secondary. For instance, in undifferentiated abdominal pain in a 12 year-old male patient, an independent physical examination for testicular torsion and appendicitis needs to be performed. In head injury cases, the neurological examination should be exhaustive, and at times, repeated.

In cases of neurological complaints, we should be focused on diagnoses of key clinical entities such as stroke, TIA, subarachnoid hemorrhage, and meningitis. The examination should reflect careful consideration of these life-threatening entities.

"Symmetrical motor and normal sensation, CN 2-12 WNL, gait normal" might be enough for an ankle sprain or GU complaint. However, when the presentation is neurological, a thorough neurological examination is required. Items such as mental status, cranial nerve assessment, motor strength, sensation, deep tendon reflexes and cerebellar function should be included.

You should ask,"Can I claim a thoughtful, careful evaluation and documentation for the possibility of serious neurological pathology? This doctor could not.

✔ **Teaching point: :** The history and exam should focus on the area of chief complaint.

Risk management/patient safety issue #3:

Error: Lack of recognition of serious neurological symptoms.

Discussion: Until we have been humbled by an unusual vascular distribution for ischemic stroke or symptoms we didn't recognize as acute cerebrovascular syndrome (ACVS), we are often quick to dismiss nonspecific neurologically-based symptoms. The operative term is "neurologically based." "Failure to diagnose" results in loss of the end-game before we even get started.

Unfortunately, the complexity of stroke syndromes is nearly endless. We have two choices:
1. Learn every possible variation in ACVS presentation
2. Recognize the complexity of the issue and our limitations

Both need to be done while resisting the temptation to explain away what we do not recognize as lacking a vascular distribution. It is the variation in presentations resulting from perforating vessel occlusion, watershed infarcts (often including the borders of multiple vascular regions), leptomeningeal artery (terminal end artery) infarcts and other partial vascular distribution strokes that are overlooked by the inexperienced or busy physician.

Adding further to confusion is ACVS caused by either internal carotid or vertebrobasilar dissection. These dissections often result in embolic phenomena, prompting symptomatology along the distribution of the dissecting vessel. A differentiating factor is pain, rarely present in traditional ischemic strokes or TIAs.

Although this patient didn't have a headache, his initial symptom was severe neck pain; such pain, followed by neurological symptoms, should prompt serious consideration for dissection. Do the neurological symptoms fit a potential vascular distribution of the vessels known to dissect in the neck? We may be able to discount the patient's report of "shakiness" and fright as too non-specific. However, upper extremity uncoordination makes sense from a posterior/cerebella circulation perspective.

✔ **Teaching point:** If there is a question about unexplained neurological symptoms, consider admission.

Risk management/patient safety issue #4:

Error: Overreliance on normal tests.

Discussion: A common error made in diagnostic data analysis is to assign more value to a test than is deserved. An excellent example is the white blood cell count (WBC) used in the decision-making process for the evaluation for appendicitis; how is a test which is only about 50% sensitive (and less in children) helpful?[1-3] Many of our surgical colleagues have assigned unwarranted importance on a normal WBC count. We've all heard the response on the other end of the phone, "Their white count is normal. They can't have appendicitis." Absurd!

Making dispositions for patients with neurological symptoms on the basis of a normal CT scan is similar. In TIA patients the CT would be expected to be normal, yet we often make the leap that a negative CT implies ischemia is excluded. We don't discharge patients at risk for acute coronary syndrome just because they have negative cardiac biomarkers; the same argument applies to a negative CT.

Even the MR is not 100% sensitive. Per Mullins, the negative predictive value of MR with diffusion-weighted imaging, standard MR and standard CT for ED patients presenting with suspected stroke is 73%, 42% and 24%, respectively.[4]

As imaging modalities improve, current thought is that many patients previously felt to have a TIA are actually experiencing a stroke in evolution. The evolution of terminology away from TIA toward ACVS reflects our understanding of the continuum of disease—a corollary to ACS.[5]

✔ **Teaching point:** Normal neuroimaging study does not rule out ACVS and should not factor into disposition decisions.

Risk management/patient safety issue #5:

Error: Using the diagnosis of anxiety without clinical basis.

Discussion: Diagnosing anxiety should make *us* anxious, even though it is such a significant part of our practice. Sometimes we pound such square diagnoses repeatedly until they fit into the round hole we are working with. Here's one for Bartlett's book of quotations, "Everyone dies, even if they have anxiety." Here's another, "Are there any patients in the process of dying who do *not* feel anxious?"

How can we avoid this? First, when considering an anxiety diagnosis, put the hammer away. If the diagnosis doesn't fit, then don't force it:

- If a patient doesn't have a previous anxiety diagnosis with history of similar symptoms in the past, use caution in initiating this diagnosis.
- If a patient isn't reporting the symptom of anxiety prior to the somatic symptoms, it is unlikely that anxiety provoked the event.

- Inform patients that we do not have definitive objective testing for anxiety, so if somatic symptoms progress or change, a return visit is mandatory.

When there is an adverse outcome, the use of the diagnosis "Anxiety" is likely to weaken the defense's case. Juries do not take kindly to assigning a psychiatric diagnosis to a plaintiff with real pathology. To the lay juror, this is the equivalent of the doctor saying, "It's all in your head."

✔ **Teaching point:** Unless a patient has a known history of anxiety and has experienced previous similar symptoms, resist the temptation to attribute the symptoms to anxiety.

Risk management/patient safety issue #6:

Error: Poor medical decision making.

Discussion: The first diagnosis is: *Neck pain of undetermined etiology—suspect musculoskeletal*. Now flip back to the neck exam: *Supple; non-tender; no cervical lymphadenopathy, Full ROM and no JVD*. ... you do the math.

✔ **Teaching point:** It is hard to explain neck pain as musculoskeletal when the exam documents a neck which is non-tender with palpation and full range of motion.

Risk management/patient safety issue #7:

Error: Not formally recommending admission.

Discussion: Should our patient be admitted? Though that question can be debated, one point cannot: it is not up to the patient to make the diagnosis and decide the disposition. What's the deal with the phrase, "the patient prefers to go home?" Unless the patient has subjective pain with ureterolithiasis, the doctor should decide if the patient needs a "room at the inn."

✔ **Teaching point:** If a patient requires admission, document your recommendation.

Risk management/patient safety issue #8:

Error: Not obtaining an informed refusal.

Discussion: The doctrine of informed consent includes informed refusal. Just as patients need to have the capacity to consent to treatment or a procedure, they must also possess the capacity to refuse. If a patient is not oriented to person, place, time and situation and is not of the age of majority (18–21 years-old, depending on the jurisdiction), he or she doesn't have the capacity to consent or refuse. Use of the term "capacity" is not incidental or casual, but it is a legal term which is differentiated from "competence," assigned by legal proceeding, not healthcare providers.

In this case, it is curious that the physician's documentation includes a statement that the patient would "prefer to go home." Admission was not specifically offered. Reading between the lines, the physician is hedging his bet. He may not feel admission is warranted, but he also finds reassurance that the patient would prefer discharge. Herein lies the problem; this is a dangerous tight rope to walk. Any good plaintiff's attorney, worth the price of his penny loafers, will trap a physician in his or her own web in less than ten minutes:

Attorney: So Doctor, you discussed admission with the plaintiff.
Defendant: Yes, I did.

Attorney: So you must have felt that admission was warranted.
Defendant: Well, it was one option.

Attorney: So, Mr. Jones refused admission?
Defendant: Not exactly. He said he would prefer to go home.

Attorney: Doctor, can you advise the jury what the elements are of an informed refusal?
Defendant (option 1): No. I can't.

Attorney: Then it is clear that you could not have obtained an informed refusal from my client.
Defendant (option 2): "Yes. I can. The patient must have the capacity to refuse, must be old enough to consent or refuse, and must understand the risks and benefits of the proposed treatment, any treatment alternatives and the option of no treatment at all.

Attorney: Did you go through this process with Mr. Jones?
Defendant: No, I did not.

✔ **Teaching point:** Casual conversations about admission to "buff the chart" are ill-advised.

IV. Against Medical Advice (AMA) Documentation

The seminal decision "Against Medical Advice" (AMA), sometimes called "The Cardozo Doctrine," was made by Justice Benjamin Cardozo (1870-1938), subsequently appointed to the United States Supreme Court by President Herbert Hoover to succeed Justice Oliver Wendall Holmes; "Seldom in the history of the Court has an appointment been so universally commended." (*New York Times*, February 16, 1932, p. 1)

The case was *Schloendorff v. Society of New York Hospital*. The plaintiff, Mary Schloendorff, was admitted to New York Hospital in January 1908 suffering from "some disorder of the stomach". She consented to being examined under ether, but not to have surgery. The surgeon found a fibroid tumor and, while Mary was under the effects of the ether, proceeded to remove it. She suffered from infection and developed gangrene of her fingers with ensuing amputation and severe pain. The non-profit hospital was sued with the intention to hold the institution responsible for the actions of its employees.

The New York Court of Appeals (1914), in an opinion written by Justice Cardozo, found the action constituted medical battery. The decision established principles of informed consent and *respondeat superior* (legal obligations of an employer for the actions of its employee) in U.S. law.

Per Cardozo: "Every human being of adult years and sound mind has a right to determine what shall be done with his own body; and a surgeon who performs an operation without his patient's consent commits an assault, for which he is liable in damages. This is true except in cases of emergency where the patient is unconscious and where it is necessary to operate before consent can be obtained."

Of note, the Schloendorff Rule was another byproduct: A non-profit hospital could not be sued for the actions of its employees. This was eventually overruled in 1957 in *Bing v. Thunig*.

Five items to document when a patient leaves against medical advice (AMA):

1. Patient is adult or emancipated minor.
2. Patient is of sound mind (Documentation can include specific questioning of each component of A&OX3 and/or that the patient does understand/comprehend the implications of her or his actions).
3. Patient has been informed of potential consequences of non-treatment.
4. Family, friends and/or the patient's physician have been involved in the decision-making process.
5. There is a signature on the AMA form of patient, family member, physician and nurse.

V. The Bounceback

After discharge from the ED, Steve leaves his car on the side of the road and drives home with his wife. They plan to get up early and for Lauren to drop him at his car so he can drive to work and she can return home to get the kids to school.

The alarm rings early. Sluggish from a 5 AM arousal, Lauren rolls over to wake her husband, but he is unresponsive. Through her panic, she dials 911. The paramedics arrive and take Steve to the closest hospital, a small rural ED about 30 minutes from their home:

ED visit #2
- Presents to ED per medics at 06:03.
- Physical examination: Temp 36.6, pulse 70, RR 10, BP 150/70, sat 95%. His extremities are flaccid. He can open his eyes but is unable to speak.
- Testing: Brain CT—normal.
- A decision is made to transport to tertiary care center. Intubated prior to transport.
- He is flown to the regional tertiary care facility (the same ED where he was originally seen).

ED visit #3 (tertiary care): The patient maintains stable vitals, is unresponsive and all four extremities are flaccid.
- He is seen by vascular surgery, neurology and cardiology.
- Advanced imaging reveals a left vertebral artery dissection with brainstem infarct. There is no flow in right vertebral artery.
- The patient is admitted with prolonged hospital stay. There is only minimal improvement of motor and cognitive function.
- A G-tube is placed, and a tracheostomy is performed.

Final Diagnosis: Quadriplegia secondary to brainstem infarct, left vertebral artery dissection with non-patent right vertebral artery.

Disposition: He is discharged with need for extensive convalescent care, including ventilator support.

PART 2—LEGAL

I. The Accusation/Cause of Action

- Failure to admit.
- Failure to obtain consultation or transfer for further evaluation.
- Failure to recognize TIA or stroke in evolution.
- Failure to perform a complete diagnostic evaluation that would have identified the dissection.

At deposition, Steve's wife, Lauren, told a powerful and heart-rending story. She described how the children were now in middle and high school. They didn't go to the hospital and never got to speak with their father again.

II. Witness statements and Depositions (summary)

Deposition of the initial ED physician:

- The patient was observed for over three hours in the Emergency Department.
- The patient had a very stressful event with his employer at work, which he did not document in the medical record.
- The symptoms were best explained by stress and an anxiety reaction.
- His tests were all normal and he had no signs or symptoms of stroke or TIA while in the ED
- There was no need for admission.

Deposition of Lauren Heller (patient's spouse):

- She and her husband knew something was wrong, since he never asks for help.
- The fact that he pulled over while driving and called 911 was evidence that something out of the ordinary had occurred.
- She was "scared" to take him home, since they lived 1½ hours away from the hospital.
- She described how the loss impacted their children.

Deposition of defense expert:

- Really tough case.
- Very easy with hindsight bias to say what should have been done during ED visit #1. Unfortunately, patient presented after a profound event while driving, and rather than listening to his wife or taking into consideration the rural location and difficult access to further medical care, the ED physician chose to attribute the event to social stress and anxiety.
- If the patient had been admitted to hospital #1 for observation, he most likely would have had the same outcome.

III. What Would Greg Do (WWGD)?

Greg Henry, past president of The American College of Emergency Physicians (ACEP), Professor of Emergency Medicine at the University of Michigan, and CEO of Medical Practice Risk Assessment, has been an expert witness in over 2,000 malpractice cases.

Greg discusses diagnosis of vertebral artery dissection, differentiation of functional vs. organic complaints, settlement vs. trial and his two pet peeves.

"If you call an organic process psychiatric, we have another name for you—the defendant"

This case allows me to speak about two pet peeves: The first is the psychiatric diagnosis. If you call a psychiatric process organic, it's hard to go wrong. However, if you call an organic process psychiatric, we have another name for you—the defendant. It's interesting we have a gentleman with no psychiatric history who is given the diagnosis of anxiety when he presented with symptoms which are referable to one anatomic area. Can I find a single anatomic location for this patient's symptoms? Absolutely, it's in the posterior fossa, involves either the upper part of the vertebrals and or basilar artery. It is perfectly explainable. The fact that the symptoms waxed and waned should be supportive of a transient ischemic attack (TIA). We really don't know what we can do for posterior fossa TIA patients, except perhaps aspirin or Plavix and eventual control of blood pressure.

When a patient presents with an obvious anatomic location, referable to a specific vascular pattern, we need a specific vascular diagnosis. The tendency to call it psychiatric means that we have decided to blame the patient for the illness. No matter how anxious the patient looks at any one moment in time, the better part of valor is to assume an organic condition. This approach rarely gets anyone into trouble.

The second pet peeve is the exam. Whenever a diagnosis is potentially neurological, a neurological exam should be on the chart. I know I sound like a broken record on this issue, but nothing beats a real examination. The process forces you to think anatomically about the regions in the nervous system that may be supplied by certain vascular territories.

A negative CT scan means just that, there is not obvious disease on the film at this time. The performance of a CT scan seems to be more religious ritual than a scientific pursuit of information, similar to believing if you stay under the covers the monster under the bed can't eat you. We do not expect positive CT findings with a TIA.

Regarding settlement, it definitely needs to be explored and pursued. This case is not defensible on a standards basis; if a patient is diagnosed with TIA, the standard of care is to pursue the work-up of TIA. Check the EKG for dysrhythmias. Arrange an ECHO and carotid study. Start antiplatelet therapy, such as aspirin or Clopidogrel. A great plaintiff's expert, who actually knows how to speak to a jury, could finish this physician off in a nanosecond.

The real question of worth in this case is: was the outcome inevitable? This is very difficult to say because there is only minimal proof that anticoagulation helps in the posterior fossa for prevention of further disease. But all of this science needs to be put aside—this will be tried in front of a jury which believes that you are better off in medical hands when bad things happen.

As the advisor to the insurance company, I would push for settlement.

IV. Trial/Settlement

What did the defense decide to do? They settled following the wife's deposition. Clearly, any jury would view the plaintiff and his family sympathetically. Although the adjudication of any case should be carried out fairly without bias, a jury of the patient's peers, not the physician's, will judge the facts presented. When the jury can relate to the travails of the plaintiff and the financial need is obvious, jurors often side with plaintiff compensation rather than minimizing financial impact to the physician (which will just be paid by the insurance company anyway, right?). Many view a medical malpractice policy as a "patient compensation fund" for those who have experienced a bad outcome.

Dissecting this case and assessing the likelihood of a defense verdict reveals several additional weaknesses:

- The symptoms suggest a neurological etiology; unfortunately the physician placed too much weight on resolution of symptoms and a normal CT scan. Additionally, the neurological examination was minimal, allowing the plaintiff's attorney to discredit the physician by asserting an incomplete evaluation was the basis for misdiagnosis.

- A cursory discussion about admission occurred, implying the physician considered it and then dismissed it. He recorded that the patient preferred to be discharged, but an informed refusal was not obtained. They would contend that if the patient was told that he may have had a TIA with potential for ensuing severe neurologic consequences, he would have preferred admission.

Outcome: A non-disclosure agreement was signed at the time of settlement, therefore the exact amount is unknown, but it is estimated to have been between $100,000 and $200,000.

V. What Would Greg Do (WWGD)? (Further discussion now that he knows the legal outcome:)

I was not surprised that this case was settled by the defense; but I am surprised that the *plaintiff* was willing to settle. A case such as this could have tremendous value depending on the stupidity of the physician, the likeability of the family and the amount of rage that can be created in a jury. For the insurance company to obtain an indemnity payment of only $100K and $200K speaks to its brilliance. To try the case would have cost $100K, so the extra amount is minimal—this had the best possible outcome for the physician.

For the plaintiff to win at trial, the key is teaching the jury the anatomic basis of diagnosis. As questions about the vascular distribution are asked, the physician would be reduced to a shivering puddle of stool. This disease entity is often referred to as the Count of Monte Cristo syndrome. As it turns out, the Count of Monte Cristo didn't actually have this syndrome, but in the novel a character is described as "a corpse with living eyes"— a posterior fossa syndrome affecting the basilar artery and everything including the pons. Since the lowest cranial nerve that is functioning is the third cranial nerve, this "corpse" was able to look up and down but not side to side since that would involve the sixth nerve nuclei.

As the case progressed, the plaintiff's counsel would merely quiz the doctor as to the fact that such cases have been known for over 150 years. He could then have the doctor draw out the posterior fossa anatomy showing where the vertebral arteries joined to form the basilar artery and the posterior communicating arteries and describe how those symptoms are generally not right-or left-sided. There are other ways that this can be presented, but in all of the scenarios, the physician loses.

The defense strategy is simple: admit to stupidity regarding the anxiety diagnosis up front and concentrate on the proximate cause relationship between missing the diagnosis and the ultimate locked-in syndrome; the fact that the emergency physician saw the patient does not mean that earlier intervention would have changed the outcome.

VI. Guest Interview—The Legal Analysis: Jennifer L'Hommedieu Stankus, MD, JD

- Former medical malpractice defense attorney and military magistrate
- Member of ACEP'S Medical-Legal Committee and Ethics Committee
- Contributing writer for ACEP News
- Adjunct professor at Regis University
- Most importantly, a senior emergency medicine resident at the University of New Mexico

Authors: *Should the defense have settled this case?*
JS: Without question, this case should have been settled at the earliest possible juncture. It would not be defensible in court, and the trial costs alone are close to the settlement amount. Frankly, I'm amazed that the family settled for so little. I don't know what was going through their minds; perhaps they simply wanted an acknowledgement by the physician that there was a major failing, even gross negligence. Sadly, failure to recognize dissection is not an uncommon malpractice occurrence; when things don't add up, go back and re-examine. If there are any signs of focal neurologic deficits, at any point, something more needs to be done, be it a consult, a CTA of head and neck—something. To rule out TIA/CVA with a CT is completely inappropriate, amounting to malpractice.

Authors: *How would you defend the case?*
JS: With a Hail Mary. The only way to defend this case is causation; the outcome would have been the same regardless of timely and proper diagnosis; failing to meet the standard of care did not affect the outcome. An expert could be found to argue both sides, but it's a crap shoot. Who would the jury believe? They will almost always side with the more sympathetic party, which is the grieving family, not the "rich doctor."

Authors: *What could have been done differently at the initial ED visit to make the case more defensible?*
JS: Be very careful about diagnoses on discharge, particularly when it is unclear. Labeling this as anxiety is inappropriate at best. The patient has no history of anxiety, so you are telling the jury that you thought this was "all in his head." The funny thing is … this *was* in his head, but in a very organic way. [Authors' note: see illustration at the beginning of this case.] Nothing will turn a jury's angry eye onto you faster than labeling the patient or making judgments in the medical record, particularly without foundation. In this case, it made the physician look careless, foolish and dismissive. It is true that when patients experience the pain of a dissection or ACS, they often feel anxious or like they are going to die. Yes, a sensation of impending death is anxiety-provoking.

Authors: *If the case had proceeded to trial, how would the plaintiff approach the questioning?*
JS: Consider these potential questions from the plaintiff's attorney:

- "And clearly, doctor, you didn't even do a thorough neurologic exam. What vascular causes should one think of in a hypertensive male when there are focal neurologic deficits?

- Aren't emergency medicine doctors trained to recognize the most life-threatening problems? Isn't vertebral artery dissection such a problem?

- And tell me, doctor, why you ordered a CT scan of the head? Ah, to rule out a stroke or TIA. Can you enlighten the jury on what percentage of the time this scan would be helpful in making that diagnosis?

- "I see … so you sent Steve Heller, a husband and father to two loving children, home with a new diagnosis of "anxiety," on the basis of a CT scan which misses a stroke *most* of the time."

Authors: *How should this encounter been documented?*
JS: Even if not explicitly stated in a progress note, your differential should be reflected in the HPI and ROS. As emergency physicians, we are trained to rule out the bad things first. It is impossible to know what this physician was thinking from his scant notes, but it appears from the record and the decision to image that TIA or stroke was on the list. If that was true, the patient should have gone to OBS or have been admitted.

VII. Medical Discussion—Evaluation of Neck Pain, Diagnosis of Vertebral and Carotid Artery Dissection

Guest author: Stephen Colucciello, MD, FACEP

- Clinical Professor, Emergency Medicine, University of North Carolina Medical School, Chapel Hill, North Carolina
- Assistant Chair, Director of Clinical Services, and Trauma Coordinator, Department of Emergency Medicine, Carolinas Medical Center
- ACEP's National Speaker of the Year, 1992

A. Introduction

While I hope you will read my entire "learned" discussion regarding dissection of the vertebral and carotid arteries, you really need to remember just one thing:

> 1. Neck pain plus neurologic complaints = dissection.

For you overachievers, there are two more things to remember (not nearly as important as the first):

> 2. If the neurologic complaint is unilateral limb weakness, it's often (but not always) anterior circulation (carotid).
> 3. If symptoms are bilateral, facial, vary between right and left, are accompanied by dizziness or nausea, or if the patient's neurologic complaints are just plain confusing, its posterior circulation (vertebral).

B. A *Very* Brief Look at Demographics and Pathophysiology
1. Demographics
   a. Dissections of the carotid and vertebral arteries are rare; about 2–3 per 100,000, but they are responsible for more than a fifth of the ischemic strokes in young and middle-aged adults. Carotid dissections are several times more common than vertebral dissections.
   b. An arterial dissection begins with a tear in the vascular intima; blood then dissects within the vessel wall. There are numerous possible symptoms of cervico-vascular dissection, but their common traits are usually neck, head or facial pain *and* some combination of neurologic deficits. The deficit may be permanent, (stroke) or transient (TIA). The transient deficits are most likely to be labeled as "anxiety-related," especially if the brainstem was briefly compromised.
   c. The dissection can cause vascular occlusion from the intramural blood. Swollen pseudoaneurysms can directly compress nearby structures. Often a thrombus forms, which can obstruct blood flow through the artery, or the thrombus can shower the brain with emboli. This embolic shower can result in apparently

"non-anatomic" complaints since multiple and even bilateral vascular territories may be involved (as in the case of vertebral artery dissection).

d. Cervico-vascular dissections can occur spontaneously or as the result of trauma. Patients may not remember any recent neck injury since symptoms may occur hours to days or even weeks after the original insult. Precipitants may be as innocuous as sudden head turning (e.g., while attempting to parallel park) or prolonged neck extension (e.g., from painting a ceiling). Medical doctors love to mention the association between vascular dissection and "neck adjustments" by chiropractors; however, I recently saw a young woman who developed locked-in syndrome from vertebral artery dissection after tipping her head back to apply eye drops.

2. Carotid dissection

a. Historical features—The presentation of carotid dissection is usually more straightforward and less of a diagnostic challenge than vertebral dissection. Patients may complain of any or all of the following:
  - Trauma to the anterior neck.
  - Pain, usually head, neck or facial; about a quarter have neck pain alone.
  - Neurologic complaints contralateral to the pain. The deficit may resolve before arrival in the ED.
  - Visual symptoms including transient blindness.
  - A "whooshing" sound in the ear (these patients are hearing their own carotid bruit).

b. Physical findings—The physical exam in carotid dissection may not be helpful if the neurologic deficits were transient. While the history of neck pain and neurologic symptoms are enough to suggest the diagnosis, physical exam can be useful to detect stroke. Patients may have any or all of the following:
  - Patients in a recent MVC may have a seat belt sign to the neck (the vast majority of patients with a cervical seat belt sign do *not* have a carotid artery dissection).
  - Neuro deficit compatible with stroke (opposite the side of pain).
  - Bruit over the carotid artery, sometimes over the face or eye. Be prepared for some strange looks if you auscultate a patient's eye—it is not a common finding.
  - Partial Horner's syndrome on the affected side (occurs in less than 50% of dissections). To detect Horner's syndrome take a good look at the eyes. The affected eye will demonstrate a droopy lid with a small pupil, ptosis and miosis. Note: Anhydrosis is rare.

3. Vertebral artery dissection

a. Historical features—The neurologic picture of vertebral dissection may be extremely confusing because emboli from a dissected right vertebral artery could travel up the basilar artery and then float to either the left or right side of the brainstem. The opposite can occur with emboli from the left vertebral artery. This inconsistent pattern combined with the sometimes vague "nausea, weak and dizzy" features of brainstem ischemia make the diagnosis of vertebral artery dissection easy to miss. When a patient presents with occipital or posterior neck pain and a patchy "non-anatomic" series of complaints, think brainstem emboli. Patients with vertebral artery dissection may complain of any of the following:

- Recent major or minor trauma (twisting neck, chiropractic manipulation).
- Occipital headache, often with neck pain.
- Brainstem symptoms, such as:
  - o Nausea and vomiting
  - o Ataxia or clumsiness
  - o Facial numbness, pain, or weakness
  - o Vertigo
  - o Visual complaints including double vision
  - o Trouble swallowing or speaking

b. Physical findings
- Posterior bruit
- Cranial nerve deficits
- Cerebellar findings (past pointing, truncal or limb ataxia)
- Motor deficit
- Problems with fine motor movement and proprioception

C. Diagnosis

1. **Imaging**—The diagnosis of carotid or vertebral artery dissection rests upon vascular imaging of the head and neck; either CTA or MRA. If you don't have an institutional approach for suspected cervico-vascular dissection, talk to your neurologists, neurosurgeons, and radiologists to develop one. If you suspect intracranial blood such as a subarachnoid hemorrhage (SAH), first obtain non-contrast images of the brain (CT or MRI) followed by a contrast study of the head and neck. Acute SAH is best seen on non-contrast studies.

2. **Functional or organic?** Distinguishing between anxiety and organic pathology is an important skill. How can we avoid confusing anxiety with serious neurological issues? If in doubt, assume organic disease. But there are a few clues which increase the chance that the anxiety-related presentations are actually from anxiety:

   a. Long history of recurrent anxiety-related complaints. The first visit to an ED for a supposed functional problem is a red flag (at least a pink flag).

   b. Younger age of onset—It is not as common to first develop an anxiety disorder in middle or advanced age; only about 15% of patients develop an anxiety disorder after age 40.

   c. Classic anxiety-related complaints include:
   - Shortness of breath
   - Palpitations
   - Light-headedness
   - Trouble swallowing
   - Chest pain
   - Paresthesias

   (Of course these can also be symptoms of MI, PE or TIA).

   d. Patients with organic complaints that are mistaken for anxiety are often middle-aged or older and have no prior history of anxiety-related complaints. Paralysis, ataxia, clumsiness, unilateral weakness, visual field cuts, diplopia and (especially) incontinence are not typical anxiety-related complaints. Although all of us have seen a case of hysterical paralysis, this diagnosis is made on the basis of covert observation, serial exams or neuroimaging. Any patient with hard neurological findings should be considered to have organic disease until proven otherwise—especially if neck pain is present!

   e. Also remember that patients with anxiety disorders do get sick; *functional illness does not protect against organic disease*. You may have heard some cynical physicians profess that "Every turkey has their Thanksgiving."

3. **Would *I* have made the diagnosis of "anxiety" in this patient?** How could I possibly admit I could have missed it and still be a respected author of a Bounceback chapter? Though I knew there was a bad outcome on my initial read, I can honestly say I would have ordered a CTA of the head and neck for the following reasons:

   a. Neck pain plus neurological complaints = dissection.
   b. No history of anxiety disorder in a 46 year-old male.
   c. The patient had diaphoresis. (No one fakes diaphoresis. If the patient is sweating, the emergency physician should be sweating too.)
   d. The patient said he was going to die. At least 50% of patients who have said this to me have died in the ED (hopefully this statistic is not unique to me).

D. Treatment

Call *someone*, preferably a neurologist or neurosurgeon. Most patients with dissection get either anticoagulation or antiplatelet agents (although there is precious little hard data to support either). There are several reviews showing good outcomes with lytics in patients with cervical artery dissection, but let someone else decide upon thrombolytics for stroke in a patient with dissection.

E. Final Words

Now you know everything an emergency physician needs to know about arterial dissection in the neck. But then, you knew that by the end of the first paragraph; Neck pain plus neurologic complaints = *what?*

VIII. Authors' Summary

Wow. Is there anything more we can add?

- Nonspecific neurologic symptoms make a safe disposition tough, since "soft signs" often prompt scorn and ridicule from the admitting physician.
- Recognizing the difference between functional and organic symptoms is key.
- When this distinction is not able to be determined, admission or rapid outpatient follow-up are crucial.

References

1. Snyder BK, Hayden SR. Accuracy of leukocyte count in the diagnosis of acute appendicitis. Ann Emerg Med 1999; 33:565-74.
2. Lyons D, Waldron R, Ryan T, et al. An evaluation of the clinical value of the leucocyte count and sequential counts in suspected acute appendicitis. Br J Clin Pract 1987; 41:794-6. Prospective.
3. Miskowiak J, Burcharth F. The white cell count in acute appendicitis. A prospective blinded study. Danish Med Bull 1982; 29:210-11. Prospective, blinded.
4. Schriger DL, Kalafut M, Starkman S, et al. Cranial computed tomography interpretation in acute stroke. physician accuracy in determining eligibility for thrombolytic therapy. JAMA. 1998; 279:1293-7.
5. Uchiyama S. Transient ischemic attack, a medical emergency; Brain Nerve 2009; 61(9):1013-22.

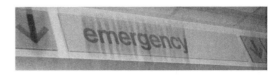

CASE 10

A 26 YEAR-OLD WOMAN WITH WEAKNESS & FALLS: A ROUGH LIFE, A TOUGH PROGNOSIS

Primary case author Michael Weinstock

PART 1—MEDICAL

    I. The Patient's Story 243

    II. The Doctor's Version (the ED Chart) 244

    III. The Errors—Risk Management/Patient Safety Issues 246

    IV. The Bounceback 248

PART 2—LEGAL

    I. The Accusation/Cause of Action 250

    II. How Does a Plaintiff's Attorney Decide if there Is a Case? 250

    III. Guest Interview: Confessions of a Hired Gun—
           Michael Redd, MD, FACEP 252

    IV. Legal analysis—Mark Kitrick, JD (plaintiff attorney) 254

    V. What Would Greg Do (WWGD)? 256

    VI. The Legal Proceedings: Depositions/Settlement vs. Trial 257

    VII. Legal Analysis: Rich Milligan, JD (defense attorney) 261

    VIII. The Legal Proceedings: Depositions/Settlement vs. Trial (continued) 262

    IX. Guest Author—Michael Weintraub, MD 264

    X. The Decision—Settlement vs. Trial 268

    XI. Therapy 268

    XII. Medical Discussion—Jerome Hoffman, MD (Interview) 269

    XIII. Authors' Summary 278

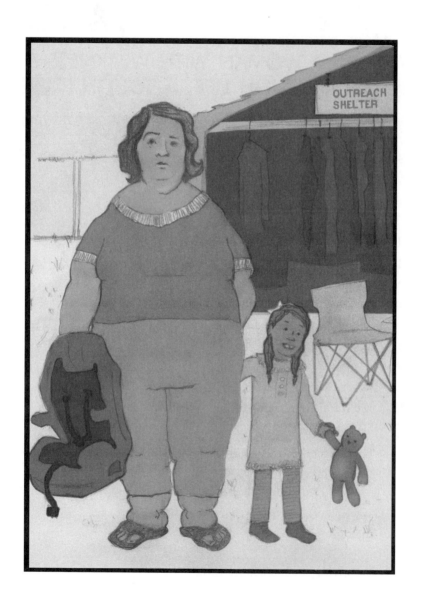

A 26 YEAR-OLD WOMAN WITH WEAKNESS & FALLS: A ROUGH LIFE, A TOUGH PROGNOSIS

How come we complain when a patient returns the next day, but the small business owner never does? "You're back *again*? Why didn't you buy everything you needed yesterday?"

And ever heard of the nurse's "punitive wait?" "*That'll* teach 'em ..."

Deep thoughts:

1. *How far should we go in evaluating transient, non-specific symptoms?*
2. *What role do risk factors play in the decision-making process?*
3. *When two providers care for a patient, how is responsibility divided when there is a bad outcome?*
4. *Why is it called a waiting "room" and an emergency "department?"*

PART 1—MEDICAL

I. The Patient's Story

Crystal does not have it easy. At the age of four, her father moves her to Louisiana. She is only to see her mother again briefly. Becoming pregnant in the 12th grade, she drops out of school and moves in with the soon-to-be father. Her pregnancy is complicated by anemia so severe that she requires a blood transfusion, but she delivers a healthy daughter by caesarian section.

It is not long before she becomes pregnant again with the same man, and on August 12, 1999, delivers another healthy daughter. Her boyfriend leaves, and Crystal moves into a mobile home, all the while working as a housekeeper at the Shifting Sands Resort Hotel. He returns and moves in next door—but they are not able to stay together due to "too much arguing." At one point in 2000 she is arrested for smashing his windshield and slashing his tires.

Crystal and her two daughters move out of the mobile home shortly after the floor in the bathroom falls through—she can now see the ground below the trailer. Bad goes to worse as she is fired from the hotel due to a misunderstanding about vacation. She wanders from job to job, first working in another hotel then in a children's daycare. Times remain rough; there is a 45-minute commute each way, and she quits work when her car breaks down.

In 2002 her children go to live with their father. Crystal is soon pregnant again from a one-night stand; it is during this pregnancy that she learns of her mother's sudden death. Depression sets in. She is admitted to a psychiatric ward for almost 10 days, but no medications are prescribed since she is pregnant. A third c-section results in a healthy baby girl at Cape Hope Hospital in 2003. Crystal calls her Joy.

With a new child, she attempts to get her two oldest children back, but their father refuses. She has a new boyfriend and finds work as a cashier at the Icy Penguin service station. One night she arrives home to find her apartment building surrounded by EMS vehicles and is told her boyfriend has burned it down. She remembers an argument from earlier in the day:

He said, "I'm moving and going to Florida." I said, "Go ahead. Then he got mad." The boyfriend is subsequently charged with arson and sent to jail.

In 2005 Crystal is stopped for a traffic violation and the police notice that her child is not in a car seat; she is cited. She does not show up for the court date, and her driver's license is revoked. She now receives government assistance with food stamps and is placed on Medicaid. With no way to get to work and a young child to care for, she moves into a shelter.

On **March 9, 2006,** she goes to a clinic across the street from the shelter with complaints of heavy menstrual cycles, sinus pain, and tension in her neck. Vitals show BP 128/70 and weight of 279 pounds (down from 331 after taking Adipex a few years earlier). She has lab work which shows a WBC count of 11.8, Hb 6.8 (MCV low at 58), and platelet count 513. She is started on Septra and Flexeril with recommendations to get a pelvic US and see a hematologist. She returns to the clinic two weeks later and is started on iron. Surgical therapy is recommended but Crystal refuses. The diagnosis: Severe anemia and menorrhagia. Appointments are made for an US and consultation with a hematologist on April 17 at 2:15 PM.

Saturday, April 7 2006 is Joy's third birthday, and the shelter helps by throwing a party at Chuck E Cheese's. While there, Crystal develops a headache which persists through the weekend.

Tuesday, April 10, 2006—Crystal is at the shelter and reaches for her daughter's car seat to put her into the daycare van. Crystal has a sudden onset of a hand cramp, then falls to the floor and cannot get up for three minutes. "[I was] standing and just fell." She calls for help but then finds that she is able to walk. There is no head trauma. She is driven to the ED.

II. The Doctor's Version (the following is the actual documentation of the providers recorded on a "T-system" chart)

Date: April 10, 2006 at 09:58

Chief complaint (per RN): "Fell/numbness to leg"

EXAM

VITAL SIGNS										
Time	Temp(F)	Rt.	Pulse	Resp	Syst	Diast	Pos.	Pain Scale		pulse ox
10:10	98.5	O	62	16	122	83	S	0		100%
15:00			60	18	140	60				

TRIAGE: Acuity 3–green. Pt ambulatory, tearful stating she fell last PM and this morning. Stating leg numbness. Pt sounds congested. Equal hand grips bilaterally.

HISTORY OF PRESENT ILLNESS (11:15) (note: all documenting, ordering, and treatment per physician assistant-PA): Right leg and arm numbness last night and today with fall X 2 – denies previous or current injury. Severity mild-moderate. Weakness RUE and RLE which is new. Numbness X 2 episodes, approx 1 minute each. No problems with vision, impaired speech, difficulty swallowing, confusion. She has approx → of prescription for Septra remaining à "makes me sick". Pt. reports prior Hb 6.7 → "taking iron."

PAST MEDICAL HISTORY:
Allergies: NKDA
Meds: Septra, zyrtec, flexeril
PMH: Anemia
PSH: C/S X 3
FH:
SH: Smoker > 2 PPD, alcohol – none, drugs – none

EXAM
PSYCH: Mood and affect are normal.
EYES: PERRL.
THROAT: Normal pharynx with no tonsillar hypertrophy.
NECK: Supple.
CARD: Regular rate and rhythm, ht. sounds nl.
RESP: No respir distress, breath sounds nl.
ABD: Nontender, no organomegaly.
SKIN: Color nl, no rash. Warm and dry.
NEURO: Cranial nerves normal as tested. EOM's intact, PERRL, cerebellar normal as tested. No motor or sensory deficit. Reflexes normal.
MS: Non-tender, normal ROM, no pedal edema.

ED COURSE:
11:15 – Orthostatic VS: Lying BP 130/43 and pulse 65 → Standing 145/80, pulse 56
12:15 – Tylenol 975mg PO—Note: Pt. refused. "I've already tried Tylenol and Motrin"
13:00 (per RN) – X-ray tech informed me pt removed IV "because it hurt"—documented on AMA (pt. was asked to sign AMA form showing knowledge of risks of removing IV)

TESTING:
WBC 9.2, Hb 7.6, plt 1,342,000
Lytes, BUN/creat – WNL, LFTs WNL, glucose 92, pregnancy test – negative
CT scan head – Indication: Head Pain. **Interpretation:** Normal per radiologist
Urine toxicology screen: Positive for marijuana

DIAGNOSIS (14:45): Sinusitis, substance abuse, paresthesias, anemia.

DISCHARGE (15:15): Per RN: Discharge instructions given. Verbalized understanding. Discharged home. Rx doxycycline 100mg Q12 hours #20, Motrin 800mg q8 hours PRN pain, F/u with PCP ASAP for recheck and further Tx, return with increased symptoms or problems.

Scott Davidson, PA
Afram Aminah, MD

III. The Errors—Risk Management/Patient Safety Issues

➤**Authors' note:** When we are faced with one problem at a time it is usually not too difficult to arrive at a diagnosis: chest pain and diaphoresis in a 50 year old man, sudden onset of flank pain and hematuria. When symptoms are nonspecific in a patient with numerous medical problems, the complexity increases …

Risk management/patient safety issue #1:

Error: Poor history of present illness (HPI).

Discussion: A common theme throughout this book: great "review of symptoms," but minimal HPIs. Our patient has concerning symptoms of numbness and weakness on one side of her body, but her age of 26 argues strongly against stroke. This type of patient requires the provider to sit down and get a thorough story. What was the exact onset and duration of the symptoms? Has this occurred in the past? Were there any associated signs or symptoms?

Did this become a legal issue? You betcha! The following is the physician answering a question from the plaintiff's attorney with information supplies by the physician assistant.

> Q. (Plaintiff's attorney): Doctor, when you reviewed Ms. Johnson's chart, did you note her history of right-sided leg and arm numbness and the fact that she had fallen within the previous 12 hours?
> A. (Doctor Aminah) Well, in terms of the fall, sir, I need—I need more information to make any assessment because it was not clear from the history about the fall as to why she fell. From [the history] she did fall twice, he [the PA] said. Whether she lost her balance, whether she was dizzy, you know, and did she actually hit the ground or just lose her balance, I don't know. So that fall, I could not make any conclusion, because she—she said that she didn't injure herself. So, whether she didn't actually hit the ground and just lost her balance, I cannot make any conclusions about that fall.

The doctor was left to defend an incomplete evaluation performed by someone else.

✔ **Teaching point:** This is not fast food—when there is diagnostic uncertainty make sure every bit of data available has been obtained.

Risk management/patient safety issue #2:

Error: Not evaluating risk factors.

Discussion: The inclusion of risk factors has lately become controversial; do risk factors really matter with a history of exertional chest pain, dyspnea and diaphoresis? The T-sheet chart had a section for family history, but it was left blank. Crystal's deposition revealed what should have been included there: history of stroke in her 16 year-old sister and in both of her parents.

✔ **Teaching point**: Sometimes, risk factors matter.

Risk management/patient safety issue #3:

Error: Not asking for help.

Discussion: This case is a good lesson for physicians as well as mid-level providers (MLPs). Just as physicians often ask for help from consultants, sometimes the MLP will need to discuss a case with the attending. Examples may include the crashing patient, the angry patient, the unusual illness patient (lupus, AIDS, methhemoglobinemia) and the patient with an uncertain diagnosis. In a more global sense, the relationship with a MLP should be fully explored and defined before clinical work begins. In some EDs all MLPs are directly supervised, with every patient being seen by a physician. In others, MLPs function autonomously without direct supervision. This decision involves a balance between cost, efficiency, safety and risk. In 2006, 12.7% of ED patients were seen by an MLP, about half also being seen by a physician.[21]

✔ **Teaching point**: The MLP-physician partnership should be a team effort.

Risk management/patient safety issue #4:

Error: Unaddressed contradiction in chart.

Discussion: The brain CT indication states "head pain," but this is not mentioned in the HPI. Did she really have head pain or was the PA forced to pick from a list of indications? If she did have head pain, questioning about onset and other symptoms, such as fever, would have been helpful. If she did *not* have head pain, documenting such in the face of other neuro symptoms was essential.

✔ **Teaching point**: All patient complaints need to be explored in the H&P.

Risk management/patient safety issue #5:

Error: Over-reliance on testing.
Discussion: It seems most likely that the brain CT was done to evaluate for TIA or CVA, not headache. During the PA's deposition, he admitted that his understanding was that a negative CT excluded TIA or CVA. Would anyone be reassured with a negative back X-ray when evaluating for spinal epidural abscess? How about a normal CBC when evaluating for appendicitis? There is a growing body of evidence that MRI will show many small strokes in evolution, previously thought to be TIAs. Reliance on a negative CT in the evaluation of cerebrovascular disease is a misapplication of data.[20]The evaluation of TIA is most commonly accomplished by admission. Though not mitigating all risk, if Crystal had been admitted … you would not be reading this chapter …

✔ **Teaching point**: Understand limitations of testing.

Risk management/patient safety issue #6:

Error: Not recognizing the dangers of thrombocytosis.

Discussion: Thrombocytosis is an uncommon diagnosis, and its acute management would exceed the bounds of most emergency physicians. However, it does not take a brain surgeon (or hematologist) to recognize that when the platelets are three times the upper limit of normal, there may be extra clotting. Faced with an overweight patient with new onset unilateral arm and leg weakness, the thrombocytosis tips the scales in favor of an acute neurologic event.

✔ **Teaching point:** If you order testing, be prepared to address abnormal results.

➤**Authors note:** If you were the attending, would you want to see this patient yourself? If you were the mid-level provider, would you want to bounce this off the attending?

Reading the history, I don't have a good idea what is going on. Why and how did she fall and was this related to the paresthesias? Why was a CT done, looking for bleed, mass, TIA/CVA—was a normal CT supposed to be reassuring? What's the deal with a diagnosis of substance abuse? (She smoked some dope behind the pews before sending her daughter to preschool, then was so "stoned" she fell and had unilateral numbness which resolved within minutes?) The "feel" of this chart is an ED staff at odds with their patient; who has a patient, soon to be discharged, sign an AMA form because her IV hurts and she refuses Tylenol?

IV. The Bounceback

Crystal is asymptomatic after ED discharge on Tuesday, but at 3AM the following morning, Wednesday April 11th, 2006, she wakes to go to the bathroom and: "I just start falling". She gets back to sleep, and then per routine is awoken by the church at 6AM. After she gets her daughter off to daycare she is driven to the Rocky Fork Department of Social Services building. While waiting to be seen, she experiences "sweat pouring down my face … I can't see nothing … slurry speech and real bad headache." Medics are called:

EMS report:
09:23 – Dispatched to Social Services building, 1236 Wahalla Street. Reason for dispatch: Breathing problems.
09:32 – Arrive on scene
09:35 – Vitals: pulse 74 regular, Resp 20, BP 126/70, sat 100%, EKG NSR. Signs and symptoms: Headache. GCS normal.
10:15 – Arrive at Cape Hope ED:
(EMS final report): 26 y/o female complaint headache with burning sensation across her nose. Pt was seen at Cape Hope yesterday and treated for sinusitis. Patient requests transport to ED for evaluation again today. Patient transported w/o incident or delay to lead charge nurse and then to triage.

ED Visit #2, Wednesday, April 11, 2006:

- 10:32 – (RN #1): Triaged and placed in waiting room.
    - "Pt. here via EMS with c/o HA. States seen here yesterday and dx with sinusitis and given Rx for same but has been unable to get filled. Pt. A&O X 3. NAD."
- 10:48 – (RN #2): One episode emesis. Pt comes to triage desk stating "I feel sick" and not answering detailed questions.
    - "Pt. dx with sinusitis yesterday and has not taken Rx. Pt. vomited in triage, clear, frothy emesis, resp easy, skin W/D." Returned to waiting room.
- 11:49 – (RN#2): Comes back to triage desk stating "I feel really sick."
    - Per RN: "Resp easy, skin W/D, no more episodes of vomiting, pt. stable." Returned to waiting room.
- 13:56 – Name is called and she is placed in an ED room (3 hours 23 minutes after arriving by squad).
- 14:45 – Initial exam by physician assistant (PA) Adam Thompson:
    - HPI: "Pt was at social services today and had syncopal episode. Came to ED c/o HA and not feeling well. Had another flaccid episode. Pt. has been aphasic and right side paralysis."
    - PE – Pt. is aphasic, will only moan. Unable to test strength due to slow or no response to commands. Will withdraw right arm from deep pain 2/5 strength.
    - The staff now responds quickly: Brain CT - Acute CVA left middle cerebral artery distribution.
- **Diagnosis:** Acute CVA with aphasia and right hand hemiparesis

HOSPITAL COURSE:

- Neuro consult: She is awake and alert but not cooperative. At times, she will move her arm in a nonspecific fashion, but most of the time has neglect. She is mute without the ability to repeat or comprehend speech. She has global aphasia.
- **Impression:** "Suspect stroke is secondary to the thrombocytosis and related hyperviscosity syndrome."
- In-hospital testing reveals 90% left carotid artery stenosis.
- **Disposition:** On April 19, 2006, after eight days in the hospital, she is discharged for outpatient rehabilitation.

Outcome: Crystal now lives with her 7 year-old daughter, Joy. With rehab, her condition has improved, and she is able to walk her daughter to the bus stop across the street, but cannot walk her as far as the park. Her speech is not clear, and her thought processes have not returned to baseline. She is embarrassed to be seen, spending most of her time at home. There are no family contacts and few friends. A nurse's aide visits the house for several hours three times a week to help with basic activities of living.

At a five-hour deposition on February 16, 2010, she stated that the last contact with her first two daughters was in October 2009. She tried to call at Christmas, but the phone was not in service and has not been connected since.

➤**Authors' note:** Crystal's hard life just got harder. In addition to all her previous problems, she now has difficulty with speech and no use of her right upper extremity. Could her TIA have been diagnosed at the initial visit? If she had been admitted, would it have changed the outcome?

I. The Accusation/Cause of Action

- Failure to diagnose
- Failure to initiate preventive therapy for management of TIA
- Failure to recognize thrombocytosis as risk for CVA
- Failure to manage increased platelets
- Failure to arrange appropriate and timely follow-up for evaluation of TIA and prevention of CVA

II. How Does the Plaintiff's Attorney Decide if there Is a Case?

➤**Authors' note:** When a patient is initially pursuing litigation, the case is brought to the attention of the plaintiff's attorney by the patient. However, the attorney has only superficial medical expertise. So, medical experts are needed to give advice as to whether negligence occurred.

The following is the abbreviated letter from the retained plaintiff's expert, Dr. Redd, the ED physician who reviewed the case. He later was an expert witness at the legal proceeding (more below). Often, the plaintiff's attorney will have three to four "experts" review a case. They want objective information, since the plaintiff's attorney (and client) get nothing if they lose, which occurs about 85% of the time if the case goes to trial. The plaintiff's best opportunity for a financial reward is through pretrial settlement.

Michael C. Redd, MD, FACEP
ED Medical-Legal Expert
353 E. Torrence Rd.
Boca Raton, FL 33433

Catherine Lefort, Esq.
Lefort, Johnson & Pruitt
Telemark Square
Summersville, NC 28451

Dear Ms. LeFort,

I had the opportunity to review the medical records of Crystal Johnson from 4/10/06 to 4/19/06. I feel that the care and treatment provided to Ms Johnson on 4/10/06 was below the accepted standard of care.

[Omitted here are 5 paragraphs summarizing the case]

When a patient presents to the emergency department with episodic hemiparesis, weakness and two episodes of falling, the first diagnosis in the differential is TIA. Ms. Johnson's risk factors of obesity, smoking and a hypercoagulable state due to her extreme thrombocytosis make this diagnosis more likely. TIA is the diagnosis that needs to be considered first.

Since a significant number of patients who experience a TIA will have a CVA within the first week, it is imperative to treat them immediately upon presentation. In fact, many institutions admit all patients presenting with TIA symptoms, especially ones presenting with their first TIA. The extremely elevated platelet count should have raised a red flag as to both the diagnosis and need for immediate intervention.

A diagnosis of sinusitis does not make clinical sense. A normal brain CT, which likely showed a significant view of the sinuses, with right-sided numbness and falling, makes it very difficult to justify a diagnosis of sinusitis. The falls, numbness and headache were not adequately explained, when in fact a diagnosis of TIA should have been the first consideration. Reading the chart, it would seem that the diagnosis of TIA was never seriously considered. A normal exam and CT scan cannot rule it out. It is a diagnosis based upon presenting signs, symptoms and risk factors; Ms. Johnson had [all three].

She did not receive any intervention with the typical medications to prevent CVA, such as aspirin. She also had a very treatable condition that was a major risk factor for her, the extreme thrombocytosis of 1.3 million. This was more than 3 times the highest acceptable number of platelets on this lab's test normal range. This level would increase the risk for stroke significantly and was easily treatable within the time frame between this visit and the next day, when she had the left middle cerebral artery infarction. Unfortunately, she was discharged.

On her return visit to the ED, she arrived by squad with significant complaints and was sent to the waiting room after being triaged. She came to the triage nurse twice and each time was sent back to the waiting room. This seems inappropriate for someone who has come in by squad, is a return from the day before (which should be a red flag) and for someone with her symptoms.

In summary, I do feel that the care and treatment provided to Ms. Johnson on 4/10/06 did not meet the standard of care. If I may be of any further assistance in the case, please do not hesitate to contact me.

Sincerely,

Michael Redd

Michael C. Redd, MD, FACEP

III. Guest Interview: Confessions of a "Hired Gun"—Michael Redd, MD, FACEP

> **Authors' note:** I found Dr. Redd, the plaintiff's expert, and he agreed to a brief telephone interview. I asked him some uncomfortable questions, he was honest and forthcoming. I also spoke with his co-workers and they uniformly agreed, from paramedics to nurses to physicians, that he was one of the best doctors they had ever worked with: engaged, caring, smart and nonjudgmental.

Authors: *How did you get involved in testifying?*
MR: A friend of mine is a physician. He founded a company which supplies experts for legal cases. He asked me if I would do it and I agreed. That was many years ago.

Authors: *How many cases have you done? Have you worked for both sides?*
MR: Well, all the cases don't go to trial, so I have looked at probably 100 total. Many are just to give the attorney an opinion about the care received in the ED. Sometimes it involves just an ED chart and sometimes includes hundreds of pages of hospital records. Of the 100, I have been deposed on 15 or 20 but only six have actually gone to trial. Of all my cases, about 90% were for the plaintiff and the rest for the defense.

Authors: *How much do you charge for your services?*
MR: For general record review I charge $350 per hour with a two-hour minimum. Depositions are 500 bucks an hour and it's $3,500 for a trial. Of course, if I have to go out of town, travel is also paid. I like to get a retainer up front because sometimes it's difficult to get paid. Some firms don't know what to look for, small firms, looking to hit it big—they want the information but don't always have the resources to pay for it.

Authors: *What types of cases have you been involved with?*
MR: PEs are a big one. Cardiac. MIs ... a few. Abdominal pain, appendix. Pelvic problems. One case where the nurse asked further about evaluating for the compartment syndrome and the doctor said no. A number of strokes and TIAs. No missed foreign bodies, but they say this is common. One case was a patient with a splenectomy with a temp of 103 and unknown source. Poor documentation and no vaccine documented. The patient came back next day septic and died. Documentation—unless you document it, the court says you didn't do it. I've had at least two cases where the doctors went back and documented after they found the outcome; if we can't even trust you to not change the record, how can we trust anything you say?

Authors: *What's it feel like having the defense lawyer and emergency physician across from you?*
MR: Not good. The first deposition I was at, the attorney was harassing and belligerent. One of their objectives is not to see what you know but to see if they can intimidate you on the stand. They want to know this up front. They will bring up things to make you look bad, to try and get you flustered. If you stay calm and say "I don't know about that," it's much easier. Don't let 'em get to you. Depositions are easy. Being on the stand is painful— anxiety provoking. All the jurors are looking at you. People in the seats are looking at you. The defendant physicians are the ones who you feel bad for. If they tried to change records, I don't feel bad, but if they made a mistake, I do feel bad for them.

You have to be careful in what you say. Try and not to trap yourself. Memorize the chart.

Authors: *Do you know what percentage you won?*
MR: That's the interesting part. Most are settled and I never found out what actually happened. Of the ones that went to court, five of the six went for the defense. I remember at one of them [I heard] the defense lawyer say, "I can't believe we won this case." One was a missed appy. Most could have gone either way. I don't remember the one that was won by the plaintiff … not off hand.

Authors: *Do you remember the deposition in this case, Crystal Johnson?*
MR: I do. It was a video conference; the defendant physician was not there. The entire deposition took four hours, it was kind of painful. They asked me about my credentials, my medical malpractice record, my childhood—trying to discredit me as a witness. The defense attorney was combative, he didn't have a case so tried to trick me into admitting I reviewed the record for a different case. He was grasping for straws. I called it Cape Valley Hospital and not Cape Hope hospital. It was miniscule and totally irrelevant to the case.

Authors: *You read the defendant physician's testimony. How would you have answered the questions?*
MR: Well, that was the problem! At the point of the deposition, it was beyond fixing; he really didn't have an argument. As far as the PA, he was not well trained. He didn't know about thrombocytosis, he didn't even know what it meant. He thought you could rule out a TIA or stroke with a CT scan.

Authors: *Do you work with PA's? How do you avoid getting in the same situation as this doctor?*
MR: The biggest problem with this case is not realizing that every one with these findings needs to be seen by the physician. This patient passed out, has paresthesias, an elevated platelet count. I would have seen the patient—that's the responsibility of the physician. The PAs need to be trained to talk to the doctor when these symptoms are present.

Authors: *Have you ever been deposed or sued?*
MR: In 2002 I received a 180-day letter. From the minute I got the letter I was distraught. It was on my mind every day. After three months they dropped the case.

Authors: *Do you remember the case?*
MR: Yeah, the patient was seen initially by a PA. It was a baby with a cold and the vitals were fine. They were asked to see the pediatrician the next day. I later found out that the child went home and vomited and aspirated and went into respiratory arrest before they could follow up. He expired a few days later. I remember the kid, the bed number and everything. The case was dropped as they couldn't find a witness. Nothing wrong was done.

Authors: *If you had such a bad experience, how can you testify against other doctors?*
MR: One reason is that it causes me to look at certain disease patterns from someone else's mistakes. Some experts will take a case for anybody, I only take cases for the plaintiff where it is pretty clear there was malpractice. It's improved the care of my patients. I'm a better physician because of the legal work I've done.

IV. Legal Analysis: Mark Kitrick, JD

- Plaintiff's attorney, President of Kitrick, Lewis & Harris Co., L.P.A., Columbus, Ohio
- Past President of the Ohio Association of Trial Lawyers

➤**Authors' note:** The following is commentary by plaintiff's attorney Mark Kitrick (not involved with the case), discussing how cases are selected. Later, we will hear from Rich Milligan, a medical malpractice defense attorney discussing the defense strategy in this case.

How a Plaintiff Decides if there Is a Case

Initial review—the patient contacts the attorney:
A plaintiff's lawyer initially analyzes three aspects of a potential medical malpractice case.

1. Is there a strong liability case against the possible defendants?
2. What are the claimant's damages?
3. Is there adequate malpractice insurance coverage or are there collectible defendants' assets?

In conjunction with this review, we must also take into account practical business considerations:

- The firm's advancement of costs and anticipated time prosecuting the claim
- The state's statutory caps on damages for pain and suffering and economic losses
- The reputations and likeability of the potential defendants
- What subrogation amount must be reimbursed
- Past jury verdicts and settlements in the relevant locale

By the time the case is filed, the trial lawyer will need to know the medicine, be prepared to spend $50,000-$150,000 (the range on this case), and will have retained the appropriate expert witnesses, including an EM physician for the standard of care, a stroke expert and damage witnesses. Most importantly, the lawyer must be highly impassioned for the client's cause. Of the many cases lawyers review, relatively few survive this vetting process.

Liability (was there negligence in this case?)
Assuming the reviewing physician opines favorably for the plaintiff, one main fact tilts the scales toward representation: The most deadly cause of Ms. Johnson's complaint was not excluded and the doctor did not pursue further investigation. Such an approach resonates with juries because it demonstrates more than negligence; it suggests intentional or gross negligence. From a juror's perspective, such behavior is more actionable and unforgivable.

First, when the defendants treated Ms. Johnson, they did not take a detailed history. Everyone knows this is a basic failure. For example, Ms. Johnson's family history of stroke was a crucial fact, and it was ignored; one cannot separate people from their bloodline. As well, the events surrounding the fall were not adequately explored. Further, her headache history was missed. Finally, the defendants should have recognized her extremely high platelet count and compared it to results from March 9, 2006 [the clinic visit one month before the ED visit].

Second, whether true or not, most people believe that if a stroke is diagnosed early on, it can be readily treated. Though the defendants did a head CT, there was no solid analysis of the unilateral numbness. A sharp trial lawyer will make it seem obvious that Ms. Johnson was at high risk for a stroke, based on risk factors and weight, smoking two packs a day and noncompliance. Of note, all this may not convince a plaintiff's attorney to take her case since a good defense attorney can use her conduct against her.

Third, Ms. Johnson was the recipient of government assistance. Most people believe that someone on assistance receives less personal attention and fewer "expensive" tests, primarily because the doctors and hospitals don't receive as much reimbursement. A three-hour wait on return, among other facts, may cause the jurors to question whether she was the victim of the defendants' presumed prejudice.

Liability Insurance Coverage
It is noteworthy that no one seemed to be truly in charge. There did not seem to be a hospital protocol for a responsible party; discovery may uncover whether the communication failure was endemic. A concerning byproduct for the defense is that plaintiff's counsel is forced to sue more doctors, employees and agents because no one can determine who is responsible. This approach may be advantageous to the plaintiff when one defendant points a finger at another or tries to blame an "empty chair."

➤**Authors' note:** The empty chair defense is used by the defendant to place the blame on a party which is not part of the suit or no longer a part of the suit. It was used successfully in Case 6.

Damages
The defendants' combined negligence caused Ms. Johnson to suffer serious, permanent conditions, which require significant, long-term medical care. Her economic costs, even if a portion are paid back to the government vis-a-vis its statutory subrogation claim, drive up the settlement or verdict. Because of this patient's major damages (some of which will not be subject to state caps) and the jury sympathy/empathy that exists, it is more likely that a lawyer will take her case.

Conclusion
To win a plaintiff's case, it helps if a jury is outraged with the defendants. The most successful plaintiff strategies allow the jurors to think about themselves and their family and how the defendants' actions have put them in jeopardy. They should be made to feel that their verdict sends a message to the defendants and society at large. In other words, if plaintiff's counsel demonstrates that this case is not just about Ms. Johnson, but about protecting the community, a significant plaintiff's verdict is likely to follow.

V. What Would Greg Do (WWGD)?

Greg Henry, past president of The American College of Emergency Physicians (ACEP), Professor of Emergency Medicine at the University of Michigan, and CEO of Medical Practice Risk Assessment, has been an expert witness in over 2,000 malpractice cases.

Greg opines on the underserved, recommendations regarding settlement and the physician's legal strategy.

"This woman is part of the sad underclass who live an undercurrent life in America ... this plethora of social and emotional problems make her a potential disaster from moment one."

You're not a true emergency physician unless you occasionally leave the room depressed to the point of catatonia. After hearing this patient's story, I would be unsure whether I should slit my wrists or take hemlock. The entire case is an emotional downer from moment one.

This woman is part of the sad underclass who live an undercurrent life in America. Nothing goes right for her. The history is page after page of disappointment and unhappiness. This plethora of social and emotional problems make her a potential disaster from moment one. One can only take so many stories of people who are caught in the government support maelstrom before coming to the realization that this country is becoming a physiological and emotional disaster. I'm afraid our "get up and go," got up and went.

The decision to settle revolves around what reasonable people on the jury might think such a case is worth. There is no question that there is a value. Once you clear away the enormity of the history, there is a core of facts which are tough to deal with. This patient did have a one-sided specific lesion which likely resulted from an event in a specific anatomic area. Can we cure all of these people? No way. Can we affect the outcome in some? That's a debate that continues on, but even if a specific treatment is not helpful, ordinary human care is the expectation of a jury.

The physician's legal strategy is simple; he will claim that the PA should have forced him to see the patient. In reality, many physicians do not want to see such patients, but the jury believes if a physician is available, there should have been consultation. The physician will claim no remembrance of the case, and the PA will remember wanting the physician to see the case. Where is the truth? Let's be honest—do you actually remember patients you saw with a PA three or four years ago?

The legal issues surrounding mid-level providers is shaping up to be a huge arena for dispute over the next ten years. I've watched the number of PA legal cases increase logarithmically. Who is to blame? Who is in charge? If you look at the billing slip, the physician's provider number and signature are there, so we know who is legally responsible. Who is morally responsible? If physician assistants are just that, shouldn't the physicians become involved? If the physicians don't have to see certain cases, why do they get paid for them?

It is the mark of a coward to blame either the resident or the PA. Man up! If you take some of the money, you take the liability, and maybe you ought to provide some of the care. About ten years ago, physician extenders were seeing about four percent of cases. Today, that number is around 15 percent. Where did this begin, and where will it end?

If we put our prejudices aside, the profession of emergency medicine is going to need to answer these questions. Anesthesiologists were almost ruined as a profession by not initially understanding the power of nurse anesthetists. Using mid-level providers creates a sea of potential unrest, unhappiness and litigation unless we, as a profession, get control, understand the uses and limitations, and accept the responsibility that comes with charging for a case.

To ask about the defensibility of this case is to ask whether you are willing to have 12 people picked from our current jury pool decide whether this woman was treated fairly or unfairly. I think "unfair" would win. This is not the kind of case that you want in the hands of an urban jury. If you are surrounded by people who have a redistributionist philosophy of life, they'll redistribute on this case. The defensibility here is debatable; you would lose this case in front of a jury six out of ten times.

The jury is going to be unhappy with the manner in which the patient was treated. Though our only treatment for TIA is aspirin, the public believes that if we can put men on the moon, we can prevent strokes. My strong inclination would be to settle this case at a level which allows for the care of her child.

VI. The Depositions (January 2010)

>**Authors' note:** This case presents significant difficulties for the defendants; both the PA and physician were named. The PA testified that he discussed the case with the attending, but there was no notation of that on the chart. Despite signing the chart, the attending did not have any recollection of the discussion.

The cast of characters (names changed):

The patient: Crystal Johnson
ED defendant doctor: Dr. Afram Aminah
ED physician assistant (PA): Scott Davidson
Plaintiff's attorney: Alan Krause, Esq.
Plaintiff's expert witness: Michael Redd, MD (Board certified emergency medicine)
Defense attorney: Randall Scoville, Esq.

➤**Authors' note:** Watch how the plaintiff's attorney plays the PA off of the attending physician.

Deposition of physician assistant Scott Davidson by plaintiff's attorney Alan Krause:

Q. Was there always during your tenure at Cape Hope, was there always an emergency physician in the emergency department?
A. Yes, sir.

Q. All right, sir. And do I understand that always you would discuss the care and disposition with the emergency physician prior to the patient being discharged?
A. Every case.

Q. And as it pertains to Crystal Johnson, who did you discuss her care with?
A. Dr. Aminah.

Q. And you discussed her care with Dr. Aminah before Crystal was discharged?
A. That is correct.

Q. Why did you do that?
A. That's what I do. That is the requirement we have—that I have with the supervising physicians. I discuss every patient with them. They are in charge and, therefore, I discuss all patients with them.

➤**Authors' note:** What do you think the physician had to say about it?

Deposition of ED defendant doctor Afram Aminah by plaintiff's attorney Alan Krause:

A. (Dr. Aminah): Yeah. To the best of my recollection, sir, I don't remember Scott Davidson (PA) speaking to me about Ms. Johnson. If he did, I don't remember what he said.

Q. All right, sir.
A. That's to the best of my recollection.

Q. Doctor, were you in charge of Crystal Johnson's care while she was in the emergency department on April 10th of 2006?
A. To the best of my recollection, sir, I—I never did see Ms. Johnson. That's to the best of my recollection.

Q. So were you in charge of her care?
A. Well, I was a backup physician for [the PA] Scott Davidson, but to the best of my recollection Scott Davidson never did discuss Ms. Johnson. If he did, you know, I don't remember and also I did not see Ms. Johnson.

Q. So that I can make sure that your answer is clear—
A. Yes, sir.

Q. —I understand then the answer to my question to be no, you were not in charge of Crystal Johnson's care while she was in the emergency department on April the 10th of 2006. Is that correct?

Defense attorney Mr. Scoville: Objection.

A. I was—

Defense attorney, Mr. Scoville: You can answer.

A. I was the backup physician, sir, and I think to the best of my recollection Scott Davidson never discussed with me Ms. Johnson. And if he did, I don't remember, sir.

➤**Authors' note:** Ouch! Who hasn't in the course of a busy ED shift forgotten a conversation which occurred or not occurred? Who has signed charts, previously dictated/documented, without reading the whole chart? I have; we all have. Does this place us in legal jeopardy? The answer would have to be "yes," but like all of medicine, there are shades of gray. It may be one thing to fail to discuss a case, but does signing the chart of a patient you never saw or discussed ramp up the risk?

Continued deposition of ED defendant doctor Afram Aminah by plaintiff's attorney Alan Krause:

Q. Given that your initials [are] on her chart, you do believe you signed off on her chart?
A. Yes, sir. Yes, sir.

Q. Doctor, are you familiar with the provisions of [your state's] administrative code as to your duties as a backup supervising physician?
A. No, sir, I'm not aware of that, sir.

➤**Authors' note:** This may seem unusually harsh, but how many of us are aware of the administrative codes in our states? The grilling continues:

Q. Is that your signature there, Dr. Aminah?
A. Yes, sir.

Q. All right. To your knowledge, does your signature appear, initials, anywhere else in the chart, other than on this particular page?
A. My signature is on the following page after that.

Q. Are you able to tell from looking at the chart what date and time that you would have signed off on the chart?
A. The date, I mean, was the 10th, but the time, sir, I'm not able to say what time, sir.

Q. Are you able to say by looking at the chart whether you signed off on the chart before or after Ms. Johnson's discharge?
A. As to my understanding, sir, that hospital policy and regulation requires that before a patient is discharged a physician must sign off on the chart, sir, and I think we follow that policy.

Q. All right, sir. My understanding from your testimony is that you did not have any discussions with Mr. Davidson about Ms. Johnson on April 10th of 2006. Is that correct?
A. That's the best of my recollection, sir.

➤**Authors' note:** Is this doctor taking care of patients, or just following a hospital policy to sign charts? Of course, there is a reason that there is a policy to sign charts—to take ownership of the patient under your care. The onslaught continues:

Q. So who was in charge of her care on April 10th of 2006?
A. My understanding is that physician assistants are licensed, you know, health providers, and they follow the hospital policy and procedures.

Q. And so would the answer to my question be that the PA in this case, Scott Davidson, was the one that was in charge of Crystal Johnson's care on April 10th of 2006?

A. Yeah. That's my understanding, sir, because they're licensed health providers, and they follow the hospital policy and procedures governing their work. I didn't know anything about Ms. Johnson, sir, and the first time I knew anything was when I got that lawsuit in the registered mail.

➤**Authors' note:** Could this actually be true? A patient "bounces back" one day later with a horrible outcome and the doctor doesn't find out about the outcome until a letter arrives in the distant future? In our ED, it seems like you are assaulted when you walk through the double doors: "Do you remember that lady you saw yesterday in Room seven with the numbness? Well, she came back today with a stroke." Not that it has ever happened to me ... I've just heard stories ...

Did the doctor and PA discuss this case upon learning of the stroke diagnosis? Were there accusations at that time? This question is almost routine in a deposition; "Doctor, with whom did you discuss this case upon learning of the 'bad outcome'?" Oh, to be a fly on the wall.

When I was a kid, I would sometimes go fishing at a trout farm. Ever been to one? Ours had a small, stone-lined pool where the fish would come to be fed. It wasn't really fair; my dad paid a few bucks, and we threw in a line into the pool and instantly caught a healthy trout. Even through my childhood eyes, I never deluded myself into thinking I was a great fisherman, but sometimes a *real* fisherman will throw a line into the ocean and catch a big fish.

Q. All right, sir. So other than the claim that was made against a bunch of physicians at Cook County, no other—no other claims have ever been asserted against you?

A. No. No. Because the other one I mentioned in interrogatories.

Q. Yes, sir. Tell me about that.

A. Yeah. This was a patient who had chest pain for 24 hours. The patient was seen at the urgent care and was referred to our emergency department and the patient was followed by—by a PA, and then we followed the patient. The patient's chest pain had gone by then. And since the patient's pain had been gone for 24 hours, we wanted to evaluate to find out, you know, when did the patient's ischemia begin? The claim was that there was a delay in—in care of that patient and there—I was named. Physician assistant was named, hospital was named, and it was settled.

Q. And do you know who the PA was that was involved in that matter?

A. The PA has passed away, sir.

Q. Did you ever see, physically see, that patient while that patient was in the emergency department?

A. No, sir.

Q. All right, sir. Were you a backup supervising physician for that PA?

A. Yes, sir.

Q. Did you sign off on that patient's chart?

A. I discussed the patient. I discussed—the PA discussed the case with me from the beginning, so I was involved in the care of that patient from the beginning. I saw all the results and everything. Yes, sir.

Q. And—and to the best of your knowledge, that's different than the situation involving Crystal Johnson, correct?

Defense attorney Mr. Scoville: Objection.

Plaintiff's attorney Mr. Krause: You may answer the question.

A. Yeah. To the best of my knowledge I never did see Ms. Johnson and I do not remember Scott speaking me to about Ms. Johnson. If he did, as I said, I don't remember.

➤**Author's note:** Well, the doctor's favorite song is now in our heads like a broken record. His strategy is to continue to deny that he ever saw the patient, though that strategy seems a bit questionable while watching the plaintiff attorney "reel in" the big one.

Depending on state law, not all patients seen by mid-level providers need to be seen by a physician, despite the fact that the physician bills for the services. Is the "to the best of my knowledge I never saw Ms. Johnson …" approach the correct way to go? To find out, we asked Rich Milligan, a medical malpractice defense attorney and trial lawyer with over 25 years of experience.

VII. Legal Analysis: Rich Milligan, JD

- Health and Medicine Practice Group, Buckingham, Doolittle & Burroughs, LLP, Canton, Ohio

ED doctor bails out on his PA

The way this physician responded in deposition was a disaster! I am not sure if it is his lawyer's fault or his own; I suspect both. His testimony not only damages his defense, but that of the PA.

As a defense lawyer, I want a doctor that a jury likes, one who steps up to the plate and takes responsibility. The medicine is secondary. If the jury starts out by thinking you are ducking your professional responsibility, the benefit of the doubt is going to be with the patient. Medicine is complicated; jurors respect the difficulty of diagnosing conditions. If you were on a jury, would you believe that this physician has no responsibility for the care because he merely signed the chart and didn't see the patient or review the record? I don't think so!

This case presents a very difficult problem. The PA, who is required to work under physician supervision, arguably made a mistake. The ED doctor, in signing the chart, did not pick up the mistake. It can only be detrimental to the entire defense for the ED doctor and PA to point an accusatory finger at each other.

Defense strategy

As a defense lawyer, my job is to figure out how the facts can best be reconciled so the testimony is supportive, not accusatory. Part of my strategy would be for the ED doctor to accept responsibility for his role:

1. "I work with Scott Davidson regularly."
2. "He is a very competent PA. I trust his skills and judgment."
3. "I don't remember seeing Crystal Johnson or seeing her chart."
4. "As part of my standard practice, when I sign off on a chart for a patient that I have not seen, I look at the chart to make sure I am comfortable with the care that was given by the PA. If I have questions, I will talk to the PA. I may also see the patient. If necessary I will do additional testing or order different therapies."

By answering in this way, the ED physician is only admitting what he must—that he doesn't remember and that in his standard practice he would do what is reasonable, at a minimum to look at the chart. In most states, a physician is not required to see the patient or even discuss the case with the PA. But you must supervise! If you don't, you can be held legally liable. Supervision is not accomplished by blindly signing charts.

The only course for this is for the doctor to acknowledge what he doesn't remember and fall back on his standard practice, likely within the standard of care for a board-certified emergency medicine physician. Great athletes sometimes win games with horrible coaching, but one thing is true in both the sporting world and lawsuits: neither poor athletes nor bad witnesses win without good preparation. Here, we have a terrible witness, poorly prepared. To the extent that the testimony reflects a "strategy," it is a bad one, horribly executed. The witness comes off as dishonest and dismissive of his obligations as a physician.

VIII. The Depositions—Continued (January 2010)

➤**Authors' note:** The physician was obviously not coached by our two attorneys. Was he coached at all?

Is it legally defensible to perform a partial evaluation for TIA and to send the patient home without a definitive diagnosis or plan? You be the judge.

Continued deposition of ED defendant doctor Afram Aminah by plaintiff's attorney Alan Krause:

Q. From your review of her chart, would you have included TIA in your differential?

A. Well sir, to me, I'll have to see a patient, evaluate and, you know, see what the past medical history is, what treatment they received, what's the current treatment, and review their studies, and then I can formulate, you know, an opinion as to what is the problem.

Q. Yes, sir. But you've reviewed Ms. Johnson's chart of April 10th of 2006, correct?
A. Yes, sir.

Q. And you've reviewed it thoroughly, correct?
A. What do you mean by "thoroughly," sir?

Q. Well, you've been sued, doctor. I mean, I assume you've reviewed Ms. Johnson's chart given the allegations that have been made against you. I assume that you've reviewed it thoroughly, have you not?

A. I have—

Defense attorney Mr. Scoville: Objection. At the start [of the deposition] you asked him if he didn't understand the question to let you know and he told you he didn't understand "thoroughly," and so I object to your lecturing the witness.

Q. Well, do you understand the term "thoroughly?"

A. I've reviewed Ms. Johnson's chart, sir.

Q. All right. Based upon your review of her chart, would you have included TIA in her differential had you been the medical professional who saw her?

A. As I said, sir, there are a lot of conditions that cause transient neurologic symptoms and TIA is one of them.

Q. Yes, sir, and I understand that's what a differential is all about. My question is, had you seen Crystal Johnson on April 10th of 2006, would you have included TIA in your differential? And if you can answer the question with a yes or no, please answer it with a yes or no and then please feel free to explain.

Defense attorney Mr. Scoville: Objection. And if you can't answer it with a "yes" or "no," you can also tell him that.

A. As I said, sir, when I evaluate the patient, sir, I have to take a history, do, you know, a physical exam, review the medications, review the past history, past treatment, and then I can formulate an opinion as to what is the problem. And that's the normal and customary way that I follow a patient. And that's the best answer I can give you, sir.

Q. Okay. So—so my understanding is that Ms. Johnson's chart contains a history, correct?

A. Yes, sir.

Q. It contains her complaints, correct?

A. Yes, sir.

Q. It contains what medications that she was taking, correct?

A. Yes, sir.

Q. All right, sir. So my understanding is all of the things that you would do in the work-up of a patient were done with Ms. Johnson? Doctor, you've been a teacher before, correct?

A. Yes, sir.

Q. All right. And you—you do case presentations to students when you teach, correct?

A. Yes, sir.

Q. All right, sir. Now, all of the things that you indicate that would be done in the work-up of a patient, do you believe that they were done in the work-up of Crystal Johnson?

A. Yeah. Reviewing the charts, sir, Ms. Johnson was evaluated, history was obtained, personal history was obtained and those studies were done.

➤**Authors' note:** OK. Due to my benevolent nature and my pity on you, the reader, I have omitted the next several pages of testimony, which includes this question being asked again in slightly different format about 20 more times. I can attest that it is painful to read. Imagine how painful it was for those around the table. Did the plaintiff's attorney let him off the hook?

Q. Doctor, let me just say this. I don't have to be anywhere until tomorrow, and I want to see if I can get an answer to this question. It's a hypothetical question, based upon your having—being a board certified emergency physician and someone who's been involved in teaching. And so my question is, based upon your review of this chart, what would you have done—I know you didn't see her—but what would you have done had you seen this patient based upon your review of this chart?

A. As I said, sir, from my review, Ms. Johnson had transient neurologic symptoms which resolved. As I said, there are many causes of that. TIA is one of them.

➤**Authors' note:** So he finally admits that TIA is in the differential … or does he? How about hypercoagulable conditions?

Q. Now, do you know what I mean by the term "hypercoagulable condition?"
A. Yes, sir.

Q. What does that mean?
A. It means that something that can clot easy, readily.

Q. Did Ms. Johnson have a hypercoagulable condition when she presented to the emergency department on April 10th of 2006?
A. Not to the best of my knowledge, sir.

Q. All right, sir. To your knowledge, is there any relationship between an elevated platelet count and stroke?
A. To the best of my knowledge, sir, there's no correlation between the level of the platelet count and neurologic symptoms. That's to the best of my knowledge, sir.

➤**Authors' note:** Hmmm … OK. OK. I will now show off *my* ignorance (this is Weinstock here, *not* Klauer). Is there a link between elevated platelets and stroke? We asked Michael Weintraub, a neurologist who has published extensively on legal implications of using thrombolytics in acute stroke, who says an increased risk of stroke/TIA with thrombocytopenia is controversial.

IX. Guest Author—Michael Weintraub, MD, FACP, FAAN, FAHA

- Clinical Professor of Neurology, Clinical Professor Internal Medicine, New York Medical College, Valhalla, NY
- Dr. Weintraub is a neurologist who has written and lectured extensively on the legal implications associated with thrombolytics and stroke.

He first opines on our patient, including a differential diagnosis, and then on the use of tPA in stroke.

Case summary

The initial evaluation and assessment by the PA and nurse, and ultimately ER doctor, were limited, poor quality and clearly departed from quality standards of care (SOC).

A differential diagnosis of this case included:

- Thromboembolism from TIA/stroke
- Carotid dissection (at the clinic visit on March 9th she was treated for neck pain)
- Hemiplegic migraine
- Hereditary disorders (hematologic) of Protein S or Protein C deficiency
- Hereditary cerebral autosomal dominant arteriopathy[1]
- Sickle cell disease

It is important to admit patients with a TIA since this is a significant risk factor for subsequent stroke; up to 17% within 90 days, with the greatest risk in the first week.[2-4] The use of antiplatelet therapy (i.e., aspirin) has been demonstrated in individual trials and meta-analysis to reduce the risk of stroke and other vascular events in high risk patients by at least 23%.[5]

Risk stratification data has identified individuals who remain at high risk for TIA/CVA based on the Framingham Study.[6] Crystal smoked, a risk factor which has been shown to increase her risk.[7-9] However, elevated platelets remain controversial as to predisposition to thromboembolism.[10] Those who support the association suggest there is an increased risk due to up-regulation of thrombin in carotid disease. Interestingly, our patient was found to have a 90% carotid stenosis. Based on the NASCET data of increased risk of stroke with > 69% stenosis, this would suggest need for carotid angioplasty and/or stenting.[11, 12]

Continued deposition of ED defendant doctor Afram Aminah by plaintiff's attorney Alan Krause:

Q. When you signed off on this chart, I assume that you saw that Ms. Johnson's platelet count was a million, three hundred and forty-two thousand, didn't you?

A. Scott Davidson did not discuss Ms. Johnson with me, sir.

Q. Yes, sir, but you looked at her chart and you signed off on it. Did you see that her platelet count was a million, three hundred and forty-two thousand?

Defense attorney Mr. Scoville: Object to the form of the question.

A. As I said, sir, Scott Davidson never discussed Ms. Johnson with me, sir.

Q. Dr. Aminah, that wasn't my question. My question was, when you signed off on her chart, did you see that she had a platelet count of a million, three hundred and forty-two thousand?

Defense attorney Mr. Scoville: Objection.

A. As I said, sir, Scott Davidson never discussed Ms. Johnson with me, sir.

Q. Yes or no, when you signed off on her chart, did you see that she had a platelet count of a million, three hundred and forty-two thousand?

A. Scott Davidson never discussed the case with me, sir.

Q. So the answer to my question would be no, you didn't see that?

A. As I said, sir, Scott Davidson never discussed the case with me, sir.

Q. I know, Dr. Aminah. When you signed off on this patient's chart, did you see—did you look at her CBC?

A. Scott Davidson never discussed the case with me, sir.

Q. That wasn't the question I asked you, Dr. Aminah. The question I asked you is whether or not when you signed off on this patient's chart you noted that she had a platelet count of a million, three hundred and forty-two thousand, yes or no? It's a simple question. Yes or no, did you note it?

A. Scott Davidson never discussed the case with me, sir.

Q. So the answer to my question would be no, you didn't note it?

A. All I can tell you, sir, is that Scott Davidson never discussed the case with me, sir. That's my answer.

Q. Yes, sir. So your answer to the question of whether you noted it in her chart at the time you signed off on it, your answer to that question is: Scott Davidson never discussed the chart with me.

A. That's my answer to you, sir.

Q. Okay. So did you look at her chart before you signed off on it?

A. I looked at the diagnosis and I signed off.

Q. Did you look at the CBC?

A. No, sir.

Q. Why not?

A. Scott Davidson never discussed the case with me, sir.

➤**Author's note:** Certainly seems clear at this point that the doctor was coached to answer all questions the same way. Does this absolve him of responsibility? How damaging is the previous case he had with a PA where the patient died? His answers remain consistent until the end when he finally admits he did not see the platelet count. Did the plaintiff's attorney wear him down? Did his strategy crack?

Q. Do you wish he had today? As you sit here today, do you wish that Scott Davidson would have said, Dr. Aminah, I've got a patient that has transient neurologic symptoms and has a platelet count of a million, three hundred and forty-two thousand? As you sit here today, do you wish that Mr. Davidson had told you that?

A. As I said, Scott Davidson is a licensed physician assistant and follows hospital policy and procedure.

Q. Well, let's play what if. What if he had?

A. As I said, sir, I would have gone to see the patient sir, examined the patient, take the history and go through what I've described, sir, and then formulate an opinion as to the diagnosis and management.

>**Author's note:** Three and a half hours and over 100 pages of deposition testimony later, the doctor finally admits that if he knew the specifics of the case, he would have evaluated the patient himself. Would he have discharged her?

Q. You said you did not know whether you would have discharged her because you didn't have a chance to examine her?
A. Ms. Johnson had transient symptoms which are resolved. The discharge was reasonable for her.

Q. You said that you never even looked at [platelet count which was] a million three, correct?
A. Yes, sir.

Q. I understood you to tell me previously that if you had noted that her platelet count was a million, three hundred thousand-plus, my understanding is that you told me that you personally would have looked in on this patient, that you personally would have gotten more detail about the circumstances surrounding her fall. Do I understand you correctly to say that you personally would have gone to Ms. Johnson and gotten more information?
A. Yes sir.

Q. All right. That's all the questions I have.

>**Author's note:** There was an additional allegation regarding thrombolytics at the second ED visit. Remember that visit, where the patient had a stroke in the waiting room? (Not my fault, says the ED doctor. Not my fault, says the paramedic. Not my fault, says the triage nurse. Not my fault, says the hospital.)

We switch gears to the deposition of the plaintiff's emergency medicine expert, Dr. Michael Redd (the same physician who wrote the initial letter alleging negligence) by plaintiff's attorney Alan Krause:

Q. Was she a tPA candidate?
A. On the first visit, no. On the second visit, possibly.

Q. And what was it that makes it possible versus [the fact that] she was a candidate?
A. Time frame of when the stroke actually started. But I can't tell when exactly it was.

Q. Back then, it was how long before?
A. Three hours.

Q. Now, back in 2006, was that the standard in terms of what would have been done?
A. Well, 2006 was right on the cusp of when that was happening. They would have been doing inter-arterial tPA by sending her to another hospital. If the stroke happens immediately, you have a time frame in which to intervene. If you don't know when it started, you don't want to give [tPA] because that can cause a bleeding in the stroke area. So, if you know a stroke started exactly at noon, and you can see the person, they suddenly have right-sided weakness and numbness and other issues that become obvious that it's a stroke, you have a time frame to get it fixed.

Q. As of 2006, then, it's your testimony that tPA and retrieval could have been done?
A. It could have been done, yes. That certainly was an option.

➤**Author's note:** So let's get a little new age-y: before reading what happened next, put down the book, close your eyes and answer two questions:

1. Could this happen in your practice?
2. If it did, would you proceed to trial or settle?

If you are an emergency physician, would you have seen this patient?
If you are a mid-level provider (MLP), are there mechanisms in place to easily discuss difficult cases with the physician?
If you are a nurse, would you "treated" this patient with a "therapeutic wait?"
If you are a hospital administrator, does your current policy account for this scenario?

X. The Decision—Settlement vs. Trial?

This case did not go to trial, but was settled for an extremely large sum; enough to provide for life-long care of the patient, estimated to be in the millions of dollars.

Envisioning a trial, it is hard to see how the defense would proceed, particularly when faced with two providers who disagree about who had responsibility. It would be easy to play them off of each other. Would a jury sit patiently as Dr. Aminah continued to evade answering the questions? Since the PA has already admitted he was not aware a TIA could have occurred in the face of a normal CT, this would be easily rebutted with expert witnesses.

XI. Use of Thrombolytics in Acute Stroke

This is a CVA case, the hottest of hot-button issues in Emergency Medicine. Though it turns out the patient was not a tPA candidate (partially due to the prolonged amount of time spent in the waiting room), doctors *have* lost suits where they gave tPA and where they failed to give tPA.

Stroke litigation can be divided into five broad categories:[13]

1. Failure to give tPA with absence of a specific hospital protocol (e.g., the hospital does not have a protocol for giving tPA or for rapid transfer to facility that does)
2. Failure to offer tPA (e.g., patient arrives within "window" and is not offered tPA)
3. Misdiagnosis of stroke (e.g., dx of vertigo, migraine, anxiety/panic) or failure to recognize stroke in evolution
4. Complications of therapy/failure of informed consent (e.g., complication for which the patient was not aware)
5. Hemorrhagic stroke after informed consent (known but unintended consequences of treatment)

Guest Author (continued): Neurology Stroke Expert Michael Weintraub, MD, FACP, FAAN

Currently, the FDA has approved tPA use for thromboembolic strokes that conform to the three hour time window of onset and without specific contraindications. While the AHA, ASA and AAN in 2009 requested the FDA to expand the time window to 4.5 hours based on the ECASS III study, the FDA has not changed its opinion. Thus, it is considered "off-label use" after three hours, including the intra-arterial route.

The current medicolegal environment regarding tPA indicates 90% allegations for failure to administer, whereas 10% are for complications from tPA[16] (i.e., bleeding, deficits, death).

For the treatment of TIA, thrombolysis using tPA has not been studied and is to be considered an "off-label use."[14] The decision to use tPA should be guided by the clinical history, examination, lab, neuroimaging and most importantly, must follow the NINDS guidelines with a three-hour window.[15]

With regard to the use of tPA for TIA, I am not aware of any specific cases of medical malpractice for failing to give for TIA (failure to administer). While not totally protecting physicians from claims being filed (plaintiff's attorneys often consider: stroke=tPA=100% improvement irrespective of guidelines), supporters and advocates of tPA utilization in TIA or CVA would argue that the same risk factors and pathophysiology exist, as well as augmented risk for recurrence and/or worsening, and therefore tPA is warranted despite lack of evidence-based studies.[17]

XII. Guest Interview—Medical: Jerry Hoffman, MD

- Professor of Medicine and Emergency Medicine, UCLA
- Associate editor, Emergency Medical Abstracts

I had the honor of speaking with one of the foremost experts in emergency medicine, Jerry Hoffman, who opined on this case, the use of thrombolytics in stroke and a patient-oriented philosophy of practice.

Authors: *Thanks for agreeing to share your thoughts with me today.*
JH: My pleasure.

Authors: *What is your impression of Crystal's initial visit—two episodes of right sided numbness which resolved?*
JH: There are some things about the history that are quite good, but others that are missing. First of all, I have no idea how she is now; does she still feel weak? Does she still have numbness? Second thing, how long did the episodes last? Why did she fall, was it because she couldn't feel her leg? Are her symptoms ongoing?

Authors: *From the documentation, can you get an understanding of the thought process of the provider?*

JH: First of all, what is absolutely obvious is that the history screams out that this is an acute neurologic event. This is a sudden onset of weakness which causes her to fall, which is why I asked the previous question; if this was a vascular event, was it ongoing?

As you know, a TIA used to be defined purely on a clinical basis: a stroke-like event which disappeared [to clinical evaluation] within a brief period of time, 10–15 minutes in the vast majority of cases. Now, there is a lot of discussion about changing the definition of TIA to include imaging, which proves there is death of brain tissue. And the only way you prove it early on is with a MRI. TIA is a definition; this would change if from a "clinical" definition to a "clinical plus imaging" definition. That is not a terribly useful thing in the ED. What we need to know is: Does this patient continue to have a neurologic deficit clinically?

There are stroke mimics which could look like this as well. She could have a complicated migraine, hypoglycemia, hyponatremia, a CNS infection or mass lesion, but these diagnoses are more likely in ongoing neurological deficits than in a patient who gets better over minutes.

If [our patient] did get better within minutes, the only thing [besides a TIA or stroke] that is credible is a complicated migraine. Without a history of migraines and absence of headache, though this can occur, the chance is very small. In the ED, we need to exclude the more serious diagnoses. I am going to worry about stroke/TIA. I also mean hemorrhagic stroke as well as atypical causes, including dissection. But the primary thought on my differential is stroke or TIA.

Authors: *How would you approach this patient?*

JH: The first thing to do is a CT scan, to make sure there is no hemorrhage and also to look for something else surprising, such as a tumor. It is really important to understand that the CT is typically normal with a stroke or TIA, dissection, or venous sinus thrombosis. The CT is to rule out other things, not to rule in stroke.

Authors: *This brings us to the next question. If your primary consideration is stroke or TIA, is there a low risk group that can be sent home?*

JH: Now you are getting into the question, what to do with a TIA? This is a little bit controversial. Fifteen years ago, many got sent home, but recent research has shown that a TIA can be considered to equate to "unstable angina of the brain." A significant number will go on to complete a stroke within a short period of time [up to 17% within 90 days and perhaps 5% in the first couple of days]. That is a lot more than unstable angina. This finding has led to the notion that all TIA patients need admission.

Next was an attempt to sub-characterize those at high and low risk. Is that possible to do? Yes it is, but … not in a way that matters. As often is the case with scoring systems, they perform better on the first iteration than subsequent iterations. For any one of the scores, even at the lowest grade, you cannot exclude the risk of stroke in the next couple of days in a few percent. If the baseline risk is 5% and you get it down to 3%, does that really help you?

When you discover a decision instrument that seems to work, it always looks best initially, and therefore needs to be validated. When there is an attempt to validate, there is a pretty good chance it will not look as good. Why? The way in which you come up with a decision instrument is "data snooping." You look and find the best thing that fits your current data. That may turn out to be right, but it very often turns out to have occurred by chance, and the next sample or trial doesn't look as good.

What I find to be amusing is that when you look at the "ABCD2" score,[18,19] it tells you that it is no longer the one score. Why? It can't be considered a validation of the original; it's *new* data snooping. And now *it* also needs to be validated. Guess what? When they tried to validate, it didn't work so well. So, every time we have the *modified* Goldman criteria or the *modified* Wells criteria, this is new data snooping and probably isn't right either.

To summarize, none of these scoring systems actually hold up. The answer is: you can't say a person is at no risk and wash your hands of them.

Authors: *Should our patient have been hospitalized?*
JH: That leads to a separate question: is admission useful? A hospital is not a therapeutic environment. It is amusing that people think that once you go into the hospital you are safe. The real issue is: Do you have a *treatable* underlying cause of stroke, which we can identify and prevent before the big event occurs? There are a few things people worry about acutely, including hypercoaguable states, embolic causes, patent foramen ovale and carotid disease. Some of them are not that easily amenable to rapid treatment. For example, carotid disease will not be fixed within 12 hours.

[All this] has led to a standard which is not unreasonable; we need to look for these things acutely. This doesn't have to be in the hospital, but you can't come back in a week for the ECHO. Diagnostic evaluation and planning are what's needed.

Authors: *So let me give you a "rubber meets the road" question. You are in the ED, your PA comes up to you with this story, what do you tell the PA to do with this patient?*
JH: First of all, you have to go see the patient. This is the type of patient who has an overwhelmingly large chance of a neurovascular event. What would you do if a nurse came up and said you have a new cardiac arrest coming in? If you are that busy, then you need to get help. This should be planned well in advance. Your hospital should have a system for management of TIAs.

Authors: *Last question on the initial visit. How do the elevated platelets play into your decision model?*
JH: The first thing is that when a young person presents with stroke-type symptoms, you need to consider other reasons than the typical atherosclerotic stroke. [The differential]

includes mass, sympathomimetic drugs, dissection, venous sinus thrombosis or a hypercoagulable state.

I don't know that I am an expert on thrombocytosis' effect on clotting, whether it has been proven to be a cause of stroke, but I would be surprised if it weren't. I would think "oh my gosh" this is what's going on with her.

You need to figure out. Who is going to help you with this? This is a big deal. You have a vascular event in a young person. There are tremendous consequences if she would go on to complete her event.

Authors: *This brings us to an interesting point, and I will show my own bias. Who orders a CBC on a patient with unilateral numbness? They unnecessarily ordered a test, got an abnormal result, and did not act on it.*
JH: I would address this in a slightly different way. Yes, I am a big fan of asking "why did you get that test?" I don't believe, in general, a CBC has any relevance to a patient with stroke-like symptoms. On the other hand, it is frequently done. I would say that *getting* the test did not hurt them, but *failing to look at it* hurt them. It is not unreasonable to look for hematologic reasons, and when you get an abnormal result, you can think, "I am more brilliant than I thought!" One possibility is that the provider who glanced at this saw 1.3 and it didn't register. This medical decision-making does not give one a great deal of confidence in the provider.

Authors: *OK. Let's now skip down to visit number two. She arrived by EMS and was promptly hustled off into the waiting room. Despite coming to the desk several times, it was over three hours until she was seen by the doctor. It seems like there was a "punitive wait."*
JH: There are two issues. First, was this patient taken seriously? Here [we have] a large, impoverished woman with a psych history. Second, the job of the ED doctor is to rule out life threatening issues.

One of the greatest impediments to a correct diagnosis is a *prior* diagnosis. If the patient has schizophrenia, they are automatically immortal! [Laughs]. We stop thinking. That is called "premature closure." The provider [in this case] called it sinusitis because they felt uncomfortable saying, "I don't know what's going on here."

It was poor thinking to say it was not a stroke, but that's not as bad as giving it a name [sinusitis] so that no one in the future will think it is a stroke. By calling it sinusitis, they have compounded their mistakes, much in the same way that we always talk about [diagnosing] gastroenteritis when the diagnosis is appendicitis.

Authors: *On a side note, many of the patients in this book were inappropriately prescribed antibiotics at the initial visit.*
JH: That is a really great point. It is perfectly fine in the emergency department to say "I don't know." I say to patients all the time with abdominal pain, "I'm not sure what it is."

The majority of the time I see patients with abdominal pain, I don't know what it is. But what I am really saying is "I don't see something bad, and I think it is going to get better." Haven't you had abdominal pain that you didn't go to the doctor for?

But this notion of "I don't know what it is" so "I'll make up something and treat it," is bad for lots of reasons. It's not bad just because it spends lots of money for antibiotics or increases resistance or because it's intellectually dishonest and lying. It's bad because it obscures the truth. "I don't know. Come back if ..." is very different than "I know. There is nothing to worry about."

Authors: *To throw out a hypothetical, assuming the patient had not been placed in the waiting room, but seen immediately by the ED doctor with a CT confirming CVA, can you walk us through some of the pros and cons of thrombolytic therapy?*
JH: It's a really interesting question. I don't believe there's evidence thrombolytics are useful in stroke. Some of the evidence is inadequate. If I had to make my best guess, it would be that it is negative. I think it is pretty clearly not positive. On the other hand, I will admit it's not definitive. It is possible there is some subset where it would be useful and some subset where it would be harmful. This is, as yet, undefined.

If I had to make a guess, I would say it is useful very, very, very early on. I am pretty sure time doesn't matter once you are beyond 60–90 minutes because neural tissue doesn't survive very long. I'm willing to believe in the first five minutes, it would matter a lot. Who knows? Because there is harm associated with this treatment, there is always a balance.

The question of how you start the clock when there is a TIA is unanswered. I have heard deposition testimony about every permutation possible: the clock starts again when the new symptoms start; the clock starts yesterday when the symptoms started. But the answer is, since we have so little information on what to do when the patient has a TIA, I can't answer, but will say we should go back to our earlier discussion; a TIA was defined as a clinical event. But, we now know that the reason they have changed this from a clinical to an imaging event is because we know the clinical event of "I had some symptoms, they got better" has two possible causes [excluding stroke mimics]:

1. The traditional definition of TIA: they had a clot, there was no cell death, the clot got resolved, and they are better.
2. The other possibility is that they had a stroke. It wasn't a TIA. It wasn't a "non-cell death" event. It was relatively small. The rest of the brain took over. There wasn't a lot of edema, and you return to baseline even though you actually had cell death.

Why am I saying all that? Suppose she got completely better, but it wasn't really a TIA in the sense of ischemia? It really was infarction. Then we are back to the case that she had a stroke, which was completed yesterday. Now, does she have a new clot? We are making it up. There is no information about this, no evidence about this. For the most part, people would say, "You have a stroke which is getting worse. You are not a candidate for tPA." The truth is that even I would have to admit, "I don't know."

The fact that Crystal had a positive CT at the second ER suggests that she did not have her stroke while she was sitting in the waiting room. She had a previous stroke. Whether this is a new one or an extension, I cannot say. But it suggests that yesterday was a stroke, not a TIA.

The irony of the awful behavior of sending her to the waiting room, and this is really, really horrendous behavior, is that it may help to amplify the verdict exponentially. You don't want the jury to think you are a Nazi *and* a [bad doctor].

Authors: *Next topic; you have heard of "The Hoffman Effect?" Do you realize your passion on this issue has affected almost every emergency physician in the country?*
JH: I don't do it for me. I do it because I think we are harming our patients. If we had 100 patients we treated according to AHA guidelines and then went back in time, there is a chance a patient was helped. It certainly is possible. But you can't go back and only pick the one who was helped, because the evidence suggests strongly there is at least one also who would be hurt. So, on balance, we are doing at least as much harm as good.

Now [for the practical aspect], in community practice, there is *more* than one harmed for every one who has benefit. I'll bet you a nickel that in ten years, people won't be talking about lytics—it will be so obvious they don't work. [In the same way] that steroids in spinal cord injuries are dying a slow death. I knew ten years ago that giving steriods was the wrong thing to do. It took a while for everyone to acknowledge that. It might not happen quickly. They are now winning the battle, just like they won the steroid battle.

Another tragedy is how this reflects bad thinking and bad behavior. Even if it is neutral, what's the big deal? It is still harmful that we allow ourselves to believe bad things, and I think that is why my comments resonate so much with emergency doctors. I think emergency doctors don't tPA because we are being sold this for all the wrong reasons. They don't have proof … they are making it up! They expect us to do something that may be harmful to patients just because it is in somebody's interests to do.

Authors: *I hear you addressing two questions. One is whether tPA works if you give it per guidelines. The other is whether this can actually be done in the community. It's hard to give it correctly.*
JH: You are making my point; the tPA literature is moderately negative. But it's not just the small Cleveland study or the small Yale study, but it's the large databases in America of 100,000 or 250,000 patients that show a *lot* of harm. I'm not making a slur on community practices. When we are under tremendous pressure to give it in an uncontrolled environment—and that is at UCLA as well as a community hospital—when we aren't looking at a study where everything is rigorously controlled, then it is more than a little harmful. In this setting, there is substantial harm.

Authors: *Have you ever given it?*
JH: I have not personally, but two of my patients have received it from the neurology stroke team. Just so you will understand, [at UCLA] the stroke team will see every potential

stroke patient. Many of my colleagues will call the stroke team and let them do what they want to do. But I am a big believer that it is my patient. We are a huge receiver for stroke patients. I try not to be negative, but to be balanced and say, "You may have heard it is the wonder drug, but there are a lot of concerns; it has never been shown to decrease mortality and may in fact increase mortality." I say the evidence is really unclear. Over the years, very few patients or family have wanted it.

Authors: *It seems sort of strange to me pathophysiologically; when you give a lytic for an MI you see an effect right away, the STs go down or their pain resolves. How could it be with a stroke, that the lytic effect is not seen for 3—6 months? It seems the therapeutic process of clot lysis should be identical.*
JH: Of course. Of course. Absolutely! Of course it doesn't work. And the mental gyrations people go through to try to pretend it does result in more than bending the laws of physics.

There are now a bunch of articles which show that "we gave it to a bunch of patients, and they did just as well as in X-study or Y-study. And it turned out that 20% didn't have a clot and 20% were a TIA." So, there are two possible conclusions to that. The conclusions of the authors: well, we gave it to stroke mimics and they were fine. Maybe it works in stroke mimics [laughs]? We gave it to people without a clot and they did fine. That's one possible interpretation. So, maybe it doesn't work by busting a clot. Maybe it works as an antibiotic. It really is an anti-inflammatory. If this is true, then it didn't work in the randomized trials. It's remarkable. It works in stroke mimics just as well? It sounds to me like "just as poorly."

Authors: *Walk me through the three main reasons why the thrombolytic studies are deceptive?*
JH: First of all, there are only a few randomized controlled trials. There are nine or ten. Only two claim to be positive, only *slightly* positive. Many are neutral. Several are quite negative. This is consistent with chance. If you flip a coin, just because there is an occasional study that looks a little positive doesn't mean that treatment works, if there are also lots of studies that don't look positive.

Clearly, there are more negative studies than positive. The advocates will say the other studies don't count. They will say "they got the timing wrong" or "they got the drug wrong. It shouldn't be streptokinase." If those are true, you need to retest it to make sure it is not by chance. The only basis for claiming the streptokinase studies are wrong is because they didn't turn out the way they wanted them to. It's not science. It's always true that all the evidence is positive if you exclude the negative evidence.

What is ironic is that ECASS III looked a little positive. They said it proved that the timing was wrong. It probably is by chance. They throw out all the studies that said it doesn't work beyond three hours, but this one counts. What is the difference? Why are the others bad and this one good? It's because the others got the wrong result.

The second thing is that if one looks carefully at the two positive studies, there is a much stronger explanation even beyond chance. If you look at the raw data in NINDS, the effect of tPA and placebo were the same. The reason that more people ended up better in the tPA group was that more people started out better. This is the most important determinant of outcome. If you look at ECASS III, which showed an even more marginal benefit than NINDS (since it was a proprietary study I could not get the raw data, unlike NINDS, where I got the raw data ten years later), one thing they have shown is that there were 5% more people in the placebo group with more severe stroke and there were 5% better outcomes with tPA. It is perfectly reasonable to assume that out of ten studies, two would look good just by chance.

Third, say we have a new procedure for [treating] ruptured AAA. For example, Dr. Genius goes in there and does a magic trick and gets the hemorrhage to stop; it doesn't mean we can *all* do it. Maybe there is a procedure that he could eventually teach us. It turns out that the differences between effectiveness and efficacy in real practice vs. what happens in the ideal settings of a clinical trial are never the same. There are many reasons we would expect it is not the same, such as:

- Advanced imaging
- Recognizing stroke mimics
- Giving the drug to the wrong person because you are under so much pressure to give it in your community hospital (The opportunity to give tPA doesn't happen very often and your administrator wants to call you a stroke center, but can't unless you give tPA.)

If it turns out that tPA is like NINDS claims, [out of ten coin flips] it is 5¼ heads. If you give it to the wrong population so that 20% of the stroke mimics are occasionally "knocked off," you can get below '5 heads' in an awfully big hurry. As I have said, I don't think it is 5¼ heads, but even if it is, there are a lot of reasons you can get it wrong. As Dave Shroyer showed ten years ago, tiny hemorrhages are commonly not seen amongst neurologists and radiologists and emergency docs. The best evidence is that in the community, outcomes are terrible.

Authors: *Last question, another hypothetical: We hang up the phone, you walk into the beautiful Los Angeles sunshine and notice your left arm and leg are numb, your speech is slurred and you are not thinking clearly. EMS takes you to a stroke center where a CT confirms there is no head bleed. Forty-five minutes into your symptoms you are offered tPA. Do you accept?*
JH: (Laughs) That's the most ridiculous question! If I did have hemiplegia, I would know I was getting an atypical migraine. I have been hemiplegic twice in my life. It was scary as shit. I would delude myself into believing that …

As a doctor, I am a skeptic. I don't believe things because people are saying them. I am critical. I ask for evidence. But me as a *patient*? I choose a doctor I really like and trust and ask their advice. I don't want to be my own doctor. I don't want to be my wife's doctor. It would depend on whether I trusted and believed the person [pause], but overall, no, I wouldn't want it. Maybe if I came in at the first one minute [pause] … No! … I think this is bad.

What I always say is that I would want to be randomized to a trial so I could help others. If I am so out of it I cannot decide, as I am having a massive stroke, and I know the outcome will be bad whatever I did, I might do the opposite (laughs).

No, I don't want this. I don't think this is good. I've never said that before. I have always hedged. But, I have to say, no I don't want it. I think it is a bad medicine.

Authors: *On a side note, finding the exact right doctor is tough, between trying to please Press Ganey and increase throughput. It is easy to opt for testing as the easy way out.*

JH: I have two things to say about that. I don't think we should be that sorry for ourselves. We have the best job in the world and are incredibly well rewarded for it. If you are a nice person and treat people with respect, the vast majority will think the world of you. Like any other skill, you get better with this over time. I am a better doctor than I was five years ago. I am far from perfect, but I can go fast and can make decisions. I know when I don't know what I am doing. Maybe it is just grey hair that they like. We have a fabulous, fabulous job. It's intellectually interesting, we get tremendous respect for it, we get tremendous monetary benefits, its fun, and it is very hard. Yes, there are legal issues. But we are so blessed.

The fundamental nature of our work hinges upon an agreement that we will do what is in the best interests of our patients, not our own best interest. That's the critical, single most important part of being a professional. The promise to use your skills and knowledge as a learned intermediary on behalf of your patient to do what is best for them. You cannot do an unnecessary test just because it's going to make you money.

The problem is that just about every one of our incentives are not what is in the best interest of the patient. Our incentive is to go faster, not to explain things, to do the simplest thing (for example, to give them the prescription for an antibiotic and not to talk to them about why they don't need it). To do the CT scan is not only easier in every way; if little Johnny has a bleed, you're a hero. No one will call you a villain for Johnny's cancer. No one will even remember. You will get fewer complaints. [sarcastically] "Boy, that doctor was thorough, he got a CT. I thought Johnny had a cold, but he got a CT. Wow! Aren't you thorough?" And to make things worse, you get paid more for it.

Authors: *Final thoughts?*

JH: We have skirted another huge issue, which is the way in which bias and prejudice interfere with our ability to think. In retrospect, it is really important not to blame our patients. If a patient comes in with what could be a stroke, how can you pass it off? It could be meningitis, but I will pass it off as a tooth ache. These were not subtle findings; Crystal fell down, her symptoms were unilateral. The moment that a patient pushes your buttons, whether she be fat, disheveled, psychiatric or homeless, the moment I don't like the person, I say to myself, "I am about to make a mistake." It's important to be vigilant and to think of these possibilities. I would have settled this case. It was terrible care.

XIII. Authors' Summary

When two providers see a patient, who is medically and legally responsible? It is safe to say that if the attending could have seen the outcome in a crystal ball, he would have taken more ownership of the patient. If the PA had recognized he was left with diagnostic uncertainty exceeding his training or comfort level, he would have asked for help. When he told the plaintiff's attorney that he spoke with the attending and he knew this because he always speaks with the attending, it was clear the case was lost. Now the plaintiff's attorney is not fighting against two providers alone, but is assisted in his battle since they are also fighting against themselves.

This case was featured in the April edition of Risk Management Monthly, resulting in a lively discussion. One point hammered home by John Rockwood, an amazing PA that I have had the pleasure of working with for over ten years, is that this is a team effort. If the doctor is not available, the default is for the MLP to make a decision on their own, one that would be better if made with collaboration. And this goes both ways, John's skills could be equated with those of a plastic surgeon; I often ask his advice on complex cases.

Take home points:

- Use caution in ordering tests which do not have a good chance of establishing the diagnosis. An unrecognized false positive can be misleading. An unrecognized true positive can be devastating.
- When a patient is discharged without a clear diagnosis, a plan must be in place for completion of the evaluation. Though Crystal could have been discharged from the ED, but only with the understanding of the potentially worst diagnosis, and definitive plans for further testing the next day, the safest approach would have been admission.
- One approach when thrombolytics are an option is to present the patient and family with the risks and benefits and let them make the decision (of course, with your guidance). If lytics are not used, specifically document why they were not given.
- The last summary point for this case also applies to all the cases in this book; though we have the most advanced technology in the world at our fingertips, *history is still king.*

References

1. M Baudrimont, F Dubas, A Joutel, et al. Autosomal dominant leukoencephalopathy and subcortical ischemic stroke. A clinicopathological study. Stroke 1993; 24:122-5.
2. Johnston SC, Gress DR, Browner WS, Sidney S. Short-term prognosis after emergency department diagnosis of TIA. JAMA 2000; 284:2901-06.
3. Rothwell PM, Warlow CP. Timing of TIAs preceding stroke: time window for prevention is very short. *Neurology* 2005; 64:817-20.
4. Mitka M. Guideline stresses aggressive approach to reducing risk of recurrent stroke. JAMA 2010; 304:2468-9.

5. Antiplatelet Trialists' Collaboration. Collaborative overview of randomised trials of antiplatelet treatment. I. Prevention of death, myocardial infarction, and stroke by prolonged antiplatelet therapy in various categories of patients. BMJ1994; 308:81–106.
6. Kannel W, Gordon T, Wolf PA, et al. Hemoglobin and the risk of cerebral infarction: The Framingham Study Stroke, 1972; 3:409-20.
7. Wolf PA, D'Agostino RB, Kannel WB, et al. Cigarette smoking as a risk factor for stroke. The Framingham Study. JAMA 1988; 259:1025-9.
8. Shinton R, Beevers G. Meta-analysis of relation between cigarette smoking and stroke. BMJ 1989; 298:789-94.
9. Colditz GA, Bonita R, Stampfer MJ, et al. Cigarette smoking and risk of stroke in middle-aged women. NEJM 1988; 318:937-41.
10. Mayda-Domaç F, Misirli H, Yilmaz M. Prognostic role of mean platelet volume and platelet count in ischemic and hemorrhagic stroke. J Stroke Cerebrovasc Dis 2010; 19: 66-72.
11. Biller J, Feinberg WM, Castaldo JE, et al. Guidelines for Carotid Endarterectomy: A Statement for Healthcare Professionals From a Special Writing Group of the Stroke Council, American Heart Association. Stroke 1998; 29:554-62.
12. Moore W, Barnett HJM, Beebe HG, et al. Guidelines for Carotid Endarterectomy: A Multidisciplinary Consensus Statement From the Ad Hoc Committee, American Heart Association. Stroke 1995; 26:188-201.
13. Weintraub M. Thrombolysis (tissue plasminogen activator) in stroke: a medicolegal quagmire. Stroke 2006; 37:1917-22.
14. Liebeskind DS. No-go to tPA for TIA. Stroke 2010; 41:3005-6.
15. Tissue Plasminogen Activator for Acute Ischemic Stroke. The National Institute of Neurological Disorders and Stroke rt-PA Stroke Study Group. NEJM 1995; 333:1581-7.
16. Weintraub MI.Thrombolysis (tPA) in stroke: a medicolegal quagmire. Stroke 2006; 36:1917-22.
17. Kohrmann M, Schellinger PD. Pro IV tPA in stroke patients with rapid, complete recovery during evaluation (TIA) and evidence of MCA occlusion. Stroke 2010; 41:3003-4.
18. Johnston SC, Rothwell PM, Nguyen-Huynh MN, et al. Validation and refinement of scores to predict very early stroke risk after transient ischaemic attack. Lancet. 2007 27; 369(9558):283-92.
19. Rothwell PM, Giles MF, Flossmann E, et al. A simple score (ABCD) to identify individuals at high early risk of stroke after transient ischaemic attack. Lancet. 2005 2-8; 366(9479):29-36.
20. Mullins ME, Schaefer PW, Sorensen AG, et al. CT and conventional and diffusion-weighted MR Imaging in acute stroke: Study in 691 Patients at Presentation to the Emergency Department. Radiology 2002: 360-.
21. Menchine MD, Wiechmann W, Rudkin S. Trends in midlevel provider utilization in emergency departments from 1997 to 2006. Acad Emerg Med 2009;16:963–9.

So there you have it.

It was a relatively light shift—only 10 patients and you sent them all home; bronchitis, a shoulder strain, gastroenteritis, benign abdominal pain, a few headaches and a homeless lady with a diagnosis of substance abuse who refused Tylenol and was made to sign an AMA form when she complained of pain from her IV. Some patients are *so annoying!* The shift went fast; in the span of a career, this should be a completely forgettable day ...

Not the end of the story

Through the course of this project, Kevin and I have been touched by the stories within these pages and enlightened by the commentary of the national medical and legal experts who have contributed.

We would be interested in *your* thoughts; insights and criticisms, questions and commiserations. To get the story-behind-the-story, see additional deposition and trial testimony, read the thoughts of your colleagues, and post your own comments, visit our blog at:

www.embouncebacks.com

In the words of Bob Dylan:

"May your thoughts always be joyful,
May your song always be sung,"
... And may you never have a light 10-patient day in the ED ...

Michael and Kevin
September 2011

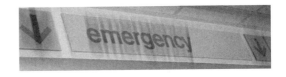

LEGAL CONSIDERATIONS
HELP! I AM BEING SUED

Kevin M. Klauer, DO, EJD, FACEP

I. The Letter 285

II. The Complaint 286

III. A Case of Failure to Report 286

IV. The Complaint Is Filed with the Court 287

V. The Complaint Moves to Discovery 287

VI. Attorney-Client Privilege and Discoverable Conversations 288

VII. Preparation of a Defense 288

    A. Duty 288

    B. Standard of Care 288

    C. Causation 289

    D. Damages 289

VIII. Preparation of a Defense: The Initial Review of a Claim 289

IX. Preparation of a Defense: Assessment of Damages 290

X. Multiple Defendants 290

XI. Preparing a Witness 291

XII. Trial v. Settlement 291

XIII. Appeals 292

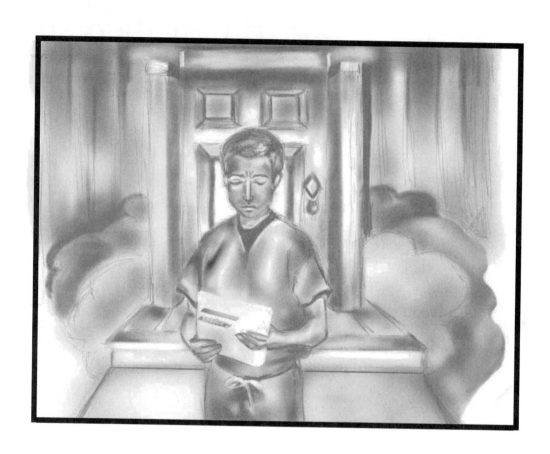

HELP! I AM BEING SUED

I. The Letter

Returning home after a busy shift, a certified letter greets you at the door. Your heart skips a beat. While opening the envelope, you are still thinking of the hypoxic young woman with breast cancer and a saddle embolus you intubated and thrombolysed a few hours earlier. Her husband was several years your junior—the case struck close to home.

Scanning down the page, there is no memory of the patient's name or her complaint.

<u>**Personal and Confidential**</u>
Timothy Madison, M.D.
365-25th Street
Canton, OH 44705

Re:	Claimant:	Anna Kamianka
	Insured(s):	Timothy Madison, M.D.
	D/I:	9-6-10
	Location:	Hilltop Hospital, Cleveland, OH
	Policy No.:	965-00032-02
	Policy Period:	7/1/2011–7/1/2012

Dear Dr. Madison:

Wind River Litigation, Inc. has been retained to assist in the management of the above-referenced matter. We have been provided with a copy a 180-day notice letter you will be receiving shortly.

This is only an incident, and to our knowledge no actual claim has been made. However, if a claim is made or suit is filed, coverage will be provided to you under the terms and conditions of the above-referenced policy, with limits of $1,000,000 per medical incident/$3,000,000 per policy aggregate.

Please do not discuss this matter with anyone other than a representative of our office. In addition, please create a personal file in order to maintain orrespondence related to this litigation and keep it separate and apart from any documentation or records you have regarding your treatment of Anna Kamianka. **If you are served with any suit papers or correspondence relating to this matter, please notify our office immediately.**

We look forward to assisting you.

Very truly yours,

Lisette Tucker, Esq.

Lisette Tucker, Esq.
Claims Attorney

PS Have a nice day

II. The Complaint

Lawsuits begin with a legal complaint. When a letter is received, a risk management incident report should be generated to track potential of formal legal action. Some providers are reluctant to do so since they feel that they are admitting to error or highlighting their inadequacy as a provider. However, a complaint that flies under the radar handicaps the risk manager's ability to mitigate risk, reduce financial liability, and to begin planning for a future defense.

In addition to the certified letter, other reasons to file a report include:

- Cases with known bad outcomes (regardless of fault or whether an error occurred)
- Complaints in which the patient or family mention potential litigation
- Cases with a known treatment complication
- Discharged patients who return with a previously-missed diagnosis (bouncebacks)

Filing an incident report will allow the risk manager to assess the level of risk and determine whether the complaint can be resolved without legal intervention, notify the insurer of a potential claim, and begin accumulating necessary documents. As in some of the cases in this book, certain pieces of the chart may turn up missing (Case 2), which is interpreted as sloppy medical care. If there is a fact in dispute, there is no doubt that the plaintiff's attorney will imply that the "mystery document" vanished into thin air to benefit the defense.

III. A Case of Failure to Report

An emergency physician who was a hospital employee evaluated a 55 year-old man with chest pain. Despite minimal risk factors and atypical, reproducible pain, he suffered an acute myocardial infarction and died. A claim was filed which progressed to a lawsuit. In addition to being unfortunate for the patient, it was also unfortunate for the physician when he discovered that his policy did not cover this act.

Why? Thirteen months prior, the hospital became self-insured and advised the employed medical staff members that all suspicious cases should be submitted to the risk manager so that these "prior acts" could be covered by the former policy. Despite the fact that the physician knew of the bad outcome two weeks after it occurred, he failed to report. The prior policy was a "claims-made" policy, covering claims identified during the policy period. (This is distinct from an "occurrence policy," which covers all claims filed during or subsequent to the policy period).

A "claims-made" policy requires tail coverage to cover claims received beyond the policy period for events that took place during the policy period. In order to save cost, the hospital elected to provide "prior acts" or "nose" coverage to cover claims during the transition period, instead of purchasing tail coverage. When this claim was received, it was discovered that the physician ignored the request to report potential claims, and the hospital refused his coverage for this "prior act" under their new captive.

IV. The Complaint Is Filed with the Court

Complaints are usually filed with the court simultaneously with the summons, advising the defendant or defendants that they are being sued. For malpractice lawsuits, delivery may be by a court courier, Sheriff's deputy or certified mail.

A summons requires a response within a proscribed period of time. The response usually consists of an answer and should address each allegation, though it is acceptable for a defendant to state that sufficient information is not possessed to confirm or deny the allegations. Do not respond to any questions without the oversight of your attorney.

In some states, additional documentation is required. For instance, in Pennsylvania, a certificate of merit must be filed within 60 days of filing a lawsuit. The certificate must confirm that a licensed physician has reviewed the case and feels that with reasonable probability, the care rendered fell below the standard of care.

If there is a clear and compelling reason why the suit should not be allowed to continue, for example, if an emergency physician not involved in the care was erroneously named in a lawsuit, a motion of dismissal may be filed and the plaintiff must respond. What should you do when you receive a summons or notice of intent to sue? An all too common response is to ignore it, but like an abscess, it only gets worse until the I&D. Regardless of merit, failure to respond is a big mistake. The doctor is in control in the ED, but with a legal proceeding everyone needs to follow the legal rules of engagement, known as civil procedure. In many jurisdictions if no response is received, the default is summary judgment for the plaintiff. If your head is buried in the sand, what is the most visible anatomical part?

V. The Complaint Moves to Discovery

Discovery is a data-gathering period, providing an opportunity for the plaintiff and defendant to get the flavor of the case the other side will present. Certain disclosures are mandatory, such as hospital documents and witnesses that will be deposed or called to testify. If any items are discovered without disclosure, they will likely be perceived as an attempt to intentionally withhold them.

Examples of data provided during discovery include:

- Documents—Medical records and hospital policies
- Interrogatories—Written questions requiring a response under oath
- Depositions—Almost universally utilized in medical malpractice cases
- Admissions—Narrowly-focused questions to which the opposing side must deny or admit. Such questions help to clarify if a party is uncertain of a fact or what position the other side will take

VI. Attorney-Client Privilege and Discoverable Conversations

The communication known as attorney-client privilege is granted the greatest power of any professional-client relationship. However, it is human nature to vent and seek validation by asking the opinion of others we trust. Unfortunately, casual conversations with colleagues are open to discovery. One of the first questions asked in a deposition is whether you have spoken to anyone about the case ... guess who gets deposed next week? One exception is spousal privilege; however, if the spouse speaks with others, those conversations are non-privileged and discoverable.

VII. Preparation of a Defense—Necessary elements of a lawsuit (Tort of Negligence):

- Duty to treat
- Breach of the standard of care (SOC)
- Causation (direct and proximate)
- Damages

A. **Duty:** The element of duty is critical, but is rarely a factor in medical malpractice claims when a physician-patient relationship clearly exists. The nature of our work and EMTALA establish a duty owed by the emergency physician to everyone who presents to the ED. There are some circumstances in which a duty does not exist, such as with "Good Samaritans," but be careful. Even if you render care voluntarily, such as to the syncope patient on a flight, if you receive any compensation, it can be deemed that a duty is now owed and the "Good Samaritan" protection may disappear. Though appealing, decline the bottle of champagne offered by the patient's family or the first-class upgrade from the airline.

B. **Standard of care:** The standard of care in medical practice is almost always a national standard, defined as *what a reasonable provider with similar training under* *similar circumstances would do.* If the provider's actions are deemed to have fallen below the standard of care, negligence will be found; if not, then no liability is assigned.

C. Causation: Many cases pivot on the merits of causation, another very common defense strategy. To prove causation, the plaintiff's injury (damages) must be the *direct cause* of the defendant physician's negligence.

However, the defendant's negligence must also be the *proximate* cause of the injury. Proximate cause requires that there be no disruption in the chain of causation between the negligent act and the injury to the plaintiff. Also, there can be no superseding or intervening events that break the chain of causation. If some other event occurred after the defendant's negligence that may have resulted in the plaintiff's injury or damages, this may relieve the defendant of liability.

For example, if a patient is seen at Blue Hospital's Emergency Department for abdominal pain due to an undetected abdominal aortic aneurysm (AAA) and is inappropriately discharged and dies, Blue Hospital and its providers will likely be found negligent; a duty to treat was owed the patient, the care was below the standard of care and their negligence was the direct and proximate cause of the patient's death.

Let's throw a causation twist into this scenario. What if the patient had a CT of the abdomen and pelvis that was misinterpreted as normal, missing the AAA? Of course, the hospital and radiologist will have substantial exposure. However, the emergency physician's alleged negligent act of discharging the patient is defensible under the theory of causation and standard of care. The misinterpreted CT was the superseding act that relieves the emergency physician of his or her liability. Furthermore, it would be argued that discharging the patient with a normal CT was not a violation of the standard of care.

D. Damages: Without damages, negligence carries no liability and there are no grounds for a lawsuit. While standard of care and causation are the cornerstones of any defense, *damages* are what strengthen a plaintiff's case. The more injured a plaintiff, the greater a jury's sympathy and the more likely a large verdict.

VIII. Preparation of a Defense: The initial review of a claim

The initial review will often provide a good sense of the cause of action (allegations), and what acts, either of commission or omission, constitute the plaintiff's claim. Review of the medical care can be accomplished by an expert panel or commissioned experts. The summary should identify strengths and weaknesses of the care, focusing on standard of care and causation issues, damages and potential defense strategies.

The primary documents utilized are the defendant's own words as documented in the medical record. The medical record is usually taken at face value unless there is documentation to cast doubt about its accuracy. For instance, if the nurse documents that the patient had syncope and the physician stated the patient didn't, such discrepancies may lead to a weakness in a case if left unaddressed. (This also emphasizes how important it is to read the nurse's notes.) Consider how the outcome of Case 4 may have changed if the doctor had read the nurse and paramedic notes.

Unfortunately, many cases focus on undocumented provider claims, such as:

- "I told the patient about the possibility of appendicitis."
- "I offered admission but the patient refused."
- "I re-examined the abdomen twice."

Plaintiff's attorney:

- "Would you consider these items important to the care of a patient with abdominal pain? (The obvious answer would have to be yes; otherwise, the physician wouldn't be claiming that they were done.)
- "If they are that important, why didn't you document them? You took the time to document the social history. Did you really re-examine the abdomen twice or just wish you had?"

It's easy to see how this will play out.

IX. Preparation of a Defense: Assessment of damages

The next step is to assess the alleged damages, which helps to set reserves for the case. Reserves are an estimate of the potential judgment should an adverse verdict be rendered. If the case is settled or the judgment is less than expected, the excess reserves will be returned to the insurer's general funds.

X. Multiple Defendants

The strengths and weaknesses of a given case may be viewed differently by co-defendants. Although "we are all in this together," each may not have the same exposure or share the same goals and defense strategy. It is important to assess the defense provided by your insurer and any conflicts of interest.

For instance, if you and the hospital are co-defendants, insured by the same company, this may create an inequity in the defense. The hospital may have a large amount of exposure, and you may have very little. However, if the hospital's strategy is to avoid an excess limits judgment, it may be willing to settle and take you along for the ride, even if your exposure is disproportionately small. Under such circumstances, it may be worthwhile to consider obtaining independent counsel. This may be at your own expense, but in the right circumstances, money well spent.

XI. Preparing a Witness

Once the case has been assessed, reserves have been set, and a defense strategy initiated, every defendant must be prepared to be a witness. This can be a long and painful process, since the average lawsuit takes 45 months to resolve. Many a defendant physician is lulled into complacency in the preparation phase, with the thought that no attorney could possibly triumph when debating medicine. This is a critical error, and one that the plaintiff's attorneys hope you make. They will never debate the medicine; they will let their experts do that. They will use language and the subtleties of law to spin the facts to their advantage, while using your own words, documented or spoken, to discredit you. Consider the final questions of the plaintiff's attorney in Case 1. There was only one way to answer, and it didn't reflect well on the ED physician.

This journey isn't about finding the truth; it's about winning. This assessment may seem harsh, but these are the ground rules. Therefore, *every* defendant needs to be trained in conduct during a deposition and courtroom proceedings. This is foreign to most of us. Your best foot must be forward from the beginning of the case, not just for your courtroom appearance. It is important to be vigilant about appearance, mannerisms, attire and attitude. It is important to be vigilant about appearance, mannerisms, attire and attitude. If you make a good showing as a credible defendant during the deposition, the plaintiff will be more apt to move toward settlement or even dismiss you altogether.

Emotional support is necessary but infrequently provided. The prolonged legal process causes us to question the core of our existence. Ensure that social, emotional and even mental health resources are available.

XII. Trial v. Settlement

The decision to go to trial is a complex one, based on the merits as well as the economics. To the physician, this is personal; our pride and professional credibility are at stake. Should an inappropriate lawsuit without negligence be fought to deter subsequent cases? The answer: yes and maybe.

We all have a responsibility to fight frivolous lawsuits, and the defendant should always be consulted about a decision to settle; however, when the damages are potentially high and the defense weak, settlement is a reasonable consideration. Losses can be minimized, expenses reduced and the defendant spared the emotional, personal and professional hardship of enduring a lengthy adjudication process.

What if the insurance company wants to settle and you don't? Well, your goals are pride and justice, whereas the insurer's are economic. Most insurers will align your goals and reassess your position. In other words, if they can settle the case for $100,000, but could be at risk for a $500,000 jury verdict, they won't be too excited about taking this risk to protect your honor. If the insurer requires your consent to settle, it will ask you to sign a "bad faith letter" if you are unwilling to give your consent, and you will be responsible for paying the portion of a jury verdict that could have been avoided by the proposed settlement. In this scenario, the defendant would be personally responsible for $400,000. Oftentimes, when a defendant has to consider the true economic risk of the case, settlement is agreed to as the best option.

All is not lost. Bad faith claims cut both ways. There are many instances in which defendants just want out, preferring to avoid the emotional strain of a lengthy legal battle. They don't want to testify in court, or they feel the settlement offer is just compensation for the patient's injury. Consider that a settlement offer for $600,000 is received, but the insurer wants to try the case to avoid any and all indemnity loss. A "bad faith letter" should be sent to the insurer, protecting the defendant against an excess limits judgment. If the case is eventually lost for excess of policy limits, let's say $1.5 million, the defendant would have grounds for a bad faith claim against the insurer and would not be responsible for the portion outside the policy limits.

Medical malpractice trials typically take a week or two, though they can last longer; the fireman's trial in Case 2 lasted four weeks. The good news is that if the decision is made to take a case to trial, the majority of cases result in a defense verdict.

XIII. Appeals

Although appeals are often more publicized in criminal cases, they may be filed in tort cases as well. The grounds for an appeal are procedural error, not retrying the facts of the case. For example:

- The Judge gave the jury an inappropriate instruction
- The court abused its power in disallowing a critical defense expert to testify

Appeals can take years to resolve. Filing an appellate motion without proper grounds is time consuming, costly, and ultimately futile.

NOTES

NOTES

NOTES

NOTES